T0259449

Advances in Cardiac and Aortic Surgery

Guest Editors

JOHN A. KERN, MD
IRVING L. KRON, MD

SURGICAL CLINICS OF NORTH AMERICA

www.surgical.theclinics.com

Consulting Editor
RONALD F. MARTIN, MD

August 2009 • Volume 89 • Number 4

SAUNDERS an imprint of ELSEVIER, Inc.

W.B. SAUNDERS COMPANY

A Division of Elsevier Inc.

1600 John F. Kennedy Blvd., Suite 1800, Philadelphia, PA 19103-2899

http://www.theclinics.com

SURGICAL CLINICS OF NORTH AMERICA Volume 89, Number 4

August 2009 ISSN 0039–6109, ISBN-10: 1-4377-1387-4, ISBN-13: 978-1-4377-1387-9

Editor: Catherine Bewick

Developmental Editor: Donald Mumford

Surgical Clinics of North America (ISSN 0039–6109) is published bimonthly by Elsevier Inc., 360 Park Avenue South, New York, NY 10010-1710. Months of publication are February, April, June, August, October, and December. Business and Editorial Offices: 1600 John F. Kennedy Blvd., Suite 1800, Philadelphia, PA 19103-2899. Periodicals postage paid at New York, NY and additional mailing offices. Subscription prices are $269.00 per year for US individuals, $432.00 per year for US institutions, $134.00 per year for US students and residents, $330.00 per year for Canadian individuals, $537.00 per year for Canadian institutions, $371.00 for international individuals, $537.00 per year for international institutions and $185.00 per year for Canadian and foreign students/residents. To receive student/resident rate, orders must be accompanied by name of affiliated institution, date of term, and the *signature* of program/residency coordinator on institution letterhead. Orders will be billed at individual rate until proof of status is received. Foreign air speed delivery is included in all *Clinics* subscription prices. All prices are subject to change without notice. POSTMASTER: Send address changes to *Surgical Clinics*, Elsevier Health Sciences Division, Subscription Customer Service, 3251 Riverport Lane, Maryland Heights, MO 63043. **Customer Service (orders, claims, online, change of address): Telephone: 1-800-654-2452 (U.S. and Canada); 314-447-8871 (outside U.S. and Canada). Fax: 314-447-8029. E-mail: journalscustomerservice-usa@elsevier.com (for print support); journalsonlinesupport-usa@elsevier.com (for online support).**

Reprints. For copies of 100 or more, of articles in this publication, please contact the Commercial Reprints Department, Elsevier Inc., 360 Park Avenue South, New York, New York 10010-1710. Tel. (212) 633-3812, Fax: (212) 462-1935, e-mail: reprints@elsevier.com.

The *Surgical Clinics of North America* is also published in Spanish by McGraw-Hill Interamericana Editores S.A., P.O. Box 5-237 06500 Mexico D.F. Mexico; and in Portuguese by Interlivros Edicoes Ltda., Rua Comandante Coelho 1085, CEP 21250, Rio de Janeiro, Brazil; and in Greek by Paschalidis Medical Publications, Athens Greece.

The *Surgical Clinics of North America* is covered in *MEDLINE/PubMed (Index Medicus), EMBASE/Excerpta Medica, Current Contents/Clinical Medicine, Current Contents/Life Sciences, Science Citation Index,* and *ISI/BIOMED.*

Printed and bound in the United Kingdom

Transferred to Digital Print 2011

Contributors

CONSULTING EDITOR

RONALD F. MARTIN, MD
Staff Surgeon, Marshfield Clinic, Marshfield; and Clinical Associate Professor, University of Wisconsin School of Medicine and Public Health, Madison, Wisconsin; Colonel, Medical Corps, United States Army Reserve

GUEST EDITORS

JOHN A. KERN, MD
Associate Professor of Surgery, Division of Thoracic and Cardiovascular Surgery; Surgical Director, Heart and Vascular Center, University of Virginia Health System, Charlottesville, Virginia

IRVING L. KRON, MD
S. Hurt Watts Professor and Chairman, Department of Surgery, Division of Thoracic and Cardiovascular Surgery; University of Virginia Health System, Charlottesville, Virginia

AUTHORS

JOSHUA D. ADAMS, MD
Fellow Vascular Surgery and Interventional Radiology, University of Virginia Health System, Charlottesville, Virginia

GORAV AILAWADI, MD
Assistant Professor, Division of Thoracic and Cardiovascular Surgery, Department of Surgery, University of Virginia, Charlottesville, Virginia

JAMES D. BERGIN, MD
Professor of Internal Medicine, University of Virginia Health System, Charlottesville, Virginia; Medical Director, Heart Failure/Cardiac Transplant Program, University of Virginia Health System, Charlottesville, Virginia

DONALD M. BOTTA, Jr, MD
Assistant Professor, Section of Cardiac Surgery, Yale University School of Medicine, New Haven, Connecticut

WILLIAM T. BRINKMAN, MD
Cardiothoracic Surgeon, The Heart Hospital Baylor Plano, Plano, Texas

KENNETH J. CHERRY, MD
Professor of Surgery, Program Director, Fellowship in Vascular Surgery, Chief, Division of Vascular Surgery, University of Virginia, Charlottesville, Virginia

CHRIS C. COOK, MD
Resident, Department of Cardiothoracic Surgery, University of Pittsburgh Medical Center Heart, Lung, and Esophageal Surgery Institute, Pittsburgh, Pennsylvania

RALPH J. DAMIANO, Jr, MD
John M. Schoenberg Professor of Surgery, Chief of Cardiac Surgery, Division of Cardiothoracic Surgery, Washington University School of Medicine, Barnes-Jewish Hospital, St. Louis, Missouri

MANI A. DANESHMAND, MD
Senior Assistant Resident, Department of General and Thoracic Surgery, Duke University Medical Center, Durham, North Carolina

JOHN A. ELEFTERIADES, MD
William W. L. Glenn Professor of Cardiothoracic Surgery, Chief, Section of Cardiac Surgery, Yale University School of Medicine, New Haven, Connecticut

LLEOWELL M. GARCIA, MD
Fellow Vascular Surgery, University of Virginia Health System, Charlottesville, Virginia

THOMAS G. GLEASON, MD
Associate Professor, Department of Cardiothoracic Surgery, Division of Cardiac Surgery, University of Pittsburgh Medical Center Heart, Lung, and Esophageal Surgery Institute, Pittsburgh, Pennsylvania; Director, Center for Thoracic Aortic Diseases, University of Pittsburgh Medical Center, Pittsburgh, Pennsylvania

MICHAEL E. HALKOS, MD
Division of Cardiothoracic Surgery, Department of Surgery, Emory University School of Medicine, Decatur, Georgia

JOHN A. KERN, MD
Associate Professor of Surgery, University of Virginia Health System, Charlottesville, Virginia

CHRISTOPHER M. KRAMER, MD
Director, Cardiovascular Imaging Center, Professor of Medicine, Division of Cardiovascular Medicine, Professor of Radiology, University of Virginia Health System, Charlottesville, Virginia

IRVING L. KRON, MD
Professor of Surgery and Chairman, Division of Thoracic and Cardiovascular Surgery, Department of Surgery, University of Virginia Health System, Charlottesville, Virginia

ANSON M. LEE, MD
Research Fellow, Division of Cardiothoracic Surgery, Washington University School of Medicine, Barnes-Jewish Hospital, St. Louis, Missouri

MICHAEL J. MACK, MD
Medical Director, Cardiothoracic Surgeon, Cardiovascular Surgery Baylor Health Care System, Dallas, Texas; and The Heart Hospital Baylor Plano, Plano, Texas

SPENCER J. MELBY, MD
Fellow, Division of Cardiothoracic Surgery, Washington University School of Medicine, Barnes-Jewish Hospital, St. Louis, Missouri

BRET A. METTLER, MD
Thoracic Surgery Resident, Division of Thoracic and Cardiovascular Surgery, University of Virginia Medical Center, Charlottesville, Virginia

CARMELO A. MILANO, MD
Department of General and Thoracic Surgery, Duke University Medical Center, Durham, North Carolina

MARC R. MOON, MD
Joseph C. Bancroft Professor of Surgery, Division of Cardiothoracic Surgery, Director, Center for Diseases of the Thoracic Aorta, Washington University School of Medicine, Saint Louis, Missouri

BENJAMIN B. PEELER, MD
Associate Professor of Surgery, Division of Thoracic and Cardiovascular Surgery, University of Virginia Medical Center, Charlottesville, Virginia; Director, Virginia Children's Heart Center, University of Virginia Medical Center, Charlottesville, Virginia

JOHN D. PUSKAS, MD
Professor, Crawford Long Hospital, Emory University School of Medicine, Atlanta, Georgia

ROBERT L. SMITH, MD
Cardiothoracic Chief Resident, Division of Thoracic and Cardiovascular Surgery, Department of Surgery, University of Virginia Health System, Charlottesville, Virginia

MARGARET C. TRACCI, MD, JD
Fellow, Department of Surgery, Division of Vascular Surgery, University of Virginia, Charlottesville, Virginia

AMY M. WEST, MD
Fellow Physician, Division of Cardiovascular Medicine, Department of Medicine, University of Virginia Health System, Charlottesville, Virginia

FREDDIE M. WILLIAMS, MD
Fellow, Cardiovascular Medicine, University of Virginia Health System, Charlottesville, Virginia

Y. JOSEPH WOO, MD
Assistant Professor of Surgery, Director of Minimally Invasive and Robotic Cardiac Surgery Program, Associate Surgical Director of Thoracic Transplantation, Division of Cardiovascular Surgery, Department of Surgery, University of Pennsylvania, Philadelphia, Pennsylvania

RICHARD K. ZACOUR, BS, CCP
Chief Perfusionist, Thoracic-Cardiovascular Perfusion, Department of Surgery, University of Virginia Health System, Charlottesville, Virginia

Contents

> Cardiovascular complications are infrequent but can result in significant morbidity following noncardiac surgery, especially in patients with peripheral vascular disease or increased age. All patients require some level of preoperative screening to identify and minimize immediate and future risk, with a careful focus on known coronary artery disease or risks for coronary artery disease and functional capacity. The 2007 American College of Cardiology/ American Heart Association Guidelines are clear that noninvasive and invasive testing should be limited to circumstances in which results will clearly affect patient management or in which testing would otherwise be indicated. β-Blocker therapy has become controversial in light of recent publications but should be continued in patients already on therapy, and started in patients with high cardiac risk undergoing intermediate- or high-risk surgery.

> There are multiple imaging modalities currently available to noninvasively evaluate the heart and coronary arteries. Choosing the most appropriate modality depends on the pertinent clinical question and the underlying patient characteristics. This article provides an overview of the fields of echocardiography, myocardial perfusion imaging, cardiac computed tomography, and cardiac magnetic resonance imaging, with particular attention to specific clinical applications for cardiac surgery patients.

> Cardiopulmonary bypass has revolutionized the ability to provide cardiorespiratory support and has advanced the field of cardiac surgery. This invention has given surgeons the ability to perform many procedures that were not possible previously. The concept and development of cardiopulmonary bypass has been pioneered by numerous legendary surgeons. Cardiopulmonary bypass, extracorporeal membrane oxygenation, and left heart bypass have revolutionized our ability to operate on

the heart, great vessels, and aorta in addition to providing means of short-term support for reversible causes of cardiac and/or respiratory failure. The success of these approaches is dependent upon excellent communication between the surgeon, perfusionist, and anesthesiologist as well as constant vigilance and troubleshooting by the caregivers.

Thoracic great vessel and cardiac trauma are characterized by anatomic location and mechanism of injury: blunt or penetrating. Management strategies are also directed by the extent and mechanism of injury. Advances in imaging and catheter-based technologies have allowed easier and more accurate diagnosis and less-invasive treatments. Although the advantages of endovascular techniques are attractive, open surgical repair remains the definitive treatment for many of these thoracic injuries. Given the increasing sophistication of these technologies and the demonstrated usefulness of a disease-oriented approach toward patient management, trauma centers have adopted a multidisciplinary team model for management of multitrauma victims. In this review, the authors detail the diagnosis and management of blunt aortic, nonaortic great vessel, blunt cardiac, and penetrating cardiac injuries.

Occlusive disease of the supra-aortic trunks remains a diagnostic and therapeutic challenge to the surgeon. Although most cases in Western series are attributable to atherosclerotic disease, other entities such as Takayasu arteritis and radiation arteritis account for a substantial subset of patients in whom choice of therapy and clinical response may be significantly affected by the peculiarities of the disease process involved. This article reviews the anatomy, causes, and diagnosis of occlusive disease of the supra-aortic trunks. The indications, techniques, and outcomes of reconstruction are also discussed.

The aortic valve–sparing root reconstruction procedure remains an ideal concept, but it has not yet become an ideal operation. There is still great variation and evolution in techniques, which mirrors the increasing understanding of the aortic root's functional anatomy and the disease processes that affect it. These operations remain complex, and the surgeons who perform them well are often times best armed with an experienced eye for what looks right more than a mathematical model that can predetermine who will do well, with what repair type and with what percentage chance of long-term success. Because of this, it will likely still be a while before these operations are more routinely used by a broader group of surgeons, as compared with the very reproducible Bentall and De Bono repair.

In an era of increasingly common and detailed imaging of the thorax, thoracic aortic aneurysms are being discovered in their precomplicated state with increasing frequency. At the same time, the list of potential treatments for thoracic aneurysms is beginning to expand. Deciding which treatment method to employ and which aneurysm to treat is often difficult. The risk of aneurysm complications must be balanced against the risks of the treatment. This work explores the behavior of thoracic aneurysms, the state-of-the-art in treatment, and a rational approach to the treatment decision is proposed.

Acute aortic dissection is a fatal disease if early diagnosis and institution of appropriate therapy are delayed. Unfortunately, the presentation of a dissection can be diabolical, leading to an initial misdiagnosis in more than 25% of patients. For type A dissections, surgical repair is essential because mortality rates approach 50% at 48 hours with expectant therapy alone. For type B dissections, medical management is successful in most patients, although a subset with complications or early dilation may benefit from newer endovascular techniques. The goal of this review is to summarize the diagnostic algorithm, initial therapeutic options, and long-term management regimen that offer patients with an acute aortic dissection the best chance for short-term and long-term survival. There is an emphasis on the specific practical approach that is applied at Washington University to patients who present with an aortic dissection.

The use of endovascular stent grafts for treatment of the descending thoracic aorta is reviewed. Currently, 3 devices have been approved by the US Food and Drug Administration for the treatment of descending thoracic aneurysms, and multiple studies are ongoing to investigate the efficacy of endovascular treatment in such pathologies as traumatic aortic injury and Stanford type B dissection. Outcomes are highly dependent on good case planning and patient selection and will likely continue to improve as newer-generation devices and delivery systems are designed and made available.

Off-pump coronary artery bypass is a safe and effective method of coronary revascularization that avoids the use of cardiopulmonary bypass. Randomized trials, typically enrolling low-risk patients, have shown comparable mortality and reduced morbidity between off-pump and on-pump coronary artery bypass. Larger retrospective analyses suggest improved mortality and a lower incidence of adverse events in patients undergoing off-pump coronary artery bypass. This article reviews the available literature comparing outcomes of patients undergoing on- and off-pump coronary artery bypass surgery.

lesion sets and approaches were introduced over the last decade which has made the operative treatment of atrial fibrillation less invasive and more confusing.

As a result of improved treatment of congenital heart disease (CHD) over the last half century, the number of patients reaching adulthood continues to grow. With increased success a challenging group of adults with unique anatomy and physiology, in addition to the usual effects of aging, has been created. All of these patients present unique and fascinating challenges, and their best care requires bridging pediatric and adult medical and surgical care. This review is a discussion of some of the more common surgical issues that arise in this evolving group of patients.

THE CLINICS ARE NOW AVAILABLE ONLINE!

Access your subscription at:
www.theclinics.com

Foreword

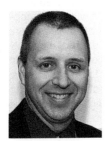

Ronald F. Martin, MD
Consulting Editor

For most general surgeons, operations involving the great vessels, aortic arch, or heart are not part of our everyday routine—in fact, these operations are rarely part of our routine on any day. But a working knowledge of the problems and solutions dealt with by cardiac surgeons is, in my opinion, potentially invaluable to any surgeon.

Cardiac surgery has afforded us with one of the best models for scientific inquiry and practical adaptation that medicine has known, second perhaps only to the study of gastric pathology and its solutions, although I will admit my bias in this matter. Cardiac surgery may also serve us even better as a model of the trajectory of surgical intervention within many fields, as it is also an example of a "canary in a coal mine."

Historically, cardiac surgery has been afforded tremendous visibility in the public eye and a great deal of latitude in development (experimentation) because of the devastating consequences associated with myocardial infarction and acute heart failure. In the 1960s, cardiac surgeons were as famous as astronauts and were celebrated figures in public life. Drs. Christiaan Barnard, Michael DeBakey, Norman Shumway, and Denton Cooley were celebrities and well known to many members of the public. In the days of the first cardiac transplants and rapid promulgation of cardio-pulmonary bypass, cardiac surgery as a discipline was well funded, was revered by the public, and became increasingly clinically effective at phenomenal rates. Over time, cardiac surgery has somewhat become a victim of its own profound success. Very few people today are astounded that someone can undergo an emergent coronary artery bypass grafting (CABG) and go home in well under a week. Cardiac surgeons are still valued members of society, but they are not looked upon as the giants they used to be—they have rejoined the ranks of the mortals. And perhaps most impor-tantly, cardiac surgeons have now taken a place as a valued, but not necessarily domi-nant, member of a more varied and complex team of professionals.

One of the great lessons that we can learn from cardiac surgery is that if one wants to improve outcomes, one must design valid questions and metrics, then measure them correctly, and share that information in a way that it can be used effectively (non-punitively). The early work of the Northern New England Cardiovascular Study Group has served as a model for outcomes analysis and collaborative effort. Without doubt,

Surg Clin N Am 89 (2009) xiii–xiv
doi:10.1016/j.suc.2009.07.002
0039-6109/09/$ – see front matter © 2009 Elsevier Inc. All rights reserved.

surgical.theclinics.com

CABG procedures are more straightforward in measurable variables than some other procedures, but the principle still holds.

Cardiac surgery also teaches us that the future of surgery ain't what it used to be (apologies to Yogi Berra). The advent of statins and stents, combined with the exceptional success of cardiac surgeons themselves, have created circumstances where the focus of cardiac surgery has shifted somewhat away from the care of the acutely ill patient to the care of the patient with chronic disease. This is likely to happen in many disciplines. The impact of these observations as regards work force projections, health care cost per patient-year, and shift from predominantly inpatient expense to chronic outpatient expense (especially pharmaceutical) is something we will all face at some point.

Cardiac surgeons have had to develop effective service line models to remain competitive in the market place. Globally priced procedures for cardiac-related services are common. Cardiac surgery in some respects is highly compartmentalized and therefore easier to offer in either boutique settings or "medical tourism" models, thus increasing the pressure on established programs. Add in highly developed clinical pathways and narrow variation in costs for many patients, and one has a "medical product" that lends itself well to bargaining pressure from government or third party payers.

The development of these service line products does create new, or newer, versions of problems for us also. Although turf battles have been around for as long as there has been turf, once a group is sharing the same limited (and getting more so) pie, the turf battles intensify. With developments in cardiac imaging, interventional cardiology, and interventional radiology causing significant overlap in what one discipline can offer that used to be the sole province of another discipline, these matters have become increasingly problematic on an administrative and reimbursement level. Cardiac surgeons may find it difficult to remain free of these entanglements also.

If all of the developmental issues, historical interests, political considerations, and scientific examples were to suddenly resolve, we general surgeons should still have great interest in the knowledge of cardiac surgery and surgery of the great vessels. The concordance of symptoms between acute cardiac and great vessel problems and problems requiring the services of a general surgeon are substantial. The need for knowledge of evaluation of cardiac performance before noncardiac operation is essential for every general surgeon. And lastly, the ability to recognize and manage the patient who has perioperative cardiac problems is absolutely necessary for every general surgeon.

We are indebted to Drs Kron and Kern and their collaborators for this excellent issue of the *Surgical Clinics of North America*. They are consummate professionals in every sense of the word. We will all be well served to learn from the successes and challenges that our brethren in cardiac surgery face as we develop through these interesting times. For several decades they have been at the front line of innovation—and that alone might earn them the revered position they once had.

Ronald F. Martin, MD
Department of Surgery
Marshfield Clinic
1000 North Oak Avenue
Marshfield, WI 54449, USA

E-mail address:
martin.ronald@marshfieldclinic.org

Preface

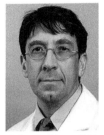 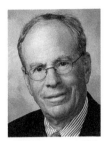

John A. Kern, MD   Irving L. Kron, MD
Guest Editors

As with most surgical specialties, surgery of the heart, aorta, and great vessels is constantly changing with the advent of new diagnostic and therapeutic technologies. Today's practice of cardiac surgery is vastly different from what it was even 10 years ago, and today's cardiac surgeons, although looking forward with excitement to what tomorrow will bring, sometimes struggle with the decision of what new techniques and technologies to embrace. For those not closely associated with the practice of cardiac surgery, keeping up to date with this rapidly changing landscape is difficult, to say the least. New treatments for atrial fibrillation, aortic dissections, valvular heart disease, and heart failure are often completely unknown to those outside of our specialty. However, it is important for all surgeons to be at least familiar with how the specialty of cardiac surgery is changing and what treatment options are presently available for patients with heart disease and diseases of the aorta and great vessels. The ability to perform coronary artery bypass without the morbidity associated with cardiopulmonary bypass or the ability to repair or replace heart valves without a sternotomy or cardiotomy are just a few examples of how drastically our specialty has changed over the past decade, to the benefit of the patient. Left ventricular assist device (LVAD) technology has improved significantly in just a very short time and is now an option for many patients with end stage heart failure, as "destination" LVAD therapy has become a reality. This issue of *Surgical Clinics of North America* includes updates on all of the most rapidly changing aspects of diagnosis and treatment of common cardiac, aortic, and great vessel pathologies. We hope you find this issue a valuable resource.

John A. Kern, MD
Irving L. Kron, MD

both: Division of Thoracic and Cardiovascular Surgery
University of Virginia Health System
PO Box 800679
Charlottesville, VA 22908-0679, USA

E-mail addresses:
jak3r@hscmail.mcc.virginia.edu (J.A. Kern)
ilk@hscmail.mcc.virginia.edu (I.L. Kron)

Surg Clin N Am 89 (2009) xv
doi:10.1016/j.suc.2009.07.001
0039-6109/09/$ – see front matter

Cardiac Screening Before Noncardiac Surgery

Freddie M. Williams, MD[a], James D. Bergin, MD[b,c],*

KEYWORDS

- Perioperative cardiac screening • Noncardiac surgery
- Revascularization • Stress imaging

Cardiovascular complications are responsible for roughly one-half of all the mortality experienced by patients undergoing noncardiac surgical procedures and occur in 1% to 5% of unselected patients undergoing vascular surgery.[1,2] Of the cardiovascular complications experienced during the perioperative period, 5% to 10% are myocardial infarctions (MI), with most of the events occurring within the first 3 days following surgery.[3–6] Those patients suffering a perioperative MI have too high a mortality rate, ranging from 32% to 69%.[5,7–13] This is due to the increased hemodynamic stress caused by surgery and the difficulty in establishing reperfusion in the coronary arteries, due to the potential for bleeding complications in a newly operated patient. Cardiac risk also remains high in the subsequent months for patients suffering a perioperative event. In a prospective study of 173 patients with coronary artery disease (CAD) or at high-risk of CAD undergoing major noncardiac surgery, patients with elevated cardiac troponin I had an odds ratio (OR) of 9.8 (95% CI 3.0–32) for death within 1 year.[14] Mangano and colleagues[15] found that patients surviving a postoperative in-hospital MI had a 28-fold increase in the rate of subsequent cardiac complications within 6 months following surgery.

GENERAL CONCEPTS

All patients need some level of screening before any surgical procedure. The goals of screening are to ensure the perioperative period is free of adverse cardiac events and to identify those patients with a poor long-term prognosis, in whom treatment and risk

[a] Cardiovascular Medicine, University of Virginia Health System, 1215 Lee Street, Box 800158, Charlottesville, VA 22908, USA
[b] Department of Internal Medicine, University of Virginia Health System, 1215 Lee Street, Box 800158, Charlottesville, VA 22908, USA
[c] Heart Failure/Cardiac Transplant Program, University of Virginia Health System, 1215 Lee Street, Box 800158, Charlottesville, VA 22908, USA
* Corresponding author. Department of Internal Medicine, University of Virginia Health System, 1215 Lee Street, Box 800158, Charlottesville, VA 22908.
E-mail address: jdb5r@hscmail.mcc.virginia.edu (J.D. Bergin).

Surg Clin N Am 89 (2009) 747–762
doi:10.1016/j.suc.2009.05.001
0039-6109/09/$ – see front matter © 2009 Elsevier Inc. All rights reserved.
surgical.theclinics.com

factor modification may improve their outcome. Patients can be grouped into low-, medium-, and high-risk. Several important factors need to be considered at the time of screening patients, including: (1) urgent/emergent nature of the surgery, (2) effect of canceling the surgery on a patient, (3) presence of a cardiovascular problem that would make deferral of the procedure and treatment of the underlying cardiovascular problem the safest approach, (4) whether a planned procedure warrants a more aggressive workup for the presence of CAD, (5) how results of the workup will alter therapy, and (6) the presence of any underlying risk factors that would predispose the patient to CAD.

Surgical procedures can be grouped into low-, medium-, and high-risk (see **Table 1**), and it is essential to keep in mind the type of procedure that is planned. High-risk procedures carry a risk of nonfatal MI or cardiac death of $\geq 5\%$, intermediate-risk of 1% to 4%, and low-risk <1%.[16,17] For a variety of reasons, patients undergoing urgent/emergent surgery have a 2- to 5-fold increased rate of cardiovascular complications than patients undergoing comparable surgery on an elective basis.[1,18–21] Such patients may simply require more aggressive monitoring but no additional screening beyond history and physical. Results of screening may not affect the decision to operate but may alert the anesthesia and surgical team to the degree of risk and facilitate communication of potential outcomes to the family.

It is important to consider the impact of cancellation of surgery on the patient and their quality of life. Some patients requiring noncardiac surgery will not benefit sufficiently from revascularization to warrant further workup and delay. Alternatively, cancellation or deferral of the procedure may be the safest option under certain circumstances (see **Table 2**).

Several studies have suggested that a recent MI places the patient at a significant risk for a cardiovascular complication during elective surgery.[7,18–20,22,23] In the Goldman series, patients with a MI within 4 weeks of the noncardiac surgical procedure had a perioperative MI and death rate of 33%, although only 12 patients were included in this group.[19] Patients with a MI between 6 weeks and 6 months of the noncardiac procedure had an event rate of 20%, although only 10 patients were included. Despite these small numbers, Tarhan noted similar rates of cardiovascular events in two

Table 1
Cardiac risk*stratification for noncardiac surgical procedures

Risk Stratification	Procedure Examples
Vascular (reported cardiac risk often more than 5%)	Aortic and other major vascular surgery Peripheral vascular surgery
Intermediate (reported cardiac risk generally 1%–5%)	Intraperitoneal and intrathoracic surgery Carotid endarterectomy Head and neck surgery Orthopedic surgery Prostate surgery
Low[a] (reported cardiac risk generally less than 1%)	Endoscopic procedures Superficial procedure Cataract surgery Breast surgery Ambulatory surgery

* Combined incidence of cardiac death and nonfatal myocardial infarction.
[a] These procedures do not generally require further preoperative cardiac testing.
From Fleisher LA, Beckman JA, Brown KA, et al. ACC/AHA 2007 guidelines on perioperative cardiovascular evaluation and care for noncardiac surgery. J Am Coll Cardiol 2007;50:1707–32. Reprinted with permission. Copyright © 2007, American Heart Association, Inc.

Table 2
Active cardiac conditions for which the patient should undergo evaluation and treatment before noncardiac surgery (Class I, level of evidence: B)

Condition	Examples
Unstable coronary syndromes	Unstable or server angina[a] (CCS Class III or IV)[b] Recent MI[c]
Decompensated HF (NYHA functional Class IV; worsening or new-onset HF)	—
Significant arrhythmias	High-grade atrioventricular block Third-degree atrioventricular heart block Symptomatic ventricular arrhythmias Supraventricular arrhythmias (including atrial fibrillation) with uncontrolled ventricular rate (heart rate greater than 100 beats per minute at rest) Symptomatic bradycardia Newly recognized ventricular tachycardia
Severe valvular disease	Severe aortic stenosis (mean pressure gradient greater than 40 mm Hg. Aortic valve area less than 1.0 cm², or symptomatic) Symptomatic mitral stenosis (progressive dyspnea on exertion, exertional presyncope, or HF)

Abbreviations: CCS, Canadian Cardiovascular Society; HF, heart failure; MI, myocardial infarction; NYHA, New York Heart Association.
[a] According to Campeau.[9]
[b] May include stable angina in patients who are unusually sedentary.
[c] The American College of Cardiology National Database Library Defines recent MI as more than 7 days but less than or equal to 1 month (within 30 days).
From Fleisher LA, Beckman JA, Brown KA, et al. ACC/AHA 2007 guidelines on perioperative cardiovascular evaluation and care for noncardiac surgery. J Am Coll Cardiol 2007;50:1707–32. Reprinted with permission. Copyright © 2007, American Heart Association, Inc.

studies.[7,22] However, all of these studies are two to three decades old, and modern methods of anesthesia and postoperative care may have a significant impact on the magnitude of the events.

Patients with unstable angina (USA), heart failure (HF), severe valvular stenosis, and significant arrhythmias are also at high-risk for a perioperative cardiovascular event.[18–20] Using the Medicare database, Hernandez and colleagues[24] identified 1532 HF patients who underwent major noncardiac surgery from 1997 to 1998. The authors adjusted for demographic characteristics, type of surgery, and comorbid conditions. They reported that patients with HF had a risk-adjusted operative mortality (death before discharge or within 30 days of surgery) of 11.7%, compared with 6.6% in patients with CAD ($P < .001$) and 6.2% in a control population. The risk-adjusted 30-day readmission rate was also significantly higher with HF.

Aortic stenosis also poses a strong risk for perioperative complications, with an independent relative risk for perioperative death or nonfatal MI of 5.2 for gradients 25 to 50 mm Hg and 6.8 for gradients >50 mm Hg, compared with patients without aortic stenosis.[25–27]

Ventricular and atrial arrhythmias may not be independent predictors of risk but may simply identify a group of patients with more severe underlying ischemic heart disease and HF.[28]

Noncardiac surgery is also high-risk for patients with pulmonary hypertension. In a group of 145 patients undergoing surgery in a pulmonary hypertension database, the mean right ventricular systolic pressure was 68 mm Hg by echocardiogram, and 30-day mortality rate was 7%, although a control group was not identified.[29]

Aggressively treating the patient and allowing a cooling down period may improve the outcomes for those with USA. Similarly, aggressive treatment of decompensated HF may allow most surgeries to be performed at an acceptable mortality and morbidity rate, although patients with New York Heart Association Class IV may never be candidates unless the situation is life-threatening. Avoiding all procedures except emergency surgery may also be reasonable for the majority of patients with symptomatic critical aortic stenosis, unless the patient can undergo aortic valve surgery first.

A complete history and physical examination is invaluable in estimating perioperative cardiac risk and determining which patients require further screening. In addition to identifying the serious cardiac conditions described above, the history and physical should also identify other significant comorbidities (cerebrovascular disease, diabetes mellitus (DM), chronic kidney disease), and elicit any recent change in symptoms. It is important to determine a pre-test probability for the presence of CAD and the extent of the disease process. All the traditional risk factors for CAD, ie, hypertension, hyperlipidemia, DM, family history of premature CAD, and tobacco use, should be considered. The history should also clarify functional capacity by ascertaining the patient's ability to perform common daily tasks, which has been proven to correlate significantly with maximum oxygen uptake by treadmill testing (see **Table 3**).[30] Reilly and colleagues[31] looked at 600 patients and found that those reporting good exercise tolerance had a low event rate (myocardial and neurologic events) during major noncardiac surgery, compared with patients with poor exercise tolerance (20.4% vs 10.4%; $P < .001$). In this study, the perioperative event rate was inversely related to the number of blocks walked or flights climbed.

In a study from 1977, Goldman and colleagues[18] elaborated the first multifactorial risk index specifically for cardiac complications, which included 9 independent risk factors. Detsky and colleagues[20] updated this index in 1986 with the addition of a pre-test probability of CAD, angina stratification, and a time course for MI and HF. Lee and colleagues[28] derived and validated a Revised Cardiac Risk Index (RCRI) for the prediction of cardiac risk in stable patients undergoing nonurgent major noncardiac surgery. At the present time, it is the most often used model of risk assessment in noncardiac surgery. The authors measured major cardiac complications (MI, pulmonary edema, ventricular fibrillation or primary cardiac arrest, and complete heart block) in 4315 patients aged ≥ 50 years. Six independent predictors of complications were identified: high-risk type of surgery (intrathoracic, intraabdominal, suprapubic vascular), history of ischemic heart disease, history of congestive heart failure (CHF), history of cerebrovascular disease, preoperative treatment with insulin, and preoperative serum creatinine >2.0 mg/dL. Rates of major cardiac complications with 0, 1, 2, or ≥ 3 of these factors were 0.5%, 1.3%, 4%, and 9%, respectively, in the derivation cohort and 0.4%, 0.9%, 7%, and 11%, respectively, between 1422 patients in the validation cohort.

RISK STRATIFICATION

Based on the widespread use of the RCRI, the American College of Cardiology (ACC)/ American Heart Association (AHA) 2007 Perioperative Guidelines replaced the intermediate-risk category from the 2002 version of the guidelines with the clinical risk factors from the index (history of CAD, history of compensated or prior HF, history of cerebrovascular disease, DM, renal insufficiency), excluding the type of surgery.[32]

Table 3
Estimated energy requirements for various activities

	Can You ...		
1 MET	Take care of yourself?	4 METs	Climb a flight of stairs or walk up a hill?
	Eat, dress, or use the toilet?		Walk on level ground at 4 mph (6.4 kph)?
	Walk indoors around the house?		Run a short distance?
	Walk a block or 2 on level ground at 2 to 3 mph (3.2–4.8 kph)?		Do heavy work around the house like scrubbing floors or lifting or moving heavy furniture?
4 METs	Do light work around the house like dusting or washing dishes?		Participate in moderate recreational activities like golf, bowling, dancing, doubles tennis, or throwing a baseball or football?
		Greater than 10 METs	Participate in strenuous sports like swimming, singles tennis, football, basketball, or skiing?

Abbreviations: kph, kilometers per hour; MET, metabolic equivalent; mph, miles per hour.
From Fleisher LA, Beckman JA, Brown KA, et al. ACC/AHA 2007 guidelines on perioperative cardiovascular evaluation and care for noncardiac surgery. J Am Coll Cardiol 2007;50:1707–32. Reprinted with permission. Copyright © 2007, American Heart Association, Inc.

*If the patient being considered for elective surgery has 1 of the active cardiac conditions described above and in **Table 2**, the Guidelines recommend further evaluation and treatment of the underlying cardiac problem as a Class I recommendation (should be done), with level of evidence (LOE) B (limited population risk studies evaluated).*

Next, the level of surgical risk should be determined, and if low-risk, it is acceptable to proceed with the planned procedure (Class I, LOE B).

For patients undergoing nonlow-risk surgery, the patient's functional capacity, based on the ability to perform activities of daily living, should subsequently be determined. Functional capacity has been classified as excellent (greater than 10 metabolic equivalents [METs]), good (7–10 METs), moderate (4–7 METs), poor (less than 4 METs), or unknown.

If the patient can achieve ≥4 METs without symptoms, then it is acceptable to proceed with surgery (Class I, LOE B).

In patients with poor functional capacity, symptoms, or unknown functional capacity, the number of active clinical risk factors will guide the need for further testing.

In patients with no clinical risk factors, proceeding with surgery is appropriate (Class I, LOE B).
    In patients with 1 to 2 risk factors, options are to proceed with surgery with heart rate control with β-blockade (Class IIa, LOE B) or to consider noninvasive testing if it will change management (Class IIb, LOE B). (Class IIa recommendation is reasonable or probably indicated. Class IIb has unknown usefulness/effectiveness.)

*In patients with ≥3 risk factors undergoing intermediate-risk surgery, options are the same as above, given insufficient data to guide choice. In patients with ≥3 risk factors undergoing vascular surgery, further cardiac testing should be considered if it will change management (Class IIa, LOE B). See **Table 1** for further details.[32]*

The usefulness of preoperative stress testing may depend on the population being studied and their background medical therapy. Poldermans and colleagues[33] performed dobutamine stress echocardiography (DSE) in 316 patients undergoing major vascular surgery and quantified extent and severity of stress-induced new wall motion abnormalities (WMA). Of note, only 23% of patients were treated with β-blockers. Patients with evidence of extensive ischemia (three or more segments of stress-induced new WMA) had a 6.5-fold increase in late cardiac events, whereas patients with limited ischemia (one or two segments) had a 2.9-fold increase, compared with those without stress-induced WMA. Dipyridamole thallium imaging was used in a similar fashion by Cohen and colleagues[34] for patients with DM and peripheral vascular disease. They found a similar ability to stratify patients into high-risk groups with an average postsurgical survival of only 1.8 years, compared with low-risk patients with an average survival of 9.4 years. However, in the Dutch Echocardiographic Cardiac Risk Evaluation Applying Stress Echocardiography-II (DECREASE-II) study, Poldermans and colleagues[35] revisited preoperative cardiac testing in intermediate-risk patients undergoing major vascular surgery and found similar incidences of cardiac death or MI at 30 days in patients with, and without, stress testing (OR 0.78; 95% CI 0.28–2.1; $P = .62$). Importantly, all patients were treated with β-blockers with tight heart rate control. The authors concluded that intermediate-risk patients might safely proceed without cardiac testing, if they are receiving β-blockers with tight heart rate control.

CARDIAC STRESS TESTING

Stress testing can be performed with exercise, vasodilators, or adrenergic stimulation in combination with radionuclide or echocardiographic cardiac imaging. Exercise and pharmacologic stress testing have negative predictive values between 90% and 100% but lower positive predictive values between 60% and 67%, resulting in a better ability to decrease risk when negative, than to identify high-risk when positive.[36] Exercise testing is preferable, as it provides an estimate of exercise capacity and hemodynamic response. However, many patients are unable to exercise secondary to arthritis, claudication, obstructive lung disease, and diminished functional capacity. In these patients, options include DSE or myocardial perfusion scintigraphy (MPS) with dipyridamole or adenosine.

Studies directly comparing stress echocardiography and MPS have been limited by small numbers of patients. Beattie and colleagues[37] performed a meta-analysis of 68 studies of 10,049 patients undergoing noncardiac surgery (25 echo studies and 50 MPS studies, seven studies with a direct comparison of the two). Stress echo had better negative predicative characteristics than MPS, owing to fewer false–negative stress echocardiograms. The likelihood ratio (LR) for stress echo was more indicative of a postoperative cardiac event than MPS (LR 4.09; 95% CI 3.21–6.56 vs 1.83; 1.59–2.10; $P = .001$). The authors found that a moderate-to-large defect, seen in 14%, by either method predicts a postoperative cardiac event (LR 8.35; 95% CI 5.6–12.45). Kertai and colleagues[38] also performed a meta-analysis of studies looking at perioperative cardiac risk stratification in patients undergoing major vascular surgery (8119 patients). They concluded that there was a trend for DSE to perform better than other stress testing modalities. However, ACC/AHA guidelines emphasize that the choice of test should be based on the center's experience.[32]

REVASCULARIZATION

Prophylactic preoperative coronary revascularization, through either bypass grafting or percutaneous coronary intervention (PCI), to decrease perioperative complications is controversial. Previous coronary artery bypass grafting (CABG) may be protective of perioperative events. Eagle and colleagues[39] looked at patients in the Coronary Artery Surgery Study registry, who had undergone CABG within the previous 5 years. They found perioperative rates of MI or death of 1% to 2%, if no intervening cardiac events had occurred (USA or MI). When comparing patients with known CAD treated medically, patients, who had undergone previous bypass surgery, had rates of death and MI less than half of those treated medically. However, this benefit was offset by the 1.4% mortality associated with the CABG procedure itself.[40] A similar post hoc analysis was performed by the Bypass Angioplasty Revascularization Investigation group, in which patients with multivessel CAD were randomized to bypass grafting or angioplasty.[41] A total of 501 patients had noncardiac surgery at a median of 29 months after their most recent coronary revascularization procedure. Rates of 30-day postoperative MI or death were similarly low in groups, with an overall event rate of 1.4%.

The Coronary Artery Revascularization Prophylaxis trial (CARP) was the first large, randomized trial to assess the long-term benefit of preoperative coronary artery revascularization in patients with stable CAD undergoing elective vascular surgery.[42] The authors recruited 510 patients with significant artery stenosis (1 or more major coronary arteries with stenosis $\geq 70\%$), who were undergoing elective surgery for expanding abdominal aortic aneurysm (33%) or arterial occlusive disease of the legs (67%), and randomized them to coronary artery revascularization before surgery or no revascularization. (Of note, patients with left main disease, left ventricular ejection fraction <20%, USA pectoris, aortic stenosis, or prior revascularization without evidence of recurrent ischemia were excluded.) Of the patients assigned to revascularization, PCI was performed in 59% and bypass surgery in 41%, with most of the patients having single-vessel or two-vessel disease. At 30 days, patients undergoing revascularization had no decrease in the number of MIs or deaths or in lengths of hospital stay. At 2.7 years after randomization, mortality in the revascularization group was 22% and in the no revascularization group 23% (relative risk 0.98; 95% CI 0.70–1.37; $P = .92$).

The DECREASE-V pilot study reported similar results in a high-risk cohort of patients undergoing vascular surgery.[43] In this study, 430 patients were identified as being high-risk, due to ≥ 3 cardiac risk factors (similar to risk factors from the RCRI), and underwent DSE or MPS. Of these patients, 101 (23%) had extensive stress-induced ischemia (≥ 5 segments on dobutamine echo or ≥ 3 walls on stress nuclear imaging), and were randomized to best medical therapy and revascularization (49 patients) or best medical therapy alone. Coronary angiography demonstrated two-vessel disease in 12 patients (24%), three-vessel disease in 33 (67%), and left main disease in four (8%). Revascularization did not improve outcomes at 30 days or 1 year. The incidence of the composite end point of all-cause mortality and MI at 30 days was 43% versus 33% (OR 1.4; 95% CI 0.7–2.8; $P = .30$), and at 1 year was 49% versus 44% (OR 1.2; 95% CI 0.7–2.3; $P = .48$) in the revascularization and no revascularization groups, respectively.

CARP and DECREASE-V pilot suggest that postoperative outcome is unchanged by prophylactic coronary revascularization in stable patients, although it should be noted that neither study was significantly powered to detect differences in outcome. CARP may have also created a selection bias, due to the screening criteria used.

The 2007 ACC/AHA Perioperative Guidelines do not recommend preoperative PCI, except in those patients in whom PCI is independently indicated for an acute coronary syndrome.[32]

Timing of elective noncardiac surgery after PCI is also controversial. Delaying surgery for at least 2 to 4 weeks after balloon angioplasty may be reasonable, as the three perioperative events between 350 patients in one study occurred in those undergoing surgery within 2 weeks of angioplasty.[44] However, postponing noncardiac surgery for more than 8 weeks after balloon angioplasty may raise the likelihood of restenosis at the angioplasty site, thus theoretically raising the chances of perioperative ischemia or MI.[32] In the current era, most of the PCI procedures involve either bare metal stents (BMS) or drug-eluting stents (DES).

Kaluza and colleagues[45,46] first described the high-risk of noncardiac surgery soon after intervention with BMS in 2000. Of the 25 patients undergoing surgery within 2 weeks of BMS placement, eight patients died (32%; 95% CI 15–54) versus none of the 15 patients who underwent surgery 15 to 39 days after stenting. Seven patients had an acute MI that was probably or definitely caused by stent thrombosis, and 6 of them died. An analysis of the Mayo Clinic database looked at 207 patients who underwent surgery in the 2 months following successful BMS placement.[47] Eight patients died or suffered a MI or stent thrombosis (3.9%; 95% CI 1.7–7.5). In contrast to the study by Kaluza and colleagues, the risk of death, MI, or stent thrombosis was considerably less, but risk remained elevated for 6 weeks, not just 2 weeks.

In a larger, more recent study from the Mayo Clinic, Nuttall and colleagues[48] looked at major adverse cardiac events (MACE: death, MI, stent thrombosis, or repeat target vessel revascularization) in 899 patients with BMS undergoing elective noncardiac surgery. The frequency of MACEs was 10.5% when surgery was performed less than 30 days after PCI with BMS, 3.8% at 30 to 90 days, and 2.8% at more than 90 days. In multivariate analysis, a shorter time interval between PCI with BMS and surgery was significantly associated with increased incidence of MACEs (OR 3.2; 95% CI 1.5–6.9; $P = .006$). Bleeding events were not associated with time between PCI and surgery.

Stent thrombosis is a catastrophic event resulting in ST segment elevation MI or death and seems to be most common in the first 2 weeks after BMS placement.[49,50] Rapid re-endothelialization of BMS occurs; therefore, dual antiplatelet therapy with thienopyridine (ticlopidine or clopidogrel) plus aspirin is recommended for only 4 weeks after BMS placement.[51]

ACC/AHA guidelines recommend delaying elective noncardiac surgery for 4 to 6 weeks after BMS placement to allow endothelialization of stent and proper thienopyridine use to decrease the risk of stent thrombosis, but not for more than 12 weeks, when restenosis may begin to occur. Continuation of daily aspirin therapy during the perioperative period is also recommended.[32]

With DES, stent thrombosis may occur late (>1 year after implantation), particularly in setting of discontinuation of antiplatelet agents before noncardiac surgery.[52,53] Compton and colleagues[54] reported the experience of a single-center with 41 major and 18 minor noncardiac surgeries at a median of 9 months from DES implantation. No MACE or deaths occurred after the major or minor procedures. Schouten and colleagues[55] described stent thrombosis in 3 of the 99 patients (3%), who underwent surgery within 2 years of DES implantation. These authors did not find a difference in the rate of MACEs in patients with DES compared with BMS.

Rabbits and colleagues looked at 520 patients who underwent noncardiac surgery within 2 years after DES placement. Unlike the results reported by this same group of authors with BMS,[48] the frequency of MACEs was not found to be significantly associated with time between PCI and surgery (rate of MACEs 6.4%, 5.7%, 5.9%, and 3.3% at 0–90, 91–180, 181–365, and 366–730 days after PCI with DES; P = .727 for comparison across groups). Observed rates of MACEs were lowest after 1 year; however, the authors note that their study was underpowered to detect a difference between groups. Additionally, the rate of bleeding complications or transfusion requirements did not seem to be related to antiplatelet therapy use.[56]

In January 2007, an AHA/ACC/Society for Cardiovascular Angiography and Interventions, American College of Surgeons, American Diabetes Association science advisory recommended deferring elective procedures until patients have completed 12 months of thienopyridine therapy after DES placement, continuing aspirin if at all possible in the perioperative period, and restarting thienopyridine as early as possible after noncardiac surgery.[51]

Currently, no evidence is available that warfarin, antithrombotics, or glycoprotein IIb/IIIa agents will reduce the occurrence of stent thrombosis after discontinuation of oral antiplatelet agents, and the optimal duration of clopidogrel to prevent late stent thrombosis is unknown.[32,46]

For patients who require revascularization before noncardiac surgery, the timing and bleeding risk of surgery needs to be carefully considered before catheterization.

For urgent surgery (within 2–4 weeks) or surgery carrying a high bleeding risk, balloon angioplasty and provisional BMS placement may be the safest option (Class IIb, LOE C). (Level C signifies that a limited number of population risk studies were available for evaluation.)

*   For surgery that can be delayed for 1 to 12 months, BMS placement and 4 to 6 weeks of dual antiplatet therapy is reasonable (Class IIa, LOE C). The risk of restenosis is higher with BMS as compared with DES, but restenosis is usually not life-threatening and occurs 2 to 3 months after stenting.*

*   If surgery can be deferred for more than 12 months, DES placement may be reasonable, depending on the patient and lesion characteristics (Class IIb, LOE C).[32,57]*

β ADRENERGIC BLOCKADE

After decisions are made regarding preoperative risk stratification and the need for further cardiac evaluation, emphasis shifts toward perioperative medical therapy to prevent cardiac ischemia. β-blockers reduce myocardial oxygen demand by decreasing the force of contraction and heart rate, and have been used for several years to prevent cardiovascular events in patients undergoing noncardiac surgery.[58] In fact, the Physicians Consortium for Performance Improvement and the Surgical Care Improvement Project have identified perioperative β-blockade as a quality measure.[59,60] Two small studies in the 1990s demonstrated a benefit with β-blocker use.[61,62] However, other studies have failed to replicate these findings, and the Perioperative Ischemia Evaluation (POISE) trial actually demonstrated increased mortality in the group receiving β-blockers.[63–65] Additionally, the ACC/AHA Update on β-Blocker Therapy points out that studies have not addressed "how, when, how long, and by whom perioperative β-blocker therapy is ideally or practically implemented."[59]

Mangano and colleagues[61] published the first randomized, double-blind, placebo-controlled trial evaluating the effect of atenolol on overall survival and cardiovascular morbidity. They randomized 200 patients with known CAD or established risk factors to atenolol orally and intravenously or placebo before the induction of anesthesia, immediately after surgery, and daily throughout their hospital stay (up to 7 days). There was no difference in perioperative cardiac events; however, overall mortality was significantly lower among the atenolol-treated patients in the 6 months after hospital discharge (0% vs 8%, $P < .001$), over the first year (3% vs 14%, $P = .005$), and more than 2 years postoperative (10% vs 21%, $P = .019$). Cardiovascular complications were also significantly reduced with a 2-year event-free survival of 68% in the placebo group and 83% in the atenolol group ($P = .008$). In the placebo group, there were slight trends toward higher frequencies of prior MI and DM, and in the atenolol group, trends toward greater use of β-blockers and angiotensin converting enzyme-inhibitors at discharge and follow-up.[66]

The unblinded DECREASE-I trial evaluated bisoprolol versus placebo in 112 vascular surgery patients with abnormal dobutamine echocardiograms (out of an initial cohort of 1351 consecutive patients).[62] Importantly, bisoprolol was initiated at an average of 37 days (range 7–89) before surgery; patients were reevaluated before surgery to titrate bisoprolol to a goal heart rate of less than 60 beats per minute; and bisoprolol was continued for another 30 days. Patients on bisoprolol had a 10-fold reduction in incidence of perioperative cardiac death and MI versus placebo (3.4% vs 34%; $P < .001$), and the safety committee stopped the study early after the first planned interim analysis. The authors in an accompanying editorial postulated that the effect of β-blockade was seen earlier in this study compared with the one by Mangano and colleagues,[61] because this study looked at a population with extremely high baseline risk.[67] Boersma and colleagues[68] reanalyzed the entire cohort of 1351 patients in a follow-up study. They identified 83% of patients as having less than three clinical risk factors. Among this subgroup, patients receiving β-blockers had a lower risk of cardiac complications (0.8%) than those not receiving β-blockers (2.3%).

Lindenauer and colleagues[69] performed a retrospective cohort study of more than 780,000 patients who underwent noncardiac surgery and used propensity-score matching to adjust for differences between patients who did and did not receive perioperative β-blockers. β-Blocker therapy was associated with no benefit and possible harm in patients with RCRI score of 0 or 1[28] and associated with mortality benefit in patients with RCRI score ≥ 2. The adjusted ORs for in-hospital death was 0.88 (95% CI 0.80–0.98) in patients with RCRI score of 2, 0.71 (95% CI 0.63–0.80) with RCRI score of 3, and 0.58 (95% CI 0.50–0.67) with RCRI score of ≥ 4. This study must be interpreted cautiously, given its retrospective design and reliance on administrative databases to discern risk index conditions and treatment.

Yang and colleagues[63] reported that metoprolol was not effective in reducing 30-day and 6-month postoperative cardiac event rates in 496 vascular surgery patients, randomized to metoprolol or placebo starting 2 hours preoperatively and continued for a maximum of 5 days postoperatively. Likewise, Brady and colleagues[64] showed no decrease in cardiovascular events in 103 vascular surgery patients, receiving metoprolol or placebo from admission until 7 days after surgery. A meta-analysis of 22 randomized controlled trials suggested that β-blockers might prevent major cardiovascular events but raise the risk of hypotension and bradycardia.[70]

POISE was the first large trial of perioperative β-blockade and randomized 8351 patients with, or at risk of, atherosclerotic disease to receive either extended release metoprolol succinate or placebo. Treatment was started 2 to 4 hours before surgery and continued for 30 days. The primary composite end point (cardiovascular death, nonfatal MI, and nonfatal cardiac arrest) was lower at 30 days in the metoprolol group than in the placebo group (5.8% vs 6.9%; hazard ratio [HR] 0.84; 95% CI 0.70–0.99;

$P = .04$), driven primarily by a reduction in nonfatal MI. However, there were more deaths in the metoprolol group (3.1% vs 2.3%; HR 1.33; 95% CI 1.03–1.74; $P = .03$) and more strokes (1.0% vs 0.5%; HR 2.17; 95% CI 1.26–3.74; $P = .005$). The increased mortality seems to have been secondary to sepsis, but the mechanism by which β-blockers increase death in the setting of sepsis is not entirely clear. Additionally, clinically significant hypotension and bradycardia were increased in the metoprolol group. The authors concluded that, for every 1000 patients with a similar risk profile, extended release metoprolol in the perioperative period would prevent 15 MIs but result in an excess of 8 deaths and 5 strokes. The POISE trial has been criticized for the aggressiveness of its regimen, with patients receiving 400 mg of metoprolol within the first day of surgery and 200 mg daily afterwards. The ongoing DECREASE-IV study of bisoprolol may provide additional information on perioperative risk reduction with β-blockers.[71]

The 2006 ACC/AHA Update on β-Blocker Therapy recommends continuation of β-blockers perioperatively in patients already receiving them (Class I, LOE C) and initiation of β-blockers in patients with ischemia on preoperative testing (Class I, LOE B).[59]

β-Blockers are recommended for vascular surgery patients in whom preoperative assessment identifies coronary heart disease (Class IIa, LOE B) or high cardiac risk as defined by the presence of multiple clinical risk factors (Class IIa, LOE B).

In addition, β-blockers are a Class IIa recommendation in patients undergoing intermediate- or high-risk procedures and in whom preoperative assessment either identifies coronary heart disease or high cardiac risk.

β-Blockers may be considered in patients undergoing vascular surgery with low cardiac risk (Class IIb, LOE C) or in patients undergoing intermediate- or high-risk procedures with intermediate cardiac risk (Class IIb, LOE C).

HYDROXYMETHYLGLUTARYL-COA REDUCTASE INHIBITORS

Evidence is emerging that hydroxymethylglutaryl-CoA reductase inhibitors, also known as statins, may reduce perioperative ischemia. Numerous large clinical trials of statins in patients with CAD have demonstrated their low density lipoprotein-lowering ability and mortality benefit.[72] Beyond low density lipoprotein reduction, statins have pleiotrophic effects, which include improvement of endothelial function, atherosclerotic plaque stabilization, decreased oxidative stress, and decreased vascular inflammation.[73] These effects may prevent plaque rupture and MI in the perioperative period.

Multiple retrospective studies have looked at the potential benefits of statins in patients undergoing major noncardiac vascular surgery. Kertai and colleagues[74] retrospectively evaluated 570 patients undergoing open repair for infrarenal abdominal aortic aneurysm. On multivariate analysis, statins reduced the incidence of the composite end point (perioperative mortality and MI) with OR of 0.24 (95% CI 0.11–0.54). The Statins for Risk Reduction in Surgery study was a retrospective cohort study of 1163 patients.[75] After multivariate analysis, statin users had a significantly lower perioperative complication rate (OR 0.52; 95% CI 0.35–0.77; $P = .001$), and protective effect persisted after adjusting for propensity of statin use.

Liakopoulos and colleagues[76] performed a meta-analysis of preoperative statin use in more than 30,000 patients included in 19 studies. Statin pretreated patients had a significant reduction in early all-cause mortality (2.2% vs 3.7%; $P<.0001$), atrial fibrillation (24.9% vs 29.3%; OR 0.67; 95% CI 0.51–0.88), stroke (2.1% vs 2.9%; OR 0.74; 95% CI 0.60–0.91), but not for MI (OR 1.11; 95% CI 0.93–1.33). Durazzo and colleagues[77] published the first randomized, blinded, placebo-controlled trial of statin therapy on perioperative cardiovascular complications.

They randomized 100 patients to atorvastatin 20 mg or placebo for 45 days and found that the incidence of cardiovascular events at 6 months was more than three-fold higher with placebo than with atorvastatin (26% vs 8%; $P = .031$). The results of the DECREASE-III trial were recently presented at the European Society of Cardiology meeting.[78] This study randomized 497 statin-naïve patients to fluvastatin XL 80 mg daily or placebo for a median of 37 days before noncardiac vascular surgery and continued for at least 1 month following surgery. The combined end point of cardiovascular mortality or nonfatal MI was significantly lower in the group receiving fluvastatin XL (4.8% vs 10.1%; OR 0.48; 95% CI 0.24–0.95, $P = .039$). The incidence of adverse events, including increase in creatine kinase or alanine aminotransferase elevation, was similar between the two groups, and there were no episodes of myopathy or rhabdomyolysis in either arm. Further studies will be needed to determine proper dosing and timing of preoperative statins.

The 2007 ACC/AHA Guidelines recommend continuation of statin therapy perioperatively in patients already receiving (Class I, LOE B) and suggest that prescribing a statin is reasonable in patients undergoing vascular surgery whether or not they have other risk factors (Class IIa, LOE B).[32]

SUMMARY

Cardiovascular complications are common and result in significant morbidity following noncardiac surgery, especially in patients with peripheral vascular disease or increased age.[72] All patients require some level of preoperative screening to identify and minimize immediate and future risk, with a careful focus on known CAD or risks for CAD and functional capacity. The 2007 ACC/AHA Guidelines are clear that noninvasive and invasive testing should be limited to circumstances in which results will clearly affect patient management or in which testing would otherwise be indicated. β-blocker therapy has become controversial in light of recent publications but should be continued in patients already on therapy and started in patients with high cardiac risk undergoing intermediate- or high-risk surgery. Emerging data suggests statins may reduce perioperative ischemia and mortality, but additional data is needed on patient selection, timing of therapy, and dosing.

REFERENCES

1. Hertzer N, Beven E, Young J, et al. Coronary artery disease in peripheral vascular patients. A classification of 1000 coronary angiograms and results of surgical management. Ann Surg 1984;199:223–33.
2. Mangano D. Perioperative cardiac morbidity. Anesthesiology 1990;72:153–84.
3. Charlson ME, McKenzie CR, Ales KL, et al. The postoperative electrocardiogram and creatine kinase: implications for diagnosis of myocardial infarction after noncardiac surgery. J Clin Epidemiol 1989;42:25–34.
4. von Knorring J. Postoperative myocardial infarction: a prospective study in a risk group of surgical patients. Surgery 1981;90:55–60.
5. Ashton CM, Petersen NJ, Wray NP, et al. The incidence of perioperative myocardial infarction in men undergoing noncardiac surgery. Ann Intern Med 1993;118:504–10.
6. Shah KB, Kleinman BS, Sami H, et al. Reevaluation of perioperative myocardial infarction in patients with prior myocardial infarction undergoing noncardiac operations. Anesth Analg 1990;71:231–5.
7. Tarhan S, Moffitt EA, Taylor WE, et al. Myocardial infarction after general anesthesia. JAMA 1972;220:1451–4.

8. Diehl JT, Cali RF, Hertzer NR, et al. Complications of abdominal aortic reconstruction. Ann Surg 1983;197:49–56.
9. Hertzer NR. Fatal myocardial infarction following abdominal aortic aneurysm resection. Three hundred forty-three patients followed 6–11 years postoperatively. Ann Surg 1980;192:667–73.
10. Hertzer NR. Fatal myocardial infarction following lower extremity revascularization. Two hundred seventy-three patients followed six to eleven postoperative years. Ann Surg 1981;193:492–8.
11. Hertzer NR, Lees CD. Fatal myocardial infarction following carotid endarterectomy. Three hundred thirty-five patients followed 6–11 years after operation. Ann Surg 1981;194:212–8.
12. Yeager RA, Moneta GL, Edwards JM, et al. Late survival after perioperative myocardial infarction complicating vascular surgery. J Vasc Surg 1994;20:598–606.
13. Charlson M, Peterson J, Szatrowski TP, et al. Long-term prognosis after peri-operative cardiac complications. J Clin Epidemiol 1994;47:1389–400.
14. Filipovic J, Jeger R, Probst C, et al. Heart rate variability and cardiac troponin I are incremental and independent predictors of one-year all-cause mortality after major noncardiac surgery in patients at risk of coronary artery disease. J Am Coll Cardiol 2003;42:1767–76.
15. Mangano DT, Browner WS, Hollenberg M, et al. Long-term cardiac prognosis following noncardiac surgery. JAMA 1992;268:233–9.
16. Eagle KA, Brundage BH, Chaitman BR, et al. Guidelines for perioperative cardiovascular evaluation for noncardiac surgery. Report of the American College of Cardiology/American Heart Association Task Force on Practice Guidelines (committee on perioperative cardiovascular evaluation for noncardiac surgery). J Am Coll Cardiol 1996;27:910–48.
17. Eagle KA, Brundage BH, Chaitman BR, et al. Guidelines for perioperative cardiovascular evaluation for noncardiac surgery. Report of the American College of Cardiology/American Heart Association Task Force on Practice Guidelines (committee on perioperative cardiovascular evaluation for noncardiac surgery). Circulation 1996;93:1278–317.
18. Goldman L, Caldera DL, Nussbaum SR, et al. Multifactorial index of cardiac risk in noncardiac surgical procedures. N Engl J Med 1977;297:845–50.
19. Goldman L, Caldera DL, Southwick FS, et al. Cardiac risk factors and complications in non-cardiac surgery. Medicine 1978;57:357–70.
20. Detsky AS, Abrams HB, Forbath N, et al. Cardiac assessment for patients undergoing noncardiac surgery. A multifactorial clinical risk index. Arch Intern Med 1986;146:2131–4.
21. Baron JF, Mundler O, Bertrand M, et al. Dipyridamole-thallium scintigraphy and gated radionuclide angiography to assess cardiac risk before abdominal aortic surgery. N Engl J Med 1994;330:663–9.
22. Steen PA, Tinker JH, Tarhan S. Myocardial reinfarction after anesthesia and surgery. JAMA 1978;239:2566–70.
23. Rao TL, Jacobs KH, El-Etr AA. Reinfarction following anesthesia in patients with myocardial infarction. Anesthesiology 1983;59:499–505.
24. Hernandez AF, Whellan DJ, Stroud S, et al. Outcomes in heart failure patients after major noncardiac surgery. J Am Coll Cardiol 2004;44:1446–53.
25. Kertai MD, Bountioukos M, Boersma E, et al. Aortic stenosis: an underestimated risk factor for perioperative complications in patients undergoing noncardiac surgery. Am J Med 2004;116:8–13.

26. Sprung J, Abdelmalak B, Gottlieb A, et al. Analysis of risk factors for myocardial infarction and cardiac mortality after major vascular surgery. Anesthesiology 2000;93:129–40.
27. Goldman L. Aortic stenosis in noncardiac surgery: underappreciated in more ways than one? Am J Med 2004;116:60–2.
28. Lee TH, Marcantonio ER, Mangione CM, et al. Derivation and prospective validation of a simple index for prediction of cardiac risk of major noncardiac surgery. Circulation 1999;100:1043–9.
29. Ramakrishna G, Sprung J, Ravi BS, et al. Impact of pulmonary hypertension on the outcomes of noncardiac surgery. J Am Coll Cardiol 2005;45:1691–9.
30. Hlatky MA, Boineau RE, Higginbotham MB, et al. A brief self-administered questionnaire to determine functional capacity (the Duke Activity Status Index). Am J Cardiol 1989;64:651–4.
31. Reilly DF, McNeely MJ, Doerner D, et al. Self-reported exercise tolerance and the risk of serious perioperative complications. Arch Intern Med 1999;159:2185–92.
32. Fleisher LA, Beckman JA, Brown KA, et al. ACC/AHA 2007 guidelines on perioperative cardiovascular evaluation and care for noncardiac surgery: executive summary: a report of the American College of Cardiology/American Heart Association Task Force on Practice Guidelines (writing committee to revise the 2002 guidelines on perioperative cardiovascular evaluation for noncardiac surgery). J Am Coll Cardiol 2007;50:1707–32.
33. Poldermans D, Arnese M, Fioretti P, et al. Sustained prognostic value of dobutamine stress echocardiography for late cardiac events after major noncardiac vascular surgery. Circulation 1997;95:53–8.
34. Cohen MC, Curran PJ, L'Italien GJ, et al. Long-term prognostic value of preoperative dipyridamole thallium imaging and clinical indexes in patients with diabetes mellitus undergoing peripheral vascular surgery. Am J Cardiol 1999;297:845–50.
35. Poldermans D, Bax JJ, Schouten O, et al. Should major vascular surgery be delayed because of preoperative cardiac testing in intermediate-risk patients receiving beta-blocker therapy with tight heart rate control? J Am Coll Cardiol 2006;48:964–9.
36. Auerbach A, Goldman L. Assessing and reducing the cardiac risk of noncardiac surgery. Circulation 2006;113:1361–76.
37. Beattie WS, Abdelnaem F, Wijeysundera DN, et al. A meta-analytic comparison of preoperative stress echocardiography and nuclear scintigraphy imaging. Anesth Analg 2006;102:8–16.
38. Kertai MD, Boersma E, Bax JJ, et al. A meta-analysis comparing the prognostic accuracy of six diagnostic tests for predicting perioperative cardiac risk in patients undergoing major vascular surgery. Heart 2003;89:1327–34.
39. Eagle KA, Rihal CS, Mickel MC, et al. Cardiac risk of noncardiac surgery, influence of coronary disease and type of surgery in 3,368 operations. Circulation 1997;96:1882–7.
40. Domanski M, Ellis S, Eagle KA. Does preoperative coronary revascularization before noncardiac surgery reduce the risk of coronary events in patients with known coronary artery disease? Am J Cardiol 1995;75:829–31.
41. Hassan SA, Hlatky MA, Boothroyd DB, et al. Outcomes of noncardiac surgery after coronary bypass surgery or coronary angioplasty in the Bypass Angioplasty Revascularization Investigation (BARI). Am J Med 2001;110:260–6.
42. McFalls EO, Ward HG, Moritz TE, et al. Coronary-artery revascularization before elective major vascular surgery. N Engl J Med 2004;351:2795–804.

43. Poldermans D, Schouten O, Vidakovic R, et al. A clinical randomized trial to evaluate the safety of a noninvasive approach in high-risk patients undergoing major vascular surgery: the DECREASE-V pilot study. J Am Coll Cardiol 2007;49:1763–9.

44. Brilakis ES, Orford JL, Fasseas P, et al. Outcome of patients undergoing balloon angioplasty in the two months prior to noncardiac surgery. Am J Cardiol 2005;96:512–45.

45. Kaluza GL, Joseph J, Lee JR, et al. Catastrophic outcomes of noncardiac surgery soon after coronary stenting. J Am Coll Cardiol 2000;35:1288–94.

46. Brilakis ES, Banerjee S, Berger PB. Perioperative management of patients with coronary stents. J Am Coll Cardiol 2007;49:2145–50.

47. Wilson SH, Fasseas P, Orford JL, et al. Clinical outcome of patients undergoing non-cardiac surgery in the two months following coronary stenting. J Am Coll Cardiol 2003;42:234–40.

48. Nuttall GA, Brown MJ, Stombaugh JW, et al. Time and cardiac risk of surgery after bare-metal stent percutaneous coronary intervention. Anesthesiology 2008;109:588–95.

49. Wilson SH, Rihal CS, Bell MR, et al. Timing of coronary stent thrombosis in patients treated with ticlopidine and aspirin. Am J Cardiol 1999;83:1006–11.

50. Berger PB, Bell MR, Hasdai D, et al. Safety and efficacy of ticlopidine for only 2 weeks after successful intracoronary stent placement. Circulation 1999;99:248–53.

51. Grines CL, Bonow RO, Casey DE, et al. Prevention of premature discontinuation of dual antiplatelet therapy in patients with coronary artery stents. Circulation 2007;115:813–8.

52. McFadden EP, Stabile E, Regar E, et al. Late thrombosis in drug-eluting coronary stents after discontinuation of antiplatelet therapy. Lancet 2004;364:1519–21.

53. Nasser M, Kapeliovich M, Markiewicz W. Late thrombosis of sirolimus-eluting stents following noncardiac surgery. Catheter Cardiovasc Interv 2005;65:516–9.

54. Compton PA, Zankar AA, Adesanya AO, et al. Risk of noncardiac surgery after coronary drug-eluting stent implantation. Am J Cardiol 2006;98:1212–3.

55. Schouten O, vanDomburg RT, Bax JJ, et al. Noncardiac surgery after coronary stenting: early surgery and interruption of antiplatet therapy are associated with an increase in major adverse cardiac events. J Am Coll Cardiol 2007;49:122–4.

56. Rabbitts JA, Nuttall GA, Brown MJ, et al. Cardiac risk of noncardiac surgery after percutaneous coronary intervention with drug-eluting stents. Anesthesiology 2008;109:596–604.

57. Satler LF. Recommendations regarding stent selection in relation to the timing of noncardiac surgery postpercutaneous coronary intervention. Catheter Cardiovasc Interv 2004;63:146–7.

58. Siliciano D, Mangano DT. Postoperative myocardial ischemia: mechanisms and therapies. In: Estafanous FG, editor. Opioids in anesthesia II. Boston: Butterworth-Heinemann; 1991. p. 164–77.

59. Fleisher LA, Beckman JA, Brown KA, et al. ACC/AHA 2006 guideline update on perioperative cardiovascular evaluation for noncardiac surgery: focused update on perioperative beta-blocker therapy. A report of the American College of Cardiology/American Heart Association Task Force on Practice Guidelines (writing committee to update the 2002 guidelines on perioperative cardiovascular evaluation for noncardiac surgery). J Am Coll Cardiol 2006;47:2343–55.

60. Harte B, Jaffer AK. Perioperative beta-blockers in noncardiac surgery: evolution of the evidence. Cleve Clin J Med 2008;75:513–9.

61. Mangano DT, Layug EL, Wallace A, et al. Effect of atenolol on mortality and cardiovascular morbidity after noncardiac surgery. N Engl J Med 1996;335:1713–20.

62. Poldermans D, Boersma E, Bax JJ, et al. The effect of bisoprolol on perioperative mortality and myocardial infarction in high-risk patients undergoing vascular surgery. N Engl J Med 1999;341:1789–94.

63. Yang H, Raymer K, Butler R, et al. The effects of perioperative β-blockade: results of the Metoprolol after Vascular Surgery (MaVS) study, a randomized controlled trial. Am Heart J 2006;152:983–90.

64. Brady AR, Gibbs JS, Greenhalgh RM, et al. Perioperative beta-blockade (POBBLE) for patients undergoing infrarenal vascular surgery: results of a randomized double-blind controlled trial. J Vasc Surg 2005;41:602–9.

65. POISE Study Group. Effects if extended-release metoprolol succinate in patients undergoing non-cardiac surgery (POISE trial): a randomised controlled trial. Lancet 2008;371:1839–47.

66. Eagle KA, Froehlich JB. Reducing the cardiovascular risk in patients undergoing noncardiac surgery. N Engl J Med 1996;335:1761–3.

67. Lee TH. Reducing cardiac risk in noncardiac surgery. N Engl J Med 1999;341: 1838–40.

68. Boersma E, Poldermans D, Bax JJ, et al. Predictors of cardiac events after major vascular surgery. Role of clinical characteristics, dobutamine echocardiography, and β-blocker therapy. JAMA 2001;285:1865–73.

69. Lindenauer PK, Pekow P, Wang K, et al. Perioperative beta-blocker therapy and mortality after major noncardiac surgery. N Engl J Med 2005;353:349–61.

70. Devereaux PJ, Beattie WS, Choi PTL, et al. How strong is the evidence for the use of perioperative β blockers in non-cardiac surgery? Systematic review and meta-analysis of randomised controlled trials. BMJ 2005;331:313–21.

71. Schouten O, Poldermans D, Visser L, et al. Fluvastatin and bisoprolol for the reduction of perioperative cardiac mortality and morbidity in high-risk patients undergoing noncardiac surgery: rationale and design of the DECREASE-IV study. Am Heart J 2004;148:1047–52.

72. Poldermans D, Hoeks SE, Feringa HH. Pre-operative risk assessment and risk reduction before surgery. J Am Coll Cardiol 2008;51:1913–24.

73. Feldman LS, Brotman DJ. Perioperative statins: more than lipid lowering? Cleve Clin J Med 2008;75:654–62.

74. Kertai MD, Boersma E, Westerhout CM, et al. Association between long-term statin use and mortality after successful abdominal aortic aneurysm surgery. Am J Med 2004;116:96–103.

75. O'Neil-Callahan K, Katsimaglis G, Tepper MR, et al. Statins decrease perioperative cardiac complications in patients undergoing noncardiac vascular surgery: the Statins for Risk Reduction in Surgery (StaRRS) study. J Am Coll Cardiol 2005;45:336–42.

76. Liakopoulos OJ, Choi YH, Haldenwang PL, et al. Impact of preoperative statin therapy on adverse postoperative outcomes in patients undergoing cardiac surgery: a meta-analysis of over 30,000 patients. Eur Heart J 2008;29:1548–59.

77. Durazzo AE, Machado FS, Ikeoka DT, et al. Reduction in cardiovascular events after vascular surgery with atorvastatin: a randomized trial. J Vasc Surg 2004; 39:967–76.

78. Fluvastatin XL use is associated with improved cardiac outcome after major vascular surgery. Results from a Randomized Placebo-Controlled Trial: DECREASE III. Presented by Dr. Don Poldermans at the European Society of Cardiology Congress, Munich, Germany, August/September 2008.

Noninvasive Imaging of the Heart and Coronary Arteries

Amy M. West, MD[a], Christopher M. Kramer, MD[b,c,d],*

KEYWORDS

- Heart • Coronary arteries • Imaging • Echocardiography
- Cardiac magnetic resonance • Cardiac computed tomography
- Myocardial perfusion imaging

OVERVIEW OF NONINVASIVE IMAGING MODALITIES

Noninvasive imaging of the heart and coronary arteries has evolved tremendously since the 1950s when the first rudimentary echocardiogram was performed by Dr. Inge Edler who recorded echoes from the heart of Hellmuth Hertz, a physicist, using a sonar device borrowed from a shipyard.[1] The techniques available today for examination of the heart and coronary arteries include advanced imaging with echocardiography, cardiac magnetic resonance (CMR), nuclear imaging, and computed tomography (CT).

Two-dimensional Transthoracic Echocardiography

Echocardiography allows for a rapid bedside assessment of cardiac including evaluation of myocardial thickness, function, valvular disease, pericardial pathology, and chamber size. An echocardiogram includes information obtained by M-mode imaging, two-dimensional analysis, and Doppler echocardiography. The velocity of blood measured by the Doppler frequency shift can be used to estimate cardiac pressure gradients and valve areas. Obtaining a comprehensive cardiac evaluation by transthoracic echocardiography can be limited with a large patient body habitus or lung hyperinflation as seen with emphysema.

Appropriateness criteria for ordering transthoracic echocardiograms (TTE) were established in 2007, which outline indications for TTE based on several

[a] Division of Cardiovascular Medicine, Department of Medicine, University of Virginia Health System, Lee Street, Box 800158, Charlottesville, VA 22908, USA
[b] Cardiovascular Imaging Center, University of Virginia, Charlottesville, VA 22908, USA
[c] Division of Cardiovascular Medicine, Department of Medicine, University of Virginia Health System, Lee Street, Box 800170, Charlottesville, VA 22908, USA
[d] Department of Radiology, University of Virginia Health System, Lee Street, Box 800170, Charlottesville, VA 22908, USA
* Corresponding author.
E-mail address: ckramer@virginia.edu (C.M. Kramer).

Surg Clin N Am 89 (2009) 763–780
doi:10.1016/j.suc.2009.05.007
0039-6109/09/$ – see front matter © 2009 Elsevier Inc. All rights reserved.

surgical.theclinics.com

themes: general evaluation of structure and function, evaluation of valvular function, evaluation of patients with hypertension, heart failure, or cardiomyopathy.[2] In the patient preparing for cardiac surgery, TTE is commonly used for evaluation of the left ventricular (LV) and valvular function to aid in surgical planning. Advances in echocardiography include real time three-dimensional transthoracic echocardiography, the use of myocardial contrast, and strain analysis used for evaluating diastolic dysfunction.

Real time, three-dimensional, transthoracic echocardiography was developed in the 1990s by von Ramm and colleagues,[3] providing three-dimensional reconstructions of two-dimensional data. The technology was updated with a new matrix-array transducer in 2002 allowing simultaneous data acquisition and visualization of the beating heart.[4] Three-dimensional transthoracic echocardiography has several clinical applications: direct three-dimensional visualization of the cardiac chambers structure and volumes, comprehensive valvular views, and enhanced analysis of myocardial abnormalities such as atrial or ventricular septal defects or hypertrophic cardiomyopathy.[5] In particular, real time three-dimensional echocardiography is helpful in evaluating mitral valve pathology. Imaging the valve opening plane allows measurement of the mitral valve orifice area, which correlates better with the Gorlin formula estimate of mitral valve area than traditional two-dimensional echo valve planimetry.[6] There is good correlation between the surgically identified location of mitral valve prolapse and the three-dimensional echocardiographic evaluation.[7] However, there is limited application for transthoracic three-dimensional echocardiography for aortic and tricuspid valve disease. For patients with atrial or ventricular septal defects undergoing repair, real time three-dimensional echocardiography is used to evaluate the location and dimensions of the defect.[8]

Contrast echocardiography is most often used to evaluate for the presence of an intracardiac or intrapulmonary shunt.[9] The contrast agent used is agitated saline because saline bubbles are too large to cross the pulmonary vascular bed and therefore cannot gain access into the left heart chambers unless there is a shunt present. Other contrast agents have been developed using a gas bubble (perfluoropropane surrounded with either a perflutren lipid microsphere (Definity, Bristol-Myers Squibb Medical Imaging, North Billerica, Massachusetts) or perflutren protein type A microsphere (Optison, GE Healthcare, Princeton, New Jersey). These injectable contrast agents have durable microbubbles that are small enough to go through the pulmonary circulation and therefore opacify the left ventricle. The main advantage of these agents is enhancement of the endocardial border and they are most often used with stress echocardiography[10] or in TTE with limited windows.[11] A Food and Drug Administration (FDA) black box warning was issued for the use of Definity and Optison in October 2007 after reports of serious cardiopulmonary reactions within 30 minutes following administration in high-risk patients.[12] The black box warning was subsequently removed in July 2008 and the current FDA recommendation is that high-risk patients with pulmonary hypertension or unstable cardiopulmonary conditions should be monitored during contrast administration and for 30 minutes afterwards.[13] A large retrospective review of more than 18,000 patients receiving stress echocardiography with contrast showed that there was no difference in death or myocardial infarction rate at 1 hour and 30 days after the study compared with patients who received stress echocardiography without contrast.[14]

Echocardiographic evaluation of diastolic dysfunction involves assessment of the LV filling patterns using the pulsed wave Doppler mitral inflow velocities, pulmonary venous flow, and tissue Doppler imaging of mitral annular motion.[15]

Transesophageal Echocardiography

Compared with TTE, transesophageal echocardiography (TEE) offers superior views of the posterior cardiac structures due to their proximity with the esophagus. Contraindications to performing a TEE include esophageal disease including stricture, malignancy or recent ulcer, difficulty swallowing given concern of undiagnosed esophageal pathology, and altered mental status or an uncooperative patient. In 2007, the American Society of Echocardiography outlined indications for TEE as an initial test, including suspected aortic dissection, guidance during percutaneous noncoronary interventions, preoperative evaluation for regurgitant valve repair, diagnosis of endocarditis with a moderate to high pretest probability or persistent fever in the setting of an intracardiac device, and evaluation for thrombus in the left atrium before ablation or cardioversion.[2]

The most widely accepted indication for intraoperative TEE is valve surgery. Intraoperative TEE is used before initiating cardiopulmonary bypass to evaluate for any changes occurring in the interval between the decision for surgery and the actual operation, as well as to aid in the decision about feasibility of valve repair versus replacement, particularly with mitral valve pathology.

For mitral valve surgery, the intraoperative pre-bypass TEE changes the operative plan in approximately 6% to 19% of cases.[16] The severity of the mitral regurgitation or stenosis seen at the time of intraoperative echocardiogram may be different from what was found on the outpatient examination due to changes in the patient's hemodynamics due to general anesthesia.[17] The severity of mitral regurgitation is determined based on the size of the jet at its origin (vena contracta), relative area of the regurgitant jet compared with the left atrium, and the proximal isovelocity surface area (PISA) method. The mechanism of the mitral regurgitation can be established by evaluating the jet direction as well as the structure and motion of the mitral valve leaflets.[18] After mitral valve repair, TEE is repeated before the administration of protamine and removal of the cannulas to assess for the degree of mitral regurgitation and any surgical complications such as systolic motion of the anterior leaflet of the mitral valve.[19] Prosthetic heart valves are evaluated post placement with intraoperative TEE to evaluate for appropriate placement and periprosthetic or prosthetic leaks.[20]

With aortic valve replacement with either a prosthetic valve or pulmonic homograft, intraoperative TEE allows for anatomic assessment of the aortic valve and aorta as well as the degree and mechanism of aortic stenosis (AS) or regurgitation. For instance, feasibility of aortic valve repair can be determined by TEE as it is most often performed in patients with a bicuspid aortic valve and leaflet prolapse, leaflet perforation due to endocarditis, or aortic root dilation causing functional valvular regurgitation.[21] As with mitral valve surgery, postoperative TEE is used to assess for the adequacy of the aortic valve repair. In addition, regional wall motion abnormalities may arise due to technical difficulties with coronary implantation.

In patients undergoing valve surgery for endocarditis, TEE provides for assessment of whether the valvular regurgitation is transvalvular or paravalvular as well as extension of the infection to involve a ring abscess (**Figs. 1** and **2**).[22] In addition, infectious endocarditis may involve other valves not previously noted on the preoperative evaluation and, as a result, a thorough valvular examination is warranted on the intraoperative TEE.

An additional use of TEE during the intraoperative period is to evaluate for the presence of intracardiac air after routine deairing in patients undergoing cardiac surgery.[23] By identifying persistent intracardiac air with TEE, additional deairing procedures can be taken to prevent air embolism and subsequent central nervous system injury.

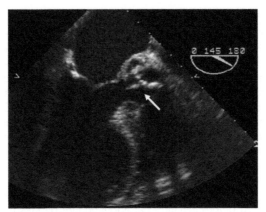

Fig. 1. TEE demonstrating the three-chamber view with a mass on the aortic valve, which is consistent with a vegetation.

Nuclear Imaging

The application of nuclear medicine in cardiac imaging is aimed at identifying myocardial perfusion as part of an ischemia evaluation, evaluating myocardial viability and measuring LV function.

ECG-gated single photon emission computed tomography (SPECT) uses a radioactive blood flow marker such as thallium-201 or technetium-99m sestamibi to enter into the cardiac myocytes in proportion with cardiac blood flow. Thallium has similar properties to potassium and accesses the myocardium through a Na-K-ATPase pump, whereas technetium-99m sestamibi is taken up by mitochondria into the cardiac myocytes.[24] As the radionuclides decay, gamma rays are emitted and detected by a gamma camera or multicrystal camera and a computer program then processes the data obtained. The reconstructed images include short-axis, horizontal long-axis, and vertical long-axis views of the heart. With the addition of a 3-lead ECG gating device, regional wall motion can be obtained. The endocardium is identified by computer analysis and cardiac volumes at end-diastole (EDV) and end-systole (ESV)

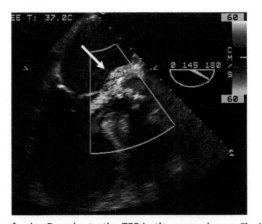

Fig. 2. The addition of color Doppler to the TEE in the same view as **Fig. 1** demonstrates the presence of moderate to severe aortic regurgitation as well as an aortic abscess.

are measured, allowing an accurate assessment of the LV ejection fraction (EDV − ESV/EDV) when compared with echocardiography.[25] Planar multigated acquisition (MUGA) with radiolabeled red blood cells is used to calculate an accurate and reproducible LV volume and ejection fraction, mostly in patients undergoing chemotherapy with potentially cardiotoxic agents.[26]

SPECT myocardial perfusion imaging identifies myocardial ischemia as a reversible defect seen on stress images that resolves with rest (**Figs. 3** and **4**). Myocardial blood flow during stress is reduced in areas supplied by vessels that have fixed stenoses and are hemodynamically significant. Fixed perfusion defects (seen at stress and rest) are indicated prior to myocardial infarction. In the setting of a mild perfusion defect that is fixed, this may be due to a small infarction or artifact due to signal attenuation.[27] In addition to obtaining perfusion and LV volume calculations, regional wall motion is assessed by gated-SPECT.

The most common pharmacologic methods for stress myocardial perfusion imaging include adenosine, regadenoson, dipyridamole, or dobutamine. If patients are able to exercise, this is the preferred method of achieving myocardial stress due to the important prognostic information gained from exercise capacity. Of the pharmacologic agents available, adenosine, regadenoson, and dipyridamole all increase myocardial perfusion by affecting adenosine receptors in the coronary vasculature leading to coronary vasodilation. As a result, side effects of these agents include flushing, nausea, chest discomfort, bronchospasm, or transient heart block. Given the potential respiratory side effects, the agents should not be used in patients with active bronchospasm, however, dobutamine remains an option.

CMR

CMR imaging at 1.5 Tesla (T) provides excellent visualization of cardiac structure and function by using steady state free procession (SSFP) cine imaging, first pass

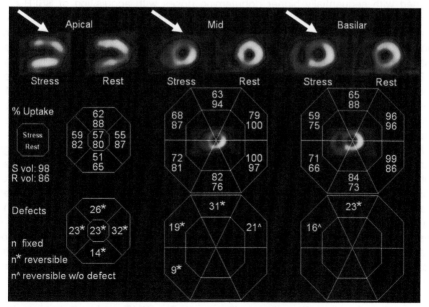

Fig. 3. There is a large region with severe reduction in uptake in the anterior, anteroseptal, and inferoseptal segments that is predominantly reversible. The defect is consistent with ischemia.

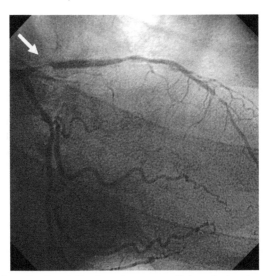

Fig. 4. Cardiac catheterization following the myocardial perfusion imaging in **Fig. 3** that demonstrates a significant proximal left anterior descending (LAD) stenosis.

contrast-enhanced perfusion, late gadolinium enhancement (LGE) for identification of fibrosis, and magnetic resonance (MR) angiography to visualize vascular anatomy. Most cardiac function and morphology information comes from the cine MRI sequences, which obtain a large number of images throughout the cardiac cycle during a breath hold, that are played in a cine mode. Dobutamine stress can be performed with sequentially higher dobutamine doses with acquisition of SSFP cine images at each stage.[28] Using a higher field strength for cardiac imaging such as 3 T allows for improved signal to noise ratios for many cardiovascular applications include perfusion, LGE and angiography. However, assessment of cardiac function with SSFP imaging is challenging at 3 T due to off-resonance artifacts.[29]

Evaluation of the coronary arteries with CMR is limited by its lower spatial resolution compared with multidetector row computed tomography (MDCT). A review of 28 MR coronary angiography studies involving more than 900 patients, done in 2006 by Schuijf and colleagues,[30] found that 83% of segments were analyzable and had a sensitivity of 72% and specificity of 87%.

Myocardial perfusion with pharmacologic stress with CMR at 1.5 T has a high sensitivity to differentiate relevant to nonrelevant coronary stenosis when compared with invasive angiography.[31] A study done in 2003 with 84 patients referred for coronary angiography who underwent adenosine stress CMR imaging demonstrated that quantitative myocardial perfusion had a sensitivity of 88%, specificity of 90%, and an accuracy of 89% for the detection of significant coronary artery disease (CAD).[32] A systematic review by Nandalur and colleagues[33] of all stress CMR studies with angiographic correlation that were done between 1990 and 2007 evaluated the diagnostic performance of CMR perfusion imaging and stress-induced wall motion abnormalities for diagnosis of CAD. There was a high prevalence of CAD in the included studies; the CMR perfusion studies had a prevalence of 57.4% compared with 70.5% in the stress-induced wall motion abnormality group. The CMR perfusion imaging had a sensitivity of 0.91 (95% CI 0.88–0.94), and specificity of 0.81 (95% CI 0.77–0.85) compared with angiography. The stress-induced wall motion abnormalities imaging had a sensitivity of 0.83 (95% CI 0.79–0.88) and specificity of 0.86 (95% CI 0.81–0.91) for detecting CAD in patients. A multicenter trial was published in 2008, which evaluated the diagnostic performance for perfusion-CMR compared with radiograph coronary angiography and SPECT myocardial perfusion imaging; more than 200 patients with known or suspected CAD were evaluated by all three modalities.[34] The difference between perfusion-CMR and gated-SPECT did not reach statistical significance, however, comparing perfusion-CMR with all SPECT studies, the area under the receiver operating characteristic curve for CMR is larger than for SPECT (0.86 + 0.06 vs 0.67 + 0.5, $P < .013$).

LGE uses gadolinium chelates to identify areas of myocardial fibrosis and necrosis. There is delayed washout of gadolinium from myocardium, which also has an increased volume of distribution in interstitial space due to loss of intact myocytes.[35] LGE allows for the accurate assessment of areas of myocardial infarction and nonviable myocardium (**Fig. 5**). Determining areas of myocardial viability is critical when deciding which patients are likely to benefit from revascularization procedures, particularly in the setting of reduced LV function. In the study by Kim and colleagues[36] evaluating 50 patients with LV dysfunction before revascularization, the likelihood of functional improvement in regions without LGE was 86% for segments with at least severe hypokinesia and 100% for segments with akinesia or dyskinesia. In addition, the transmural extent of myocardial infarction is inversely related to recovery of regional LV function after revascularization. Adding low-dose dobutamine cine CMR to LGE may increase the predictive value for regional functional recovery, particularly in cases of preserved end-diastolic wall thickness.[37] In a group of patients with chronic ischemic heart disease and LV systolic dysfunction evaluated with dobutamine CMR before and after revascularization with coronary artery bypass graft (CABG), improved function in myocardial segments with less than 50% transmural infarcts was predicted by the response to dobutamine.[38]

Compared with thallium-201 SPECT myocardial perfusion imaging, CMR using LGE has similar specificity for detecting transmural myocardial infarctions (MI; 98%

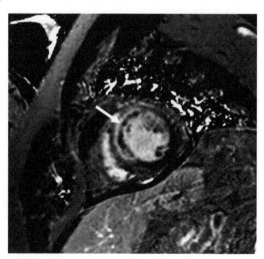

Fig. 5. Example of a patient with an ST elevation myocardial infarction imaged with CMR. The image shows a short-axis view of the left ventricle with delayed contrast enhancement to demonstrate the area of anteroseptal transmural myocardial infarction (*light gray*), and endocardial microvascular obstruction (*black*).

compared with 97%); however, LGE has higher diagnostic power to identify subendo-cardial MI not appreciated by SPECT in 47% of myocardial segments and 13% of patients.[39] LGE aids in differentiating ischemic and nonischemic cardiomyopathies based on the presence of myocardial scar in an ischemic pattern seen by LGE in patients with reduced LV function due to CAD. There are distinct patterns of LGE that aid in the identification of the cause of certain cardiomyopathies such as myocar-ditis (acute and chronic), cardiac sarcoidosis, amyloidosis, and endomyocardial fibrosis.[40]

CMR provides excellent characterization of right ventricular function and allows for the diagnosis of arrhythmogenic right ventricular cardiomyopathy based on ventricular size, wall motion abnormalities as well as the presence of LGE consistent with fibro-fatty replacement of the myocardium.[41] Accurate assessment of right ventricular func-tion and the motion of the interventricular septum during real time free breathing imaging provides a framework for evaluating pericardial constriction with CMR in addi-tion to imaging of pericardial thickness.

Valvular heart disease is most frequently evaluated by echocardiography, including Doppler techniques. The essential information needed for the diagnosis and management of patients with valvular heart disease includes data on valve morphology, valve function, ventricular function, and the presence of coexisting cardiac disease.[42] SSFP or gradient echo sequences by CMR provide visualization of the valve structure and dysfunction. Velocity-encoded cine allows for quantification of flow across valves and therefore blood flow velocities and volumes to be measured.[43] In particular, stroke volume, cardiac output, regurgitant flow through incompetent valves or high velocity jets through stenotic valves can be readily calcu-lated. The limits for regurgitation fraction for mitral regurgitation have been established using CMR and are derived by subtracting the forward flow of the aorta from the ventricular stroke volume.[44]

Cardiac Computed Tomography

Initial cardiac CT technology with electrocardiographic gating for imaging of the heart used electron beam CT (EBCT) and had limitations with spatial resolution. EBCT was mainly used for calculating a CT-based calcium score of the coronary arteries to aid in stratifying the patient's risk of coronary atherosclerosis. The temporal and spatial resolution of CT improved significantly with the development of MDCT. Since its advent in 1999, the use of MDCT with retrospective cardiac gating has steadily increased for cardiac imaging. The number of detectors used for acquiring raw data has increased geometrically. The advent of 64 detector scanners allowed for enhanced temporal and spatial resolution with short scan times. Scanners are now becoming available with as many as 256 or 320 detectors and data can be acquired during a single breath hold in as little as one heartbeat. A typical amount of intravenous iodinated contrast used for coronary CT angiography is between 60 and 100 mL de-pending on patient size and heart rate. The average dose of ionizing radiation from a 64-slice cardiac MDCT examination using ECG gating and dose modulation is 7 to 11 mSV,[45] but these doses can be reduced further with prospective gating as well as 256 or 320 detector scanners. The radiation dose is similar to that from an abdomen and pelvis CT (8–11 mSv) but higher than x-ray coronary angiography (3–6 mSv).[46]

As part of a CT coronary angiographic study, a coronary calcium score is usually obtained first. If patients have a high calcium score (greater than 400 Agaston units), there is a greater likelihood of coronary artery calcifications, which can cause a blooming artifact, obscuring the ability to analyze plaque within the vessel.[47] Excess artifact is also caused by irregular heartbeats, difficulty with breath holding, and pacing wires.

A review in the European Heart Journal from 2008 pooled the data of more than 800 patients who had CT coronary angiography using 64 detector MDCT in patients with suspected CAD.[48] The sensitivity was 89% (95% CI 87–90) with a specificity of 96% (95% CI 96–97) and a positive and negative predictive value (NPV) of 78% (95% CI 76–80) and 98% (95% CI 98–99), respectively. Another recent study of CT coronary angiography using a 64-slice multidetector scanner in patients with chest pain and low to intermediate risk of underlying CAD, showed a high NPV (99%) for detecting stenosis greater than 70%.[49] However, the positive predictive value (PPV) was low at 48%.

Given the high NPV of CT coronary angiography, the main clinical application at the present time is evaluating chest pain in patients with low to intermediate risk of CAD, especially in emergency department patients. Other clinical indications include detection of CAD with prior equivocal stress test results, suspected coronary anomalies, and evaluation of pericardial disease. In addition, cardiac CT is used before interventional and surgical procedures, including evaluation of pulmonary vein anatomy before atrial fibrillation ablation and noninvasive coronary imaging before ventricular tachycardia ablation. CT coronary angiography is not routinely used for assessing coronary stent patency as the overall accuracy is inadequate for diagnostic purposes especially in smaller stents.

Identification of occluded or stenosed bypass grafts is straightforward on cardiac CT angiography given their large diameter; however, accurate visualization can be limited by the presence of surgical metal clips. Evaluation of native coronary arteries after bypass surgery with CT angiography is limited due to coronary calcifications and advanced atherosclerosis. The European Society of Cardiology published a report in 2008 on cardiac CT, which pooled the available literature on the diagnostic accuracy of 16- and 64-slice MDCT for evaluation of patients after coronary artery bypass surgery (**Table 1**).[48]

Evaluation of the coronary vessels is usually done with images reconstructed from mid- to end-diastole (**Fig. 6**). However, LV function, volume, and wall thickness can be obtained from reconstruction of the raw data throughout the cardiac cycle.[50] When compared with cardiac MR measurements the LV ejection fraction correlates well, as do EDVs and ESVs, but there is a tendency to systematic overestimation of volumes compared with cardiac MR due to lower temporal resolution.

Table 1
Diagnostic accuracy of MDCT for evaluation of patients after coronary artery bypass surgery

Vessel	Not Evaluable (%)	Sensitivity (%)	Specificity (%)	PPV (%)	NPV (%)
Graft occlusion	0.7 (3/418) (95% CI 0.15–0.21)	100 (130/130) (95% CI 97–100)	100 (494/495) (95% CI 99–100)	99 (130/131) (95% CI 96–100)	100 (494/494) (95% CI 99–100)
Graft stenosis	6.4 (39/611) (95% CI 4.6–8.6)	97 (184/1889) (95% CI 94–99)	95 (337/354) (95% CI 92–97)	92 (184/201) (95% CI 87–95)	99 (337/342) (95% CI 97–100)
Native arteries	19.6 (333/1697) (95% CI 18–22)	95 (524/545) (95% CI 93–97)	75 (608/813) (95% CI 72–78)	67 (424/629) (95% CI 64–71)	97 (608/629) (95% CI 95–98)

From Schroeder S, Achenbach S, Bengel F, et al. Cardiac computed tomography: indications, applications, limitations and training requirements. Eur Heart J 2008;29(4):531–56; by permission of Oxford University Press/European Society of Cardiology.

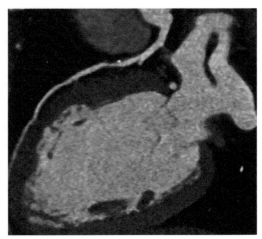

Fig. 6. Coronary CT angiogram in the two-chamber view demonstrating the CAD artery with a small amount of proximal calcium.

SPECIFIC APPLICATIONS OF CARDIAC IMAGING
Evaluation for Ischemia

Exercise ECG stress testing has a lower sensitivity than stress imaging, however, it remains useful in patients who have a normal baseline ECG and can exercise to a high level. The 2007 update to the American College of Cardiology (ACC)/American Heart Association (AHA) task force on chronic stable angina reinforced that among patients who are able to exercise and have an intermediate pretest probability of disease with resting ECG abnormalities, either exercise echocardiography or exercise radionuclide myocardial perfusion imaging is acceptable.[51]

If patients are unable to exercise, dobutamine stress echocardiography is an option. The inotropic and chronotropic effects of dobutamine elicit ischemia from regions of myocardium with impaired blood flow. Echo images are obtained throughout the dobutamine infusion and during peak stress. Exercise echo and myocardial perfusion imaging have similar NPVs for MI or cardiac death over a 3-year period: 98.4% and 98.9%, respectively.[52] In terms of ability to detect CAD, a meta-analysis demonstrated exercise echo and exercise MPI stress tests have similar sensitivities (85% and 87%, respectively), however, exercise echo has a higher specificity (77% vs 64%).[53] In terms of pharmacologic stress testing, another meta-analysis compared patients who underwent echo or SPECT stress testing with adenosine, dipyridamole, or dobutamine for diagnosis of CAD. The study found that SPECT imaging with vasodilators has the highest sensitivity, whereas the maximum combination of sensitivity and specificity is found with dobutamine echocardiography.[54]

Pharmacologic stress CMR testing uses either vasodilator therapy for perfusion imaging or dobutamine for stress functional imaging. The former has higher sensitivity but the latter has higher specificity.[33] Both have excellent NPVs over 2 to 3 years.[55]

Viability Testing

Studies suggest approximately 25% to 40% of patients with ischemic cardiomyopathy will demonstrate improved LV function with revascularization.[56] In patients with CAD and abnormal LV function, myocardial viability seen on noninvasive imaging is strongly associated with improved survival after revascularization.[57]

Given the prognostic importance of identifying viable myocardium, accurate assessment of patients likely to benefit from revascularization is a key component of the preprocedure evaluation. A pooled literature review performed by Bax and colleagues[58] in 2001 compared the sensitivity, specificity, PPV and NPV for improved LV function with revascularization of the most often used viability techniques at that time: dobutamine stress echo, SPECT with thallium- or technetium-labeled sestamibi, and positron emission tomography (PET) with [18F]fluorodeoxyglucose (FDG). For dobutamine stress echo, the mean sensitivity was 81% and the specificity was 80%, with a PPV and NPV of 77% and 85%, respectively. Dobutamine stress echo tests for contractile reserve and identifies viable myocardium based on the myocardium's response to dobutamine with either an initial improvement in LV contractility followed by worsened wall motion or an immediate decrease in LV contractility. In comparison, for technetium-labeled sestamibi SPECT viability studies, most were 1-day resting studies without the use of nitroglycerin and had a mean sensitivity of 81% and specificity of 66%, with a PPV and NPV of 71% and 77%, respectively.

CMR has been validated as an accurate method of determining viability with either LGE or low-dose dobutamine contractile reserve as discussed above. It is being increasingly used to evaluate patients before planned coronary artery bypass surgery and is especially useful to evaluate the LV apex when considering ventricular restoration surgery.

There are limited clinical data to date on the use of cardiac CT for assessment of myocardial perfusion and viability. Sixty four-slice MDCT was performed in 34 patients with acute myocardial infarction and the perfusion defects on MDCT had a moderate correlation with SPECT ($r = 0.48$, $-7\% \pm 9\%$).[59] MDCT has been shown to detect myocardial scar as late hyperenhancement compared with CMR. In a study of 28 patients with reperfused infarction by Mahnken and colleagues,[60] late myocardial enhancement seen on MDCT and CMR had good agreement.

Aortic Valve Disease

AS severity is established noninvasively by echocardiography using the continuity equation and Doppler analysis.[61] The aortic jet velocity, mean pressure gradient, and valve area stratify patients into mild, moderate, and severe AS. Indications for surgery in patients with severe AS include the presence of symptoms, LV systolic dysfunction, or planned cardiac surgery for another indication. If it is unclear whether a patient is symptomatic, exercise testing can be performed to assess for development of symptoms, degree of functional ability, decrease in blood pressure, or the presence of ventricular arrhythmia.[62]

Echocardiography provides excellent imaging of the aortic valve, particularly with TEE. Calculation of the aortic valve area (AVA) using direct planimetry with CMR has been validated in patients with severe AS against the AVA measured invasively using the Gorlin equation, the AVA from TEE with planimetry, and the AVA generated from TTE using the continuity equation.[63] The AVA measured by the continuity equation with CMR correlates well with the continuity equation measured by TTE ($r = 0.98$). In TEE and CMR, the AVA measured by planimetry is larger than that calculated by the continuity equation. CMR studies of patients with AS show the peak jet velocity measured by phase-shift velocity mapping has good agreement with measurements made by conventional Doppler ultrasound.[64]

A study by Pouleur and colleagues[65] in 2007 compared the accuracy of MDCT, TEE, and CMR measurements of the AVA in patients with severe AS preparing for valve surgery, using TTE as the reference standard. The AVA by planimetry from MDCT correlated closely with CMR ($r = 0.98$), TEE ($r = 0.98$), and TTE ($r = 0.96$). The planimetry determinations of AVA were all significantly higher than the AVA generated by the continuity equation with TTE. Echocardiography, however, remains the mainstay of aortic valve evaluation.

Mitral Valve Disease

Mitral valve regurgitation is easily assessed with TTE and information about the cause of the valve dysfunction can be obtained. Primary mitral regurgitation stems from anatomic disruption of the mitral valve apparatus and secondary mitral regurgitation occurs in the setting of LV dysfunction due to prior infarction or cardiomyopathy. The severity of mitral regurgitation can be estimated by regurgitant fraction and regurgitant orifice area. With increasing severity and duration of the valvular regurgitation, patients develop depressed LV ejection fraction and enlarged LV systolic dimensions, which are predictors of poor outcome.[66] Surgery for primary mitral valve disease is usually recommended before LV dilatation and dysfunction develops.

The gold standard for evaluation of mitral valve disease is echocardiography. However if patient body habitus or presence of lung disease precludes an adequate examination and sedation for a transesophageal study is not desired, then a viable alternative is CMR. An advantage in using CMR to characterize mitral regurgitation is obtaining accurate information about LV volume and function as well as viability and regional wall motion in patients with ischemic mitral regurgitation.[67] In addition, the location of leaflet prolapse or restriction is identified.

Pericardial Disease

The pericardium is visualized easily by echocardiography, CMR, and cardiac CT. The best diagnostic test depends on the clinical question at hand. Echocardiography is the gold standard for assessing pericardial effusions and evaluating for tamponade. CMR is an excellent modality for diagnosing constriction based on the appearance of the pericardium and ventricular interdependence demonstrated on real time cine imaging. Using CMR, normal pericardium appears as a thin, less than 3 mm, low signal rim around the heart surrounded by higher signal fat. Thickened pericardium suggests fibrinous pericarditis and CMR can also identify the presence of pericardial fluid and constriction (**Fig. 7**).[68] Cardiac CT readily demonstrates pericardial calcification, pericardial thickening, and the presence of effusion.[69]

Cardiac tamponade occurring after cardiac surgery occurs in 0.5% to 5.8% of patients and can present either early or late in the postoperative course.[70] Late tamponade has been defined in the literature as occurring 5 to 7 days postoperatively, but has been reported up to 6 months after surgery.[71] A retrospective review of 510 consecutive cardiac surgery patients was performed to identify the frequency and clinical features of postoperative cardiac tamponade, which found 10 diagnosed cases, with five or six patients having late tamponade.[72] The two-dimensional echocardiography found loculated pericardial effusions and selective chamber compression in most patients. The presence of loculated pericardial effusions or selective chamber compression due to clot can result in atypical presentations of tamponade. In addition, TTE can be technically challenging in surgical patients due to limited acoustic windows secondary to mechanical ventilation, patient position or incisional pain. In cases of suspected tamponade with nondiagnostic transthoracic images, TEE is indicated.[73]

Cardiac Masses/Thrombus

Echocardiography and CMR play a complementary role in evaluating patients suspected of cardiac masses or thrombus. Most initial evaluation of cardiac masses is done by TTE, however, it has limited acoustic windows. The clinical application of

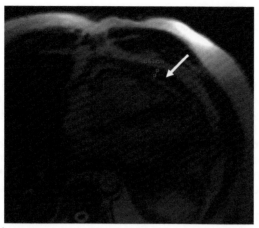

Fig. 7. Example of thickened pericardium seen on a four-chamber axial CMR image for evaluation of constrictive pericarditis. The normal thickness of pericardium is less than 0.3 cm and this patient has a pericardial thickness of 0.63 cm.

three-dimensional echocardiography for evaluation of cardiac masses or thrombi is still evolving. Intracardiac masses visualized with three-dimensional echocardiography may become a standard preoperative evaluation, complementing the traditional two-dimensional TTE and TEE.[74]

Further characterization of a cardiac mass can be done with TEE or CMR. CMR offers a complete morphologic and functional evaluation, particularly with respect to associated pericardial or extracardiac involvement.[75] Bright blood cine CMR details the morphology of a cardiac mass including the origin and involvement of surrounding structures. Additional sequences answer the questions about the presence of hemorrhage, vascularity, and calcification.[76] Cardiac CT can provide information about the involvement of the surrounding pericardium, mediastinum, and lungs; however, the widespread use of CT in evaluating cardiac masses is limited due to the superior tissue characterization by CMR and the radiation exposure of CT.

Congenital Heart Disease

Echocardiography is the primary tool used to diagnose and follow patients with congenital heart disease. CMR is used to diagnose more complex congenital heart disease as well as follow patients after surgical therapy. Transposition of the great vessels, tetralogy of Fallot, pulmonary artery stenosis, double outlet RV, truncus arteriosus, and total anomalous pulmonary venous return are just some of the conditions with excellent characterization using CMR and MR angiography.[77] Cardiac CT can diagnose anomalous coronary arteries, total anomalous pulmonary venous return, bicuspid aortic valve, and pulmonary artery anomalies but has limited experience with more complex congenital heart disease[78] and should be avoided in pediatric patients who are at higher risk from radiation exposure.

SUMMARY

The growth and development in noninvasive imaging of the heart and coronary arteries provides for an environment whereby a true multimodality approach can be taken when evaluating patients with known or suspected heart disease. The application of each imaging modality is best interpreted in the context of the specific diagnostic question and the underlying patient characteristics.

REFERENCES

1. Meyer RA. History of ultrasound in cardiology. J Ultrasound Med 2004;23(1):1–11.
2. Douglas PS, Khandheria B, Stainback RF, et al. ACCF/ASE/ACEP/ASNC/SCAI/SCCT/SCMR 2007 appropriateness criteria for transthoracic and transesophageal echocardiography. J Am Coll Cardiol 2007;50:187–204.
3. Sheikh KH, Smith SW, Von Ramm O, et al. Real-time, three-dimensional echocardiography: feasibility and initial use. Echocardiography 1991;8(1):119–25.
4. Wang X-F, Deng Y-B, Nanda NC, et al. Live three dimensional echocardiography: imaging principles and clinical application. Echocardiography 2003;20(7):593–604.
5. Correale M, Riccardo I, Di Base M. Real time three-dimensional echocardiography: an update. Eur J Intern Med 2008;19:241–8.
6. Suggeng L, Weinert L, Lammertin G, et al. Accuracy of mitral valve area measurements using trans-thoracic rapid freehand 3 dimensional scanning: comparison with invasive and non-invasive methods. J Am Soc Echocardiogr 2003;16(12):1292–300.
7. Delabays A, Jeanrenaud X, Chassot PG, et al. Localization and quantification of mitral valve prolapse using three-dimensional echocardiography. Eur J Echocardiogr 2004;5(6):422–9.
8. Cheng TO, Xie M-X, Wang X-F, et al. Real-time 3-dimensional echocardiography in assessing atrial and ventricular septal defects: an echocardiographic-surgical correlative study. Am Heart J 2004;148(6):1091–5.
9. Meerbaum S. Introduction and general background. In: Meerbaum S, Meltzer R, editors. Myocardial contrast two-dimensional echocardiography. Boston: Kluwer Academic Publishers; 1989. p. 2.
10. Dolan MS, Riad K, El-Shafei A, et al. Effect of intravenous contrast for left ventricular opacification and border definition on sensitivity and specificity of dobutamine stress echocardiography compared with coronary angiography in technically difficult patients. Am Heart J 2001;142(5):908–15.
11. Crouse LJ, Cheirif J, Hanly DE, et al. Opacification and border delineation improvement in patients with suboptimal endocardial border definition in routine echocardiography: results of the Phase III Albunex Multicenter Trial. J Am Coll Cardiol 1993;22(5):1494–500.
12. Main ML, Goldman JH, Grayburn PA. Thinking outside the "box" – the ultrasound contrast controversy. J Am Coll Cardiol 2007;50:2434–7.
13. Available at: www.FDA.gov. Accessed July 17, 2008.
14. Dolan MS, Gala SS, Dodla S, et al. Safety and efficacy of commercially available ultrasound contrast agents for rest and stress echocardiography a multicenter experience. J Am Coll Cardiol 2009;53(1):32–8.
15. Khouri SJ, Maly GT, Shuh DD, et al. A practical approach to the echocardiographic evaluation of diastolic dysfunction. J Am Soc Echocardiogr 2004;17:290–7.
16. Grimm RA, Steward WJ. The role of intraoperative echocardiography in valve surgery. Cardiol Clin 1998;16:477–87.
17. Grewal KS, Malkowski MJ, Kramer CM, et al. Multiplane transesophageal echocardiographic identification of the involved scallop in patients with flail mitral valve leaflet: intraoperative correlation. J Am Soc Echocardiogr 1998;11:966–71.

18. Stewart WJ, Currie PJ, Salcedo EE, et al. Evaluation of the mitral leaflet motion by echocardiography and jet direction by Doppler color flow mapping to determine the mechanism of mitral regurgitation. J Am Coll Cardiol 1992;20:1353–61.

19. Stewart WJ, Salcedo EE. Echocardiography in patients undergoing mitral valve surgery. Semin Thorac Cardiovasc Surg 1989;1:194–202.

20. Meloni L, Aru G, Abbruzzese PA, et al. Regurgitant flow of mitral valve prostheses: an intraoperative transesophageal echocardiographic study. J Am Soc Echocardiogr 1994;7:36–46.

21. Frank L, Aicher D, Kissinger A, et al. Aortic valve repair using a differentiated surgical strategy. Circulation 2004;110:67–73.

22. Shapiro SM, Bayer AS. Transesophageal and Doppler echocardiography in the diagnosis and management of infectious endocarditis. Chest 1991;100:1125–30.

23. Tingeleff J, Joyce FS, Pettersson G. Intraoperative echocardiographic study of air embolism during cardiac operations. Ann Thorac Surg 1995;60:673–7.

24. Baggish AL, Boucher CA. Radiopharmaceutical agents for myocardial perfusion imaging. Circulation 2008;118:1668–74.

25. Cwajg E, Cwajg J, He Z, et al. Gated myocardial perfusion tomography for the assessment of left ventricular function and volumes: comparison with echocardiography. J Nucl Med 1999;40(11):1857–65.

26. Levy WC, Cerquiera MD, Matsuoka DT, et al. Four radionuclide methods for left ventricular volume determination: comparison of a manual and an automated technique. J Nucl Med 1990;31:450–6.

27. Russell RR, Zaret BL. Nuclear cardiology: present and future. Curr Probl Cardiol 2006;31:557–629.

28. Nagel E, Lehmkuhl HB, Bocksch W, et al. Noninvasive diagnosis of ischemia-induced wall motion abnormalities with the use of high-dose dobutamine stress MRI: comparison with dobutamine stress echocardiography. Circulation 1999; 99:763–70.

29. Lohan DG, Saleh R, Tomasian A, et al. Current status of 3T cardiovascular magnetic resonance imaging. Top Magn Reson Imaging 2008;19:3–13.

30. Schuijf JD, Bax JJ, Shaw LJ, et al. Meta-analysis of comparative diagnostic performance of magnetic resonance imaging and multislice computed tomography for noninvasive coronary angiography. Am Heart J 2006;151(2):404–11.

31. Rieber J, Huber A, Erhard I, et al. Cardiac magnetic resonance perfusion imaging for the functional assessment of coronary artery disease: a comparison with coronary angiography and fractional flow reserve. Eur Heart J 2006;27:1465–71.

32. Nagel E, Klein C, Paetsch I, et al. Magnetic resonance perfusion measurements for the non-invasive detection of coronary artery disease. Circulation 2003;108: 432–7.

33. Nandalur KR, Dwamena BA, Choudri AF, et al. Diagnostic performance of stress cardiac magnetic resonance imaging in the detection of coronary artery disease: a meta-analysis. J Am Coll Cardiol 2007;50:1343–53.

34. Schwitter J, Wacker CM, van Rossum AC, et al. MR-IMPACT: comparison of perfusion-cardiac magnetic resonance with single-photon emission computed tomography for detection of coronary artery disease in a multi-center, multivendor randomized trial. Eur Heart J 2008;29:480–9.

35. Marcu CB, Ninveldt R, Beek AM, et al. Delayed contrast enhancement magnetic resonance imaging for assessment of cardiac disease. Heart Lung Circ 2007;16:70–8.

36. Kim RJ, Wu E, Rafael A, et al. The use of contrast enhanced magnetic resonance imaging to identify reversible myocardial dysfunction. N Engl J Med 2000;343: 1445–53.

37. Baer FM, Thiessen P, Schneider CA, et al. Dobutamine magnetic resonance imaging predicts contractile recovery of chronically dysfunctional myocardium after successful revascularization. J Am Coll Cardiol 1998;31:1040–8.

38. Bove CM, DiMaria JM, Voros S, et al. Dobutamine response and myocardial infarct transmurality: functional improvement after coronary artery bypass grafting – an initial experience. Radiology 2006;240:835–41.

39. Wagner A, Mahrholdt H, Holly TA, et al. Contrast-enhanced MRI and routine single photon emission computed tomography (SPECT) perfusion imaging for detection of subendocardial myocardial infarcts: an imaging study. Lancet 2003;361:374–9.

40. Isbell DC, Kramer CM. The evolving role of cardiovascular magnetic resonance imaging in non-ischemic cardiomyopathy. Semin Ultrasound CT MR 2006;27:20–31.

41. Marcu CB, Beek AM, Van Rossum AC. Cardiovascular magnetic resonance imaging for the assessment of right heart involvement in cardiac and pulmonary disease. Heart Lung Circ 2006;15:362–70.

42. Masci PG, Dymarkowski S, Bogaert J. Valvular heart disease: what does cardiovascular MRI add? Eur Radiol 2008;18:197–208.

43. Lotz J, Meier C, Leppert A, et al. Cardiovascular flow measurement with phase-contrast MR imaging: basic facts and implementation. Radiographics 2002;22: 651–71.

44. Gelfand EV, Hughes S, Hauser TH, et al. Severity of mitral and aortic regurgitation as assessed by cardiovascular magnetic resonance: imaging. J Cardiovasc Magn Reson 2006;8:503–7.

45. Hoffman U, Ferencik M, Cury RC, et al. Coronary CT angiography. J Nucl Med 2006;47:797–806.

46. Bae KT, Hong C, Whiting BR. Radiation dose in multidetector row computed tomography cardiac imaging. J Magn Reson Imaging 2004;19:859–63.

47. Roberts WT, Bax JJ, Davies LC. Cardiac CT and CT coronary angiography: technology and applications. Heart 2008;94:781–92.

48. Schroeder S, Achenbach S, Bengel F, et al. Cardiac computed tomography: indications, applications, limitations and training requirements. Eur Heart J 2008;29: 531–56.

49. Budoff MJ, Dowe D, Jollis JG, et al. Diagnostic performance of 64-multidetector row coronary computed tomographic angiography for evaluation of coronary artery stenosis in individuals without known coronary artery disease: results from the prospective multicenter ACCURACY trial. J Am Coll Cardiol 2008;52: 1724–32.

50. Schuijf JD, Bax JJ, Salm LP, et al. Noninvasive coronary imaging and assessment of left ventricular function using 16-slice computed tomography. Am J Cardiol 2005;95:571–4.

51. Fraker TD, Fihn SD, et al. 2007 Chronic angina focused update of the ACC/AHA 2002 guidelines for the management of patients with chronic stable angina. J Am Coll Cardiol 2007;50:2264–74.

52. Metz LD, Beattie M, Hom R, et al. The prognostic value of normal exercise myocardial perfusion imaging and exercise echocardiography: a meta-analysis. J Am Coll Cardiol 2007;49(2):227–37.

53. Fleischmann KE, Hunink MG, Kuntz KM, et al. Exercise echocardiography or exercise SPECT imaging? A meta-analysis of diagnostic test performance. JAMA 1998;280(10):913–20.

54. Kim C, Kwok YS, Heagerty P, et al. Pharmacologic stress test for coronary artery disease diagnosis: a meta-analysis. Am Heart J 2001;142(6):934–44.

55. Jahnke C, Nagel E, Gebker R, et al. Prognostic value of cardiac magnetic resonance stress tests. Circulation 2007;115:1769–76.
56. Bonow RO, Dilsizian V. Thallium-201 for assessing myocardial viability. Semin Nucl Med 1991;21:230–41.
57. Allman KC, Shaw LJ, Hachamovitch R, et al. Myocardial viability testing and impact of revascularization on prognosis on patients with coronary artery disease and left ventricular dysfunction: a meta-analysis. J Am Coll Cardiol 2002;39: 1151–8.
58. Bax JJ, Poldermans D, Elhendy A, et al. Sensitivity, specificity and predictive accuracies of various non-invasive techniques for detecting hibernating myocardium. Curr Probl Cardiol 2001;26(2):147–81.
59. Cury RC, Nieman K, Shapiro MD, et al. Comprehensive assessment of myocardial perfusion defects, regional wall motion, and left ventricular function by using 64-section multidetector CT. Radiology 2008;248:466–75.
60. Mahnken AH, Koos R, Katoh M, et al. Assessment of myocardial viability in reperfused acute myocardial infarction using 16 slice computed tomography in comparison to magnetic resonance imaging. J Am Coll Cardiol 2005;45:2042–7.
61. Hatle L, Angelsen BA, Tromsdal A. Non-invasive assessment of aortic stenosis by Doppler ultrasound. Br Heart J 1980;43:284–92.
62. Dal-Bianco JP, Khandheria BK, Mookadam F, et al. Management of asymptomatic severe aortic stenosis. J Am Coll Cardiol 2008;52:1279–92.
63. Pouleur AC, le Polain de Waroux JB, Pasquet A, et al. Planimetric and continuity equation assessment of aortic valve area: head to head comparison between cardiac magnetic resonance and echocardiography. J Magn Reson Imaging 2007;26(6):1436–43.
64. Kilner PJ, Manzara CC, Mohiaddin RH, et al. Magnetic resonance jet velocity mapping in mitral and aortic valve stenosis. Circulation 1993;87:1239–48.
65. Pouleur AC, le Polain de Warouix JB, Pasquet A, et al. Aortic valve area assessment: multidetector CT compared with cine MR imaging and transthoracic and transesophageal echocardiography. Radiology 2007;244(3):745–54.
66. Carabello BA. The current therapy for mitral regurgitation. J Am Coll Cardiol 2008; 52:319–26.
67. Chan JKM, Wage R, Symmonds K, et al. Towards comprehensive assessment of mitral regurgitation using cardiovascular magnetic resonance. J Cardiovasc Magn Reson 2008;10(1):61.
68. Masui T, Finck S, Higgins CB. Constrictive pericarditis and restrictive cardiomyopathy: evaluation with MR imaging. Radiology 1992;182:369–73.
69. Axel L. Assessment of pericardial disease by magnetic resonance and computed tomography. J Magn Reson Imaging 2004;19:816–26.
70. Weitzman LB, Tinker WP, Kronzon I, et al. The incidence and natural history of pericardial effusions after cardiac surgery – an echocardiographic study. Circulation 1984;69:506–11.
71. Ofori-Karkye SK, Tyberg TI, Geha AS, et al. Late cardiac tamponade after open heart surgery: incidence, role of anti-coagulants in its pathogenesis and its relationship to the postpericardiotomy syndrome. Circulation 1981;63:1323–8.
72. Russo AM, O'Connor WH, Waxman HL. Atypical presentations and echocardiographic findings in patients with cardiac tamponade occurring early and late after cardiac surgery. Chest 1993;104:71–8.
73. Cujec B, Johnson D, Bharadwaj B. Cardiac tamponade by loculated pericardial hematoma following open heart surgery: diagnosis by transesophagel echocardiography. Can J Cardiol 1990;7:37–40.

74. Badano LP, Dall'Armellina E, Monaghan MJ, et al. Real-time three-dimensional echocardiography: technological gadet or clinical tool? J Cardiovasc Med 2007;8:144–62.
75. Gulati G, Sharma S, Kothari SS, et al. Comparison of echo and MRI in the imaging evaluation of intracardiac masses. Cardiovasc Intervent Radiol 2004;27(5): 459–69.
76. Lima JAC, Desai MY. Cardiovascular magnetic resonance imaging: current and emerging applications. J Am Coll Cardiol 2004;44:1164–71.
77. Pohost GM, Hung L, Doyle M. Clinical use of cardiovascular magnetic resonance. Circulation 2003;108:647–53.
78. Boxt LM. Magnetic resonance and computed tomography evaluation of congenital heart disease. J Magn Reson 2004;19:827–47.

Cardiopulmonary Bypass/Extracorporeal Membrane Oxygenation/Left Heart Bypass: Indications, Techniques, and Complications

Gorav Ailawadi, MD[a],*, Richard K. Zacour, BS, CCP[b]

KEYWORDS

- Cardiopulmonary bypass
- Extracorporeal membrane oxygenation • Left heart bypass
- Complications • Coronary artery bypass grafting
- Valve surgery

Cardiopulmonary bypass (CPB) has revolutionized the ability to provide cardiorespiratory support and has advanced the field of cardiac surgery. This invention has given surgeons the ability to perform many procedures that were not possible previously. The concept and development of CPB has been pioneered by numerous legendary surgeons. Alexis Carrel and Charles Lindbergh developed a device that successfully perfused organs, including hearts, keeping them alive for several days.[1] John Gibbon[2] deserves credit for devising the concept of a heart-lung machine after caring for a young woman with a massive embolus in 1930. Over the next 20 years, Gibbon developed the heart-lung machine during his time at the Massachusetts General Hospital, the University of Pennsylvania, and Thomas Jefferson University. In the early 1950s, Lillehei and colleagues[3,4] at the University of Minnesota developed a technique called controlled cross-circulation by using circulatory support from another person's native circulation, usually the patient's parent or relative. By 1955,

---

[a] Division of Thoracic and Cardiovascular Surgery, Department of Surgery, University of Virginia, PO Box 800679, Charlottesville, VA 22908-0679, USA
[b] Thoracic-Cardiovascular Perfusion, Department of Surgery, University of Virginia Health System, PO Box 800677, Charlottesville, VA 22908, USA
* Corresponding author.
E-mail address: gorav@virginia.edu (G. Ailawadi).

Surg Clin N Am 89 (2009) 781–796
doi:10.1016/j.suc.2009.05.006
0039-6109/09/$ – see front matter © 2009 Elsevier Inc. All rights reserved.
surgical.theclinics.com

Lillehei abandoned cross-circulation and began using CPB; this approach was rapidly adopted by many surgical groups.

The safe use of CPB requires an understanding of the device by all members of the operative team. Specifically, the cardiac surgeon, the anesthesiologist, and the perfusionist all must be experienced and knowledgeable in their understanding of the physiology of CPB, its risks and limitations, and the potential injuries that may result from its misuse. Protocols for the use of CPB are developed collaboratively, and any deviation from a protocol should be based on the needs of the individual patient and agreed to by all team members. If the surgeon is to realize the full advantage of CPB, he or she must have knowledge of the perfusion circuit in use at their institution. This includes priming solutions, speed and ability to vary perfusate temperature, maximum and minimum flow rates, and available cannula sizes.

Before each procedure, the surgeon must develop a plan for conducting the operation, especially the use of CPB. The surgeon should review with the other team members the planned incisions, methods of cannulating the heart and great vessels, the systemic and myocardial temperatures desired, the possible need for low flow or circulatory arrest, and any anticipated pathologic or anatomic variations that may require alterations in the plan.

The surgeon should consider all potential complications during the planning of the operation—possible anatomic variants and catastrophic events. Examples of anatomic variants might include mitral regurgitation with a heavily calcified posterior mitral annulus requiring a longer and more complex operation with additional steps to protect the myocardium, a persistent left superior vena cava (SVC) accompanying an atrial septal defect, or a tetralogy of Fallot with a variant coronary artery crossing the right ventricular outflow tract. Potential catastrophic events should be reviewed frequently, since they occur suddenly, and all members of the surgical team must be prepared to deal with them rapidly and precisely. Catastrophic events during reoperative surgery include unexpected right ventriculotomy or aortotomy, or ventricular fibrillation before the sternum is open.

INDICATIONS FOR CPB

The most common indication to use CPB is to provide cardiac and respiratory support during operations on the heart or great vessels. Coronary artery bypass grafting (CABG) still remains the most frequent use for CPB.[5] Roughly 20% of CABG procedures in the United States are performed without the use of CPB (off-pump CABG) and use the patient's own heart and lungs to maintain perfusion to the body.[5] Other common procedures where CPB is used in adult and/or acquired diseases include valve operations and operations on the ascending aorta and aortic arch. In these cases, it is not uncommon to use CPB to cool the patient and allow the bypass circuit to be temporarily ceased. This allows for a bloodless field to perform critical parts of the operation while protecting the brain. CPB has revolutionized the approach to repair of congenital heart defects. Rarely, CPB is also used to provide hemodynamic support during major venous reconstruction. An additional benefit of the bypass in this instance is in cases of major venous injury or bleeding, shed blood can be collected and recirculated to maintain intravascular volume and perfusion. Occasionally, CPB is used in complex airway and pulmonary operations and reconstructions. CPB has also been used for isolated hyperthermic limb perfusion to deliver chemotherapy at supranormal temperatures to treat malignancy confined to one limb.[6] The primary goals and purposes of CPB are listed in **Box 1**.

Box 1
Purposes and goals for CPB

1) Maintain perfusion to brain and other vital organs

2) Provide a bloodless field (heart, great vessels, or other) to allow the surgeon to visualize and perform the operation

3) Maintain thermoregulation for protection of organs (cooling and warming)

4) Provide cardiac assistance/protection

5) Provide pulmonary assistance/protection

COMPONENTS OF CPB CIRCUIT

The components of the CPB circuit include venous cannula(e) typically in the right atrium or vena cavae, a venous reservoir, a membrane oxygenator, a heat exchanger, a pump, a microfilter in the arterial line, and an arterial cannula(s) (**Fig. 1**). Cannulae can be placed in the right side of the heart, into the right atrium, or into the SVC and inferior vena cava (IVC) and secured in place with 3-0 or 4-0 polypropylene (Prolene) pursestring sutures. These can be placed directly by opening the pericardium or percutaneously through the internal jugular vein and femoral vein. These latter approaches are used during minimally invasive cardiac operations. They remove lines from the operative field and allow for smaller incisions. Venous drainage can be obtained with gravity, whereby the venous reservoir is placed 40 to 70 cm below the level of the heart, or with vacuum suction. Venous cannula size is determined by the patient size, size of the right atrium and/or vena cava, and amount of flow desired.

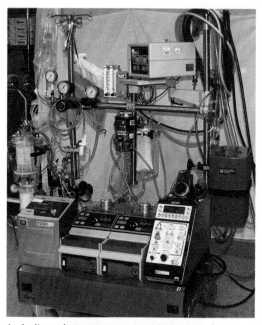

Fig. 1. CPB circuit, including the venous reservoir, pump, heat exchanger, membrane oxygenator, and arterial filter.

Venous reservoirs provide a low pressure chamber that serves as a storage chamber for venous and shed blood. The reservoir can hold an additional 2 to 3 L of blood volume to allow for uninterrupted arterial blood flow if venous return is occluded. Rigid canister reservoirs facilitate removal of venous air and are easier to prime, whereas soft plastic bags maintain a closed system and lower the risk of embolization.[7,8]

Blood in the circuit then goes through a membrane oxygenator which distributes a thin layer of blood over a large surface area with high differential gas pressures across a thin microporous (0.3–0.8 μm pores) hollow-fiber membrane layer to facilitate oxygenation. Since carbon dioxide is highly diffusible in the plasma, it is removed easily through the membrane oxygenator. Partial pressure of oxygen in arterial blood (PaO_2) is controlled by the fraction of inspired oxygen delivered to the oxygenator, whereas partial pressure of carbon dioxide in arterial blood ($PaCO_2$) is controlled by the sweep speed of gas flow. Traditional bubble oxygenators were cheap, but they had a high risk for gas embolization and are no longer manufactured.

A heat exchanger is commonly used and allows for active cooling and rewarming of blood going into the patient. The temperature differential between the patient and blood is limited to a difference of 10°C to prevent bubble emboli. Moreover, blood should not be warmed over 42°C to minimize protein denaturation and emboli.[7,8] A separate heat exchanger is used for cardioplegia and is often kept at temperatures of 4°C to 15°C.

The most recognized component of the CPB circuit is the pump (**Fig. 2**). Two options for pumps include roller pumps and centrifugal pumps. Roller pumps are independent of afterload, requiring low prime volumes, and they are cheap; however, they have a potential for air embolism, and they can cause significant positive and negative pressure, resulting in tubing rupture. Centrifugal pumps are afterload sensitive, adapt to venous return, and are superior for left heart bypass (LHB) and for long-term bypass, at the expense of large priming volumes, higher cost, and potential for passive backward flow.

The risk of embolism has been greatly decreased by the introduction of filters. Numerous sources of gaseous microemboli smaller than 500 μm are present, including loose pursestrings around venous cannulae, stopcocks in the circuit used for injection of medications, priming solutions, oxygenators, and rapid warming of

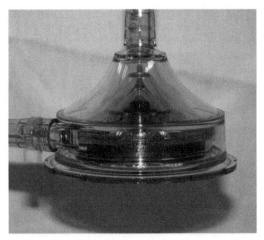

Fig. 2. Centrifugal pump used in CPB, ECMO, and LHB.

cold blood. Blood itself is the primary source for particulate emboli, including thrombin, fibrin, platelet clots, hemolyzed blood cells, and fat particles as well as shed muscle, bone, and marrow that gets aspirated into the cardiotomy reservoir.

Methods to minimize emboli to the arterial system include the use of membrane oxygenators, centrifugal pumps, and filters in the cardiotomy venous reservoir and in the arterial line. In our practice, we use two sequential arterial filters to decrease the number of microemboli in the arterial system. The temperature differential between the blood in the circuit and the body is maintained at less than 10°C to minimize emboli formation.

TECHNIQUES/CONDUCT OF CPB

Although the surgeon takes primary responsibility for the patient during the hospital course, a team of experts is required to administer anesthesia, maintain perfusion, and relay changes in the patient status during the operation. The surgeon will determine the plan of the operation, including methods of cannulation, cardioplegia, and cooling. The anesthesiologist is responsible for induction of anesthesia, endotracheal intubation, and the placement or insertion of most monitoring devices. In patients who are hemodynamically unstable, direct arterial pressure measurement should be established and a pulmonary artery catheter inserted before the induction of anesthesia. Often, the anesthesiologist provides assistance with transesophageal echocardiography (TEE) during the operation. The perfusionist helps to select the optimal cannula size, provides circulatory support and cardiac protection, and maintains anticoagulation during the operation. Further, the perfusionist is responsible for maintaining a written perfusion record and performing a series of safety checks. The surgeon, anesthesiologist, and perfusionist must have free and open communication.

Patient Positioning

Once all monitoring lines have been placed, the patient is positioned and pressure points are padded to prevent pressure necrosis. All monitoring cables and lines are secured to prevent displacement or disconnection during the operation. The traditional approach is through a median sternotomy. In this case, a padded roll is placed beneath the patient's shoulders and arms placed at the sides to avoid brachial plexus injury. Minimally invasive approaches to the mitral and tricuspid valve are often performed through a right mini-thoracotomy. In this setting, a small bump is placed under the right chest and arms are secured at the patient's sides.

Sterile preparation of the skin and draping is performed to ensure access to all aspects of the operative field. This typically includes the chest, abdomen, and both groins, as well as both lower extremities if saphenous vein is needed for CABG. In cases where the saphenous vein may be of poor quality and additional conduit for CABG is required, the nondominant arm is prepped in the field to harvest the radial artery.

The pump and cell-saving equipment are brought into position and the pump lines are passed to the field. The pump lines are located such that the operative field and surgeons are unhampered; with the pump lines in full view of the perfusionist, allowing immediate access to the lines should an event occur. The lines should be secured in a standard manner so that even excessive force cannot displace them. Inexperienced members of the team are instructed not to touch or compress the lines.

Incisions

The selection of the incision site for exposure and cannulation of the heart is based on considerations of safety, exposure, and cosmesis. Anatomic and pathologic variations, such as a large ascending aortic aneurysm pressing against the sternum or severe pectus excavatum in which the entire heart is displaced to the left chest, may require careful planning to avoid catastrophe. Obviously, variations in the incision to achieve cosmesis must not compromise safety or adequate exposure.

The pericardium is opened in the midline from its reflection on the aorta down to the diaphragm. The pericardium is released from the diaphragm with a transverse incision, with care being taken to avoid entering the pleural space or injuring the phrenic nerve. At this point, consideration is given to the specific exposure that will be required for the operation. Heavy silk sutures are placed in the cut edges of the pericardium and tied to the presternal fascia on the ipsilateral side of the incision to elevate and stabilize the appropriate cardiovascular structures.

Cannulation

Once the pericardium is opened, the aortic cannulation site is chosen. Commonly the distal ascending aorta, just proximal to the innominate artery, is used. There are many methods to cannulate and secure the arterial cannula. The authors' preference is to use two opposing diamond pursestring sutures with pledgeted 3-0 polypropylene approximately 30% larger than the size of the arterial cannula. The sutures are kept on opposing tourniquets. Venous cannulation sutures are placed using nonpledgeted 3-0 polypropylene pursestring. One or two venous cannulae are used depending on the operation. In settings where the right atrium or left atrium will be opened, 2 venous cannulae are placed into the SVC and IVC. Other operations typically can be performed with 1 large venous cannula placed through the right atrial appendage directed toward the IVC.

After ensuring systemic heparinization (200–300 units/kg, confirmed by activated clotting time [ACT] >400 sec), the aorta is cannulated by creating an aortotomy with a #15 blade and inserting the cannula. It is important to ensure that the aortotomy is large enough to admit the cannula without difficulty to avoid injuring the aorta. In addition, care must be taken to avoid cutting the cannulation sutures. After the cannula is secured to the aorta with the tourniquets, it is attached to the arterial line and deaired. The arterial line is tested to ensure that flow into the arterial system is unobstructed and line pressure on the arterial cannula is not high.

Venous cannulation is performed by creating an atriotomy with scissors or a #11 blade. The atriotomy must be made large enough to admit the cannula easily. Deairing of the venous cannula and line is only necessary if using gravity drainage and an airlock needs to be avoided.

Additional cannulae are placed depending on the plan of the operation, including cannulas for cardioplegia and venting of the heart. Typically, a small cannula for cardioplegia is placed into the ascending aorta with 4-0 pledgeted polypropylene and a retrograde cardioplegia cannula placed through the right atrium into the coronary sinus secured with 4-0 polypropylene. These will be used to administer cardioplegia to arrest the heart and protect the myocardium. The left ventricle can be vented by using a cannula placed into the right superior pulmonary vein and advanced through the left atrium and mitral valve into the left ventricle. This will allow for a bloodless field when operating on the left ventricle or aorta.

Venous return can be achieved by a passive or assisted approach. Passive venous return is more traditional, and is dependent on gravity, the height of the operating table above the venous reservoir, and large-bore tubing. Assisted venous return is achieved with the aid of vacuum being applied to the venous line or reservoir and does not require gravity drainage. Assisted venous return provides some advantages over the traditional venous drainage, such as permitting smaller venous cannula, tubing, incisions, and lowering the priming volume. It can increase the risk for gaseous microemboli if the vacuum is too great and the reservoir volume is too low to allow proper dissociation. Because of these concerns, the maximum amount of vacuum is limited to less than 80 mm Hg and maintains a venous reservoir volume that permits at least 10 second reaction time or no less than 1000 mL.

Blood Strategy During CPB

The pump is typically primed with 1.5 to 2 L of crystalloid. It is important to prime the pump before use in a patient to eliminate microemboli through the filter. The addition of this volume results in significant hemodilution. The usual hematocrit when on CPB is 20 to 25 mg/dL. The degree of hemodilution may be calculated before bypass is initiated, and if the expected priming volume would cause an unacceptable anemia, packed red blood cells may be added to the extracorporeal circuit.

Hemodilution provides an advantageous effect for perfusion by decreasing viscosity and by augmenting blood flow. Blood flow reflects the interaction of many influences; hemodilution aids in negating those inherent effects by diminishing blood's viscosity and resistance to flow and promotes increased microcirculatory flow and tissue perfusion. However, hemodilution can be deleterious by reducing oncotic pressure, resulting in tissue edema and decreasing oxygen delivery during bypass. Hypothermia also influences blood rheology and vascular geometry. A decrease in temperature provokes direct vasoconstriction and increases viscosity, creating sludging and stasis at the capillary level, and a reduced blood flow. These effects are counteracted by hemodilution.

The acceptable degree of hemodilution is highly contested. It is common to see hematocrit of 18% to 21% during CPB. Hematocrit less than 15% can also be tolerated in cases of circulatory arrest and in patients who will not accept blood transfusion. The authors use a blood conservation strategy that has established transfusion indicators during CPB, depicted in **Box 2**. A general rule of thumb is that the hematocrit in percent should not exceed the desired level of hypothermia in °C.

Initiating CPB

CPB is begun at the instruction of the surgeon. Visual inspection of the field, monitors, and bypass lines as the perfusionist initiates CPB will provide an immediate assessment of the conversion. The perfusionist initiates CPB by releasing the arterial line clamp and slowly transfusing the patient with the volume. The arterial blood flow of the extracorporeal circuit should be free-flowing and exhibit a reasonable

---

Box 2
Strategy for blood transfusion during CPB

1. During moderate hypothermic CPB, a hematocrit less than 18% is the trigger threshold for blood transfusion unless the patient exhibits a history of cerebrovascular accident and disease, carotid stenosis, or diabetes mellitus, in which case a hematocrit of 21% becomes the trigger.

2. The patient's clinical condition also determines the need for blood transfusion: age, severity of illness, cardiac function, end-organ ischemia, massive or active blood loss, mixed venous oxygen saturation (SVO_2), and so on. In this environment, a hematocrit of 21% to 24% becomes the authors' trigger.

3. Routine use of the cell saver except for patients with infection and malignancy

4. Low-prime and mini-extracorporeal bypass circuits

extracorporeal line pressure. A sudden spike in the extracorporeal line pressure may indicate an occluded arterial line, a malpositioned aortic cannula, or an aortic dissection. Should this occur, CPB should be terminated immediately and the cause identified and corrected.

As soon as it is obvious that arterial flow is unobstructed, the venous clamp is released, diverting the patient's venous blood into the CPB circuit. The right heart should be decompressed, and the central venous pressure should be less than 5 mm Hg. A high central venous pressure and poor venous drainage at the initiation of CPB may indicate a malpositioned venous cannula, a kinked venous line, an "air-lock," venous cannulas that are too large or too small, an inappropriate height between the operating table and the venous reservoir, an inappropriate amount of vacuum, or a vacuum leak.

During this transition period of 1 to 2 minutes, the perfusionist gradually increases the rate of arterial flow, the ventricles receive less blood, and the pulsatile arterial waveform diminishes and becomes "flat-lined." Once total bypass is achieved, a continued pulsatile arterial waveform signifies the left ventricle is receiving unwanted blood from aortic insufficiency, excessive bronchial venous return, or incomplete drainage of the systemic venous return.

Because of acute vasoactive substance release on initiating CPB, an acute, transient state of systemic arterial hypotension is common and can be treated with vasopressor agents if needed. Acceptable mean arterial pressure when on CPB ranges from 50 to 90 mm Hg. In the presence of cerebrovascular or renovascular disease, a perfusion pressure of 70 to 90 mm Hg is preferred. The adequacy of a mean arterial pressure in a patient is confirmed by a normal systemic vascular resistance index and mixed venous blood gas.

In patients with severe aortic regurgitation, the surgeon should be ready to cross-clamp the ascending aorta if ventricular fibrillation occurs. A distended, fibrillating left ventricle is subject to additional ischemia and injury to the myocardium. Once on full CPB support, the patient can be cooled to the desired temperature. The primary advantage of systemic hypothermia during CPB is the reduced metabolic rate and oxygen consumption of approximately 5% to 7% per °C.[9,10] In addition, hypothermia sustains intracellular reservoirs of high-energy phosphates (essential for cellular integrity) and preserves high intracellular pH and electrochemical neutrality (a constant OH^-/H^+ ratio). As a result of these associated interactions, hypothermic patients can survive periods of circulatory arrest of up to 1 hour without suffering from the effects of anoxia.[9,10]

In addition to core cooling with cold blood through the circuit, hypothermia may be augmented by surface cooling using cooling blankets and ice packs applied directly to the patient. Because tissues and organs have varying amounts of perfusion, systemic cooling is not a uniform process. To minimize this, the flows on the circuit are maintained at high rates (2.2 to 2.5 L/min/m^2), and the rate of the cooling is limited to less than 1°C per minute until the desired temperature is reached. Bladder and nasopharyngeal temperatures are monitored to ensure uniform temperatures.

In most cases, the beating heart will be arrested to cease motion and allow a bloodless field on the heart. This is achieved by administering cardioplegia antegrade through the coronary arteries or retrograde through the coronary sinus. Since there are no valves in the coronary sinus, cardioplegia is able to run retrograde into the coronary arteries and out the ostium.

In certain cases, a state of circulatory arrest may be desired where the blood flow to the patient is drained and the circuit is stopped to allow for a bloodless field. This state of "no blood flow" to the patient is achieved with extreme systemic cooling at 16°C to

22°C. Safe periods of circulatory arrest can be achieved based on the patient's core temperature (**Table 1**). Beyond these times there are risks for cerebral and other end-organ injury. The negative effects of circulatory arrest include additional time required to cool and rewarm the patient and systemic coagulopathy that often requires blood component replacement.

Systemic rewarming is instituted by gradually increasing the perfusate temperature. Rewarming is slower than cooling because of the maximum 10°C permissible temperature gradient between perfusate and nasopharyngeal temperatures, the maximum allowable blood temperature of 42°C, and the reduced thermal exchange as the temperature gradient between the patient and perfusate narrows. During this part of the procedure, warming blankets are set to 40°C, the perfusion flow rates are increased to 2.5 to 3.0 L/min/m^2, and, pressure permitting, pharmacologic vasodilation is used. When the bladder temperature reaches 32°C, the patient begins to vasodilate spontaneously and the pharmacologic vasodilator may be terminated.

Weaning Off of CPB

The heart is deaired before the cross-clamp is removed. The patient is placed in a 30° head-down (Trendelenberg) position, and the heart is filled with blood by manually restricting venous return to the pump. The right heart begins to fill, and the anesthesiologist ventilates the lungs. The heart is gently massaged. Vents in the left ventricle or in the aortic root cardioplegia cannula are used to remove air from within the heart. Once all air appears to have been evacuated, pump flow is reduced to half flow, arterial pressure is reduced to 50 mm Hg, and the aortic cross-clamp is removed while suction is maintained on the antegrade cardioplegic cannula. TEE is often used to determine if there is residual air within the heart. Maneuvers to remove any residual air include filling the heart, giving Valsalva breaths, and rocking the table from side to side when the aortic root vent is on. When echocardiography confirms that the left heart is free of air, the operating table is restored to a level position and the aortic cardioplegic/vent cannula and the retrograde cardioplegic cannula are removed.

Temporary pacing wires are sutured to the right atrium and ventricle if needed. Rewarming is continued until the patient's temperature reaches 36°C. Termination of CPB is performed gradually, with constant communication between surgeon, perfusionist, and anesthesiologist. The ventilator is turned on. The perfusionist progressively occludes the venous return line, translocating blood volume from the venous reservoir into the patient's vascular system. The patient is now on "partial" CPB, with blood flowing through the heart and pulmonary circulation. When the blood volume in the heart reaches an adequate level, the aortic valve begins to open with each heart beat, and a measurable cardiac output will be observed. The translocation of volume is continued until the arterial systolic pressure reaches 100 mm Hg. Simultaneously, the flow through the circuit is reduced. The surgeon checks for surgical

Table 1		
Definition of levels of hypothermia and approximate "safe" circulatory arrest times		
Hypothermia Level	**Patient Temperature (°C)**	**Circulatory Arrest Times (min)**
Mild	37–32	5–10
Moderate	32–28	10–15
Deep	28–18	15–60
Profound	<18	60–90

bleeding and assesses heart function, as well as checking heart and valve function by TEE. On the surgeon's approval, the perfusionist then terminates CPB by completely occluding the venous and arterial lines. Thereafter, the perfusionist transfuses volume to the patient to maintain a systolic blood pressure of 100 mm Hg unless the heart becomes distended.

If the heart does not function effectively when CPB is terminated, bypass is reinstituted to prevent overdistention or hypoxia. If heart functions appropriately with hemodynamic stability, decannulation can begin. The venous cannulae are removed but the tourniquets are still present should the need arise for rapid return to bypass. The heparin is reversed with protamine. When half of the protamine is administered, the aortic cannula should be removed to prevent arterial embolism from the cannula. Additional volume should be given to the patient as needed to fill the heart adequately though the aortic cannula before removing it. The protamine is then completed and arterial and venous cannulation sites are tied and secured. Shed blood should not be returned to the extracorporeal circuit once protamine is introduced into the patient's circulation. Thereafter, final hemostasis and surgical closure of the wound are performed.

COMPLICATIONS

Complications associated with CPB can be divided into those related to malfunction of the circuit, those related to problems with cannulation, and those related to the physiology of CPB on the body.

Complications Related to Cannulation

Cannulation of the heart must be done carefully because this can result in major catastrophes. The risk for ascending aortic dissection is less than 1% with direct cannulation; however, when it does occur, it may require circulatory arrest and complete replacement of the ascending aorta. More common is bleeding from the aortic cannulation site as a result of misplaced sutures, too small a pursestring, bites of the aorta that are full thickness (and too deep), or poor quality tissue. Many of these errors can be avoided with careful planning of the location of cannulation and meticulous suture placement. Repair of a distal aortic injury can often be performed by covering the site with an autologous pericardial patch. At this point of the operation, the patient is typically off bypass and the aortic cannula has been removed. The assistant will need to control the bleeding with direct pressure on the aortic cannulation site. The surgeon can harvest a 2 to 3 cm circular piece of autologous pericardium. Using 5-0 polypropylene the surgeon secures the pericardium to the aorta around the cannulation site, making certain to get good bites of the aortic adventitia and media. The suture is run circumferentially and tied down. This will control the bleeding in most cases. Rarely, femoral cannulation is required to go back on pump and the patient may need to be cooled and circulation arrested to fix the cannulation injury as with an aortic dissection.

Venous cannulation injuries can occur as well and are typically related to quality of the atrial tissue and location of the pursestring suture. When cannulating the right atrial appendage and the IVC, the surgeon should ensure there is enough atrial tissue to allow closure of the atriotomy without tension. A tear in the atrioventricular groove or down the IVC can be very challenging to repair but can often be repaired primary or with a large bovine pericardial patch.

Peripheral arterial and venous cannulation can also lead to complications. Femoral arterial cannulation should only be performed with some knowledge of the femoral, iliac, and aortic anatomy to avoid retrograde aortic dissection, malperfusion of the body during bypass, and aortic or iliac injury. In cases of severe peripheral vascular disease, calcification of the vessels, or the presence of an aortic or iliac aneurysm, alternative cannulation sites should be considered with a preoperative CT scan. Femoral venous cannulation can also lead to venous injury in the retroperitoneum or abdomen leading to hemorrhage and poor flows when on bypass. Cannulation of the axillary artery should be performed by sewing a Dacron graft in an end to side fashion. In this setting, the surgeon must ensure there is no obstruction or disease in the axillary or innominate arteries by CT angiogram.

Complications Related to the Effects of CPB on the Body

Although CPB has advanced heart surgery to allow us to perform complex reconstruction on the heart, it is clearly not a physiologic state with nonpulsatile flow, manipulation of core temperature, alterations in venous pressure, and increased interstitial fluid. In addition to a host of inflammatory cytokines that are released during bypass, CPB also causes dysfunction of clotting factors and platelet activation and lysis which ultimately lead to coagulopathy and bleeding. Meticulous hemostasis is the first key to minimize bleeding. Longer procedure times are associated with higher risk for bleeding and more coagulopathy. Additional topical hemostatic agents can be used to minimize nonsurgical bleeding. Blood component administration is the most common method of treating coagulopathy following CPB. Antifibrinolytic agents including aminocaproic acid are commonly used during and after CPB in long or complex cases to prevent fibrinolysis.

In addition to effects on coagulation, there are multiple effects of CPB that can lead to organ damage. It can be difficult to determine the source of postoperative cardiac injury and attribute it to CPB or to cardiac arrest/cross-clamping. Ischemic reperfusion causes myocardial edema. Lung injury has been attributed to ischemic reperfusion injury as well as changes in pulmonary capillary permeability. Renal dysfunction is thought to be because of alterations in blood flow when on CPB as well as tissue edema. Neurologic dysfunction has been the focus of many studies and is thought to be a result of nonpulsatile cerebral blood flow, microemboli to the brain, and loss of cerebral autoregulation. Neurologic sequelae include frank strokes as well as mild cognitive dysfunction often termed "pump head." Careful planning of arterial cannulation, maintenance of adequate perfusion pressure when on CPB, and avoidance of microemboli with the use of arterial filters can minimize the risk for neurologic injury.

Complications Related to Pump Malfunction

Pump malfunctions are rare events but can have devastating consequences. Massive air embolism can occur with break in the integrity of the circuit, on depletion of the venous reservoir, during opening of the left atrium or ventricle without a cross-clamp (as can occur during insertion of a left ventricular vent), or from an inadvertent bolus of air into the arterial line. Systemic air embolism is treated by stopping the CPB and placing the patient in steep Trendelenberg. The circuit is reprimed to remove the air. The surgeon then cannulates the SVC and runs flow retrograde through the cerebral circulation for 1 to 2 minutes to allow air to exit through the aorta. Once the pump is primed and visible air in the arterial system is removed, the pump is restarted antegrade and the patient is cooled to 20°C to increase the solubility of the air embolism.

Air lock in the venous line can occur with gravity drainage and can result in loss of venous drainage and depletion of the venous reservoir. This is treated by closing the source of venous entry, walking the air through the venous line into the reservoir, and adding fluid to the reservoir.

Pump failure can occur as a result of electrical or mechanical causes. This is prevented by frequent servicing of the equipment and ensuring a functioning backup battery. If the pump stops during CPB, if possible wean the patient off bypass. If this is not possible, then a manual hand crank can be used to continue perfusion through the pump.

EXTRACORPOREAL MEMBRANE OXYGENATION

The indications for extracorporeal membrane oxygenation (ECMO) are listed in **Box 3**. The ECMO circuit differs from the traditional CPB circuit in a number of ways. The ECMO circuit is a single closed system and is unable to tolerate air in the venous line. There is no separate circuit to administer cardioplegia as with the CPB circuit. ECMO is more compact than CPB, allowing for easier transportation of the patient (**Fig. 3**). Typical ECMO circuits have heparin bonded tubing allowing for lower levels of anticoagulation (ACT 180-220s).

Cannulation for ECMO can be performed with a variety of techniques. Venoarterial (VA) ECMO is performed for both circulatory and pulmonary support. VA ECMO is often performed for cardiogenic failure post cardiac surgery. In this scenario, the aorta is cannulated directly as aforementioned. If the aortic cannula is still present from CPB, it can be used as the arterial inflow for VA ECMO. In settings where the chest is not open, arterial cannulation is usually performed through the femoral artery. Venous cannulation is performed in the right atrium if the chest is open or through the femoral vein and/or internal jugular when the chest is not open. Femoral, arterial, or venous cannulation can be performed percutaneously or via a cutdown. When performed via cutdown, 5-0 pursestring suture is used to secure the cannulas. Once the cannulas are confirmed to be in good location providing good flows on ECMO, the cannulas and tubing are secured with heavy silk sutures to the skin to ensure they are not inadvertently moved during routine care of the patient.

Venovenous ECMO is used for isolated pulmonary support in cases of reversible pulmonary failure. Most often, cannulation is performed through the femoral and internal jugular veins. Inflow is from the femoral vein and outflow through a cannula in the right atrium positioned through the internal jugular vein.

Box 3
Indications for ECMO support

1. Cardiac support for reversible conditions

2. Postcardiotomy shock

3. Post myocardial infarction (MI)

4. High-risk coronary artery and intracardiac interventions (cath lab)

5. Respiratory support (reversible conditions)

    a. Acute lung injury (trauma)

    b. Post lung transplant

6. Hypothermia resuscitation

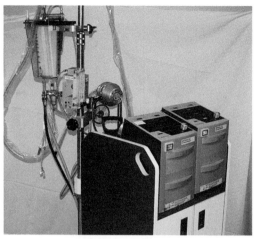

Fig. 3. ECMO circuits are smaller than CPB and are portable.

Complications

In addition to the aforementioned concerns with air embolism and microemboli, complications specifically related to ECMO are primarily because of the extended period of time in which a patient is anticoagulated while on cardiopulmonary support. This results in significant coagulopathy, especially when ECMO support is required for longer than 48 to 72 hours. Despite maintaining lower ACTs while on ECMO, the pump and circuit result in consumption of clotting factors and platelets. It is not unusual for patients on ECMO to receive several times their blood volume in blood component replacement while on support. The resultant transfusions can lead to reactions to the blood products and secondary injury to the lungs.

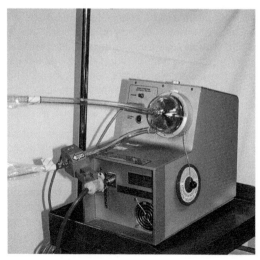

Fig. 4. LHB machine.

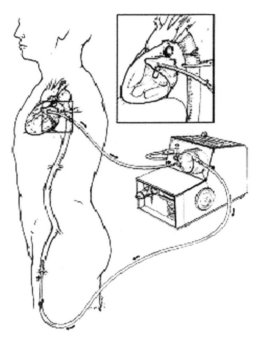

Fig. 5. Location cannulation strategy for LHB during descending and thoracoabdominal aortic surgery. *From* Szwerc M, Benckart D, Lin J, et al. Recent clinical experience with left heart bypass using a centrifugal pump for repair of traumatic aortic transection. Ann Surg 1999; 230:486; with permission.

LHB

LHB is partial heart bypass designed to provide partial blood flow to limited sections of the body during surgery (**Fig. 4**). LHB is primarily used to provide support and perfusion of the visceral vessels and lower extremities during reconstruction of the descending aorta, allowing the perfusionist to divert a portion of the patient's saturated blood from the patient's circulation after it has passed through the lungs and returns it to the arterial system by way of the distal aorta or femoral artery (**Fig. 5**). This parallel circuit technique permits the perfusionist to vary the preload of the left ventricle, controlling the volume of blood being ejected into the aorta, and it provides blood flow to the lower intercostals, lumbar, renal, and visceral arteries. The use of LHB has been shown to decrease the incidence of paraplegia and renal failure, and it limits intestinal ischemia during operations on the descending thoracic and thoracoabdominal aorta.[11–13]

Access to the thoracic and thoracoabdominal aorta is obtained through a left thoracotomy and a thoracoabdominal incision, respectively. Following exposure of the aorta, heparin is administered (100 units/kg) and ACTs are maintained at 200 sec. The femoral artery is cannulated with a 15F Bio-Medicus arterial cannula percutaneously or through femoral artery cutdown through a 5-0 polypropylene pursestring. If cannulating directly into the distal aorta, a 12F Bio-Medicus arterial cannula is used through a 4-0 polypropylene pursestring. The cannula is then attached to the outflow side of the circuit, with great care being taken to ensure the system is devoid of air bubbles. The left atrium is cannulated through the left inferior pulmonary vein with a 14F Bio-Medicus venous cannula and secured with a 5-0 polypropylene pursestring.

The inferior pulmonary ligament should be divided entirely and the inferior pulmonary vein should be isolated circumferentially. As noted on the arterial side, the cannula is secured to the circuit ensuring no air bubbles in the line.

A blood flow rate of 20 to 40 mL/kg, or a cardiac index of 1.3 m^2 (2.0–2.5 L/min) is generally acceptable for perfusing the viscera and lower extremity. Following the initiation of bypass and aortic cross-clamping, there are two parallel circulations. Circulation to the great vessels and heart is dependent upon the patient's native cardiac function and preload in the left ventricle, whereas the lower circulation is dependent on the bypass circuit. The regulation of blood flow and pressure is controlled by the rate in which the blood is removed by the bypass circuit. As the pump flow of the bypass circuit increases, the blood flow into the ascending aorta is decreased along with the upper extremity blood pressure; whereas the distal blood flow and pressure increases. By altering the flow through the circuit, the radial artery pulsatile pressure is maintained around 100/60 mm Hg, whereas the femoral artery mean pressure is maintained to roughly equal the radial diastolic pressure.

The LHB circuit is a simple circuit consisting of a centrifugal pump, tubing, and cannulae. The use of a centrifugal pump offers the advantage of providing a negative pressure on the inflow blood, allowing the pump to be close to and at table level, thus reducing the tubing length. This arrangement traps air bubbles that may entrain into the circuit, and it minimizes blood element trauma. In addition, two cell savers are used to process and return the patient's shed blood.

Complications

LHB does possess some unique hazards in addition to the aforementioned risks for CPB. Although meticulous care must be taken to avoid air embolism in other modes of CPB, this cannot be overstated using LHB. Excess flow through the circuit or relative hypovolemia will result in proximal aortic hypotension and suboptimal perfusion of the brain and upper extremities. Excessive rpm of the centrifugal pump may cause vortexing, which can generate microemboli that can be passed distally into the patient. Finally, femoral cannulation can result in limb ischemia by the arterial cannula obstructing flow in the distal femoral artery.

SUMMARY

CPB, ECMO, and LHB have revolutionized our ability to operate on the heart, great vessels, and aorta in addition to providing means of short-term support for reversible causes of cardiac and/or respiratory failure. The success of these approaches is dependent upon excellent communication between the surgeon, perfusionist, and anesthesiologist as well as constant vigilance and troubleshooting by the caregivers.

REFERENCES

1. Edwards WS, Edwards PD. Alexis Carrel: visionary surgeon. Springfield (IL): Charles C Thomas; 1974. p. 92–95.
2. Gibbon JH Jr. The gestation and birth of an idea. Phila Med 1963;59:913–6.
3. Lillehei CW, Cohen M, Warden HE, et al. The results of direct vision closure of ventricular septal defects in eight patients by means of controlled cross circulation. Surg Gynecol Obstet 1955;101:446–66.
4. Lillehei CW, Cohen M, Warden HE, et al. The direct vision intracardiac correction of congenital anomalies by controlled cross circulation. Surgery 1955;38:11–29.
5. National adult cardiac surgery database. Society of Thoracic Surgeons. Fall 2008.

6. Kroon BB, Noorda EM, Vrouenraets BC, et al. Isolated limb perfusion for melanoma. Surg Oncol Clin N Am 2008;17(4):785–94, viii–ix.

7. Mora CT, editor. Cardiopulmonary bypass: principles and techniques of extracorporeal circulation. New York: Springer-Verlag; 1995.

8. Reed CC, Kurusz MA, Lawrence AE Jr, editors. Safety and techniques in perfusion. Stafford (TX): Quali-Med; 1988.

9. Castaneda AR, Jonas RA, Mayer JE Jr, et al, editors. Cardiac surgery of the neonate and infant. Philadelphia: Saunders; 1994.

10. Casthely PA, Bregman D, editors. Cardiopulmonary bypass: physiology, related complications, and pharmacology. Mount Kisco (NY): Futura; 1991.

11. Lemaire SA, Jones MM, Conklin LD, et al. Randomized comparison of cold blood and cold crystalloid renal perfusion for renal protection during thoracoabdominal aortic aneurysm repair. J Vasc Surg 2009;49(1):11–9 [discussion 19]. Epub 2008 Nov 22.

12. Schepens M, Dossche K, Morshuis W, et al. Introduction of adjuncts and their influence on changing results in 402 consecutive thoracoabdominal aortic aneurysm repairs. Eur J Cardiothorac Surg 2004;25(5):701–7.

13. Coselli JS. The use of left heart bypass in the repair of thoracoabdominal aortic aneurysms: current techniques and results. Semin Thorac Cardiovasc Surg 2003;15(4):326–32.

Great Vessel and Cardiac Trauma

Chris C. Cook, MD[a], Thomas G. Gleason, MD[b,c],*

KEYWORDS

- Thoracic aortic injury • Aortic transection
- Aortic stent grafting • Aortic reconstruction • Cardiac trauma

Penetrating trauma often affects structures remote from a projectile's trajectory, affecting structures by cavitation and other forces created by high-velocity missiles. Low-velocity penetrating chest injuries that occur from stabbing or impalement can similarly be highly lethal because of the proximity of a large number of vital structures in the thorax. The full extent of thoracic injury may not be initially appreciated simply by the recognition of entrance and exit wounds. Epidemiologic studies demonstrate that greater than 90% of thoracic great vessel injuries are due to penetrating trauma; however, most of these injuries are lethal.[1]

Alternatively, blunt aortic injury (BAI) is the most common cardiovascular injury seen in civilian practice. In 1557, Vesalius first described a death from BAI in a patient who was thrown from a horse. Blunt trauma often occurs as a result of massive, sudden forces that can also injure the heart, venae cavae, pulmonary vessels, thoracic aorta, and brachiocephalic branches. Blunt thoracic trauma can be rapidly lethal or cause more delayed morbidity because of associated injuries to the chest wall, pulmonary parenchyma, and esophagus. Traumatic thoracic injuries can manifest up to years after the accident.

BAI
Epidemiology

Before the latter half of the 20th century, BAI was uncommon. The increase in this injury paralleled the rapidly expanding use of motor vehicles as the primary means

[a] Department of Cardiothoracic Surgery, University of Pittsburgh Medical Center Heart, Lung, and Esophageal Surgery Institute, PUH C-800, 200 Lothrop Street, Pittsburgh, PA 15213, USA
[b] Department of Cardiothoracic Surgery, Division of Cardiac Surgery, University of Pittsburgh Medical Center Heart, Lung, and Esophageal Surgery Institute, PUH C-718, 200 Lothrop Street, Pittsburgh, PA 15213, USA
[c] Center for Thoracic Aortic Diseases, University of Pittsburgh Medical Center, Pittsburgh, PA 15213, USA
* Corresponding author. Department of Cardiothoracic Surgery, Division of Cardiac Surgery, University of Pittsburgh Medical Center Heart, Lung, and Esophageal Surgery Institute, PUH C-718, 200 Lothrop Street, Pittsburgh, PA 15213.
E-mail address: gleasontg@upmc.edu (T.G. Gleason).

Surg Clin N Am 89 (2009) 797–820
doi:10.1016/j.suc.2009.05.002
0039-6109/09/$ – see front matter

of transportation, with motor vehicular trauma now accounting for greater than 70% of blunt thoracic aortic injuries. Aortic injury occurs in 1.5% to 1.9% of motor vehicle crashes.[2] It is second only to brain injury as the leading cause of death in automobile accidents and occurs in up to 15% of deaths due to motor vehicles.[3,4]

BAI follows the typical demographics of trauma patients, who tend to be younger, with an average age of 39 years.[3] Patients are intoxicated in greater than 40% of cases. Ejection from the vehicle doubles the risk for BAI, whereas the use of seatbelts decreases the risk by a factor of 4.[5,6] However, 81% of deaths resulting from BAI have been reported to occur in patients who were restrained with seatbelts or by an air bag.[7] Seatbelts (active restraints) are more effective than air bags (passive restraints) at preventing aortic injury.[8] Airbags have been implicated as a cause of BAI in cars travelling less than 10 mph in some cases.[9-11] Overall, it does appear that the use of seatbelts, airbags, and chest protectors has decreased the number of fatalities, the number of associated injuries, and the size of aortic defects in motor vehicle and cycle crashes.[12,13] Frontal and side-impact crashes carry the highest risk of aortic injury.[2] Other causes of aortic rupture include crush injuries, cave-ins, airplane accidents, and falls, which are typically from heights greater than 3 m.[14-16]

Natural History

Death from BAI occurs at the scene in 75% to 90% of cases.[4,17] Approximately 8% survive for more than 4 hours. There is a short latent period in which to intervene in most instances. Of those who arrive to the hospital alive, 75% are initially hemodynamically stable.[3] However, up to 50% die before repair.[12,18] It is estimated that 2% to 5% of patients survive without intervention or even detection of their injury to form a chronic false aneurysm.[19] Some injuries certainly go unnoticed, making it difficult to ascertain the true incidence of injury, the number and character of injuries that heal spontaneously, and the number of undiagnosed chronic pseudoaneurysms.

Nearly all patients have other associated serious injuries. Survivors typically have 2 other serious injuries, whereas nonsurvivors have four or more.[3,17] Data collected prospectively from the American Association for the Surgery of Trauma (AAST) trial from the 1970s to the 1990s indicate that closed head injury occurs in 51%, multiple rib fractures in 46%, pulmonary contusions in 38%, and orthopedic injuries in 20% to 35%.[3] In contrast to Parmley and colleagues' paper[17] in 1958, which reported a 42% incidence of associated cardiac injury, the AAST database reported cardiac contusion in only 4% of patients.[3] There are fewer associated injuries at the initial trauma in patients who later present with chronic pseudoaneurysms.[20-22]

Pathology

Most injuries occur at the aortic isthmus, just distal to the takeoff of the left subclavian artery. Autopsy series have shown that injuries occur at the isthmus in 36% to 54% of cases, 8% to 27% in ascending aorta, 8% to 18% in the arch, and 11% to 21% in the distal descending aorta.[23,24] The percentage of injuries that occur at the isthmus is even higher in surgical series, with 84% to 97% occurring in this location and only 3% to 10% occurring in the ascending, arch, or distal descending aorta.[3,4,23,24] This implies that a greater number of patients with injury occurring at the isthmus survive longer, owing to the protective effect that may be provided by the mediastinal periadventitial tissues surrounding the isthmus. Injuries to more than one area of the aorta in a single patient are rare but have been reported.[25]

Typically, the aorta is completely transected in a transverse fashion, with all three layers of the vessel wall disrupted and the edges separated by several centimeters.[17,23] Partial disruptions and spiral injuries occur less frequently and are associated with intramural hematomas and focal dissections, unlike complete transections.[17] Partial tears are usually posterior and involve the vessel intima and media, leaving the adventitia intact. Initial survivors usually have an incomplete transection, with disruption of the media and intima only, although patients have survived circumferential, full-thickness disruptions. The integrity of the periadventitial tissues prevents free rupture and can maintain distal perfusion in survivors. Aortic wall structure at the site of injury is the same as the uninjured adjacent aorta. Although the greatest number of injuries occur at the isthmus, there is no evidence to suggest that the aorta is weaker in this area.[26] Atherosclerosis is generally not present at the site of injury or the adjacent aorta.[17,23]

In the case of chronic pseudoaneurysms, there is blood flow in the false aneurysm that later thromboses and organizes into a fibrous wall, which then tends to calcify.[19,27,28] Posttraumatic aneurysms have been known to fistulize to the pulmonary artery or bronchus.[29-31] Symptomatic compression of the left main bronchus has also been reported.[32]

Pathogenesis

No single theory regarding the pathogenesis of BAI has emerged as a universally accepted mechanism of injury, because this continues to be an area of debate. Held in place by the ligamentum arteriosum, the left mainstem bronchus, and the paired intercostal arteries, the aortic isthmus is situated at the junction between the more mobile aortic arch and the relatively fixed descending thoracic aorta. Experimental data suggest that the aorta can be displaced longitudinally with sufficient force to cause traction tears at the isthmus.[33] Deceleration forces can reach several hundred times the force of gravity, and can produce injury without direct impact on the chest.[34,35]

Several theories have been proposed, including a "shoveling mechanism," whereby cranially directed traction stresses occur in drivers and front seat passengers in motor vehicle accidents.[36] BAI has also been believed to occur as a result of sudden increases in blood pressure. Review of tensile data from Mohan and Melvin[37] demonstrates that aortic wall samples rupture transversely. In 1956, Zehnder calculated that an intravascular pressure of greater than 2000 mm Hg is required to cause aortic rupture.[38]

Another hypothesis is the "water-hammer effect." When flow of a noncompressible fluid is suddenly obstructed, as might occur at the diaphragm with rapid deceleration, a reflected high-pressure wave is generated. The pulse pressure generated by the reflected wave is greatest at the aortic arch from amplification that occurs because of the curvature of the arch.[39] Symbas concluded that this mechanism may play a greater role in injuries of the ascending aorta, whereas injuries at the isthmus are more likely the result of bending and shear.[40]

Finally, Crass and Cohen[41-43] have argued that forces of differential deceleration, torsion, or hydrostatics alone are of insufficient magnitude to cause aortic rupture, given the inherent properties of the aorta. They proposed the "osseous pinch" hypothesis, which surmises that the aorta is directly sheared between the bony structures of the anterior thorax (manubrium, first ribs, and clavicular heads) and the posterior vertebral column. This theory has been supported by clinical data.[44,45]

CLINICAL PRESENTATION

Fewer than 50% of the patients with BAI present with specific signs or symptoms of the injury.[46-50] Although patients may complain of dyspnea, chest pain, or back pain, these symptoms are common among trauma patients and can be because of several other injuries. Therefore, it is imperative to obtain a thorough trauma history when possible and to consider the diagnosis of aortic injury when patients have sustained a sudden deceleration, fall, or crush injury.

Physical examination signs that increase the suspicion for aortic injury include shock, steering wheel deformity of the anterior chest, cardiac murmurs, hoarseness, paraplegia, or unequal extremity pressures. Fractures of the sternum, clavicles, first rib, scapula, or multiple ribs are also commonly seen. Long-bone fractures are frequently associated and can be extremely painful and distracting. They should be stabilized for comfort and hemorrhage control, but definitive management should be delayed until aortic injury or other potentially life-threatening injuries have been ruled out. Details from the history and physical that should increase the index of suspicion for aortic injury are provided in **Box 1**.

Time to diagnosis of aortic injury is critical, because the leading cause of death in these patients is still exsanguination from the aorta, which occurs in at least 20% of patients who make it to the hospital alive. Even among those who are initially hemodynamically stable, 4% will die in the hospital before surgical repair can be accomplished.[3]

Box 1
Clues that suggest aortic disruption

History

    Motor vehicle crash greater than 50 km/h

    Motor vehicle crash into fixed barrier

    No seat belt

    Ejection from vehicle

    Broken steering wheel

    Motorcycle or airplane crash

    Pedestrian hit by motor vehicle

    Falls from heights greater than 3 m

    Crush or cave-in injuries

    Loss of consciousness

Physical Signs

    Hemodynamic shock

    Fracture of sternum, first rib, clavicle, scapula, or multiple ribs

    Steering wheel imprint on chest

    Cardiac murmurs

    Hoarseness

    Dyspnea

    Back pain

    Hemothorax

    Unequal extremity blood pressures

    Paraplegia

Diagnosis

Although BAI should be suspected based on the history, physical examination, and associated injuries, the aortic disruption must be imaged to secure the diagnosis. Standard portable chest radiographs can suggest the injury, but they are insufficient to make the diagnosis or rule it out.[51,52] Classic chest radiograph findings seen in BAI are provided in **Box 2**.[51] The collective impression of chest radiograph abnormalities seems to be more sensitive than any single finding with regards to predicting aortic injury.[53]

Historically, aortography was the gold standard for diagnosis of aortic injury. Its sensitivity and specificity approach 100% in experienced hands.[54] The rates of contrast reactions, contrast-induced nephropathy, groin hematomas, and pseudoaneurysm formation are low. Disadvantages of aortography include the need for a skilled team to perform the study, and a majority (85%–95%) of these diagnostic aortograms are negative.[47,54–57] Helical computed tomography angiography (CTA) has supplanted aortography as the diagnostic modality of choice, with sensitivity and negative predictive values approaching 100%.[58–60] Approximately 1% of blunt trauma patients have a thoracic aortic injury identified by CT.[60] Besides superb diagnostic accuracy, other advantages of CT include widespread availability, speed, and reasonable cost. Unlike other diagnostic modalities, CT has the unique ability to readily identify associated injuries, with the capability to scan the brain, facial bones, neck, chest, abdomen, and pelvis in the same diagnostic setting. CT identifies direct signs of aortic injury, which include contrast extravasation, intimal flaps, pseudoaneurysm formation, and filling defects, such as mural thrombus. Indirect signs of BAI include periaortic and mediastinal hematomas.[61,62] Typical CTA findings of BAI are demonstrated in **Fig. 1**.

Box 2
Chest radiograph findings associated with blunt aortic disruption

1. Widened mediastinum (>8.0 cm)
2. Mediastinum-to-chest width ratio greater than 0.25
3. Tracheal shift to the right
4. Blurring of the aortic contour
5. Loss of the aortic knob
6. Left apical pleural cap
7. Depression of the left mainstem bronchus
8. Opacification of the aortopulmonary window
9. Rightward deviation of the nasogastric tube
10. Wide paraspinal lines
11. First rib fracture
12. Other rib fractures
13. Clavicle fracture
14. Pulmonary contusion
15. Thoracic spine fracture

Data from Cook A, Klein J, Rogers F, et al. Chest radiographs of limited utility in the diagnosis of blunt traumatic aortic laceration. J Trauma 2001;50:843.

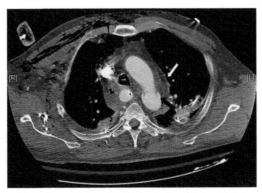

Fig. 1. CTA demonstrating characteristic findings of intimal disruption at the aortic isthmus (*black arrow*) with associated mediastinal hematoma (*white arrow*). Common findings of rib fractures and subcutaneous emphysema are also seen.

False positives can be seen with CT when failing to recognize a ductus diverticulum remnant.[60] However, a ductus diverticulum has no associated intimal disruption or periaortic hematoma, unlike a true aortic injury.

Transesophageal echocardiography (TEE) is now readily available at all cardiac surgery centers and has the ability to identify injuries of the thoracic aorta with a sensitivity and specificity approaching 100%.[63,64] It is portable and can be performed in the emergency department or operating room concomitantly with other procedures. The risk of complications from TEE is low.[63,64] However, TEE is highly operator dependent and lacks the ability to visualize the distal ascending aorta and proximal aortic arch because of the artifact created by the intervening air of the trachea and bronchus. TEE is contraindicated in many trauma patients who have associated injuries of the cervical spine, oropharynx, esophagus, or maxillofacial bones. The greatest use of TEE may be in the patient who requires emergent laparotomy to control ongoing hemorrhage and in whom aortic injury is suspected.

MRI has little application in the evaluation of acute aortic trauma because of long examination times and limited access. It can be used, however, in the follow-up of aortic injuries treated nonoperatively.[65,66]

Management

In 1958, Parmley and colleagues[17] reported on a series of patients with nonpenetrating aortic injury, which shaped the management of BAI for the next 3 decades. Because the percentage of death was 85% in this report, and most survivors died within a few days, immediate angiography for suspicious findings followed by repair, regardless of associated injuries, was touted. The management of these injuries has since evolved. It is now apparent that there is a spectrum of severity of BAI and, in the context of other associated injuries, morbidity of intervention must also be considered. It is now clear that minimal injuries often heal and can be followed safely with effective medical management.[67] Finally, the revolution of endovascular aortic stent grafting has greatly simplified repair of many BAIs.

Initial assessment and timing of intervention

As with any trauma patient, the initial assessment begins with principles of the Advanced Trauma Life Support protocol. This includes a rapid assessment of airway, breathing, and circulation, followed by a thorough secondary survey that includes obtaining adjunctive laboratory and radiographic data. There are 3 broad categories of patients with BAI: (1) those who die at the scene (70%–80% of the whole); (2) those who present unstable or become unstable (2%–5% of the whole, with a mortality of 90%–98%); and (3) those who are hemodynamically stable and are diagnosed 4 to 18 hours after injury (15%–25% of the whole, with a mortality of 25%, largely caused by associated injuries).[68]

In unstable patients, repair of a contained aortic rupture is third in the hierarchy of addressing life-threatening injuries. Ongoing hemorrhage must be controlled first regardless of the source. This may include chest tube drainage of hemopneumothorax, temporary stabilization of long-bone fractures, temporary reduction of unstable pelvic injuries, exploratory laparotomy or thoracotomy, and coil embolization of ongoing pelvic bleeding. TEE can be used to evaluate the aorta for possible injury while performing other procedures. Secondly, intracranial hemorrhage causing mass effect must be identified and drained. Aortic injuries should be subsequently addressed. Ongoing resuscitation should continue and antiimpulse therapy should be instituted as dictated by the patient's hemodynamic status in preparation for definitive treatment of the aortic injury. Antiimpulse therapy is synonymous with short-acting beta-blockade to reduce wall stress by reducing blood pressure and heart rate. Antiimpulse therapy has been shown to reduce in-hospital aortic rupture rates without adversely affecting the outcome of other injuries.[69,70]

Patients with severe associated injuries and contained aortic disruption can often have their aortic injury treated in delayed fashion with continued antiimpulse therapy. Considerations for initial medical therapy followed by delayed repair are outlined in **Box 3**.[71–73] Brain injury remains the leading cause of death in trauma patients. Delaying intervention for an aortic injury in hemodynamically stable patients may allow time to determine the neurologic prognosis and to allow for reversible causes of depressed level of consciousness to be treated. Studies have reported on the safety of delayed repair in patients with multiple severe injuries.[71–73] The optimal extent of delay has not been clearly determined.

Nonoperative management in extremely comorbid patients has been extended for prolonged periods of time with acceptable mortality. Holmes and colleagues[74] reported on 30 patients managed in a delayed fashion (>24 hours) or nonoperatively, with 15 patients in each group. In the delayed group, progression of the aortic injury was seen within 5 days in three patients, two of whom died. There were three total deaths in this group, with one rupture and two intraoperative arrests. In the 15 patients who were treated nonoperatively, there were five deaths, all resulting from brain injury.

Box 3
High-risk patients who may benefit from delayed repair

1. Brain injury with significant hemorrhage or edema on CT scan.

2. Pulmonary contusion with PaO_2/FiO_2 ratio less than 300, positive end-expiratory pressure requirements of 7.5 cm H_2O, or inability to tolerate single-lung ventilation.

3. Preexisting cardiac disease: recent angina, earlier coronary artery bypass surgery, requires inotropic support.

4. Coagulopathy: nonsurgical bleeding, international normalized ratio greater than 1.5, platelets less than 400,000.

5. Intraabdominal solid organ injury.

6. Severe pelvic fracture.

Of the 10 survivors, five had complete radiographic resolution of their injury and five developed stable pseudoaneurysms. No patient in this group required surgery after an average follow-up of 2.5 years.

The need to intervene during a period of delayed or nonoperative management is indicated with an expanding mediastinal hematoma, hemothorax, free extravasation of contrast on follow-up CT scan, or signs of distal malperfusion (anuria lasting more than 6 hours, limb ischemia, or persistent acidosis).[75]

Stable patients who do not require other resuscitative procedures to address hemorrhagic shock and who have no indication of a potentially devastating neurologic injury can proceed directly to definitive aortic repair. Early institution of beta-blockade in these patients provides an increased margin of safety during the interim to surgical intervention. Non–life-threatening injuries should be addressed after definitive repair of the aortic injury.

Open repair

Conventional open repair of traumatic aortic disruption with interposition grafting is the standard with which all other management strategies should be compared. It has proven to be safe, effective, and durable. Simple aortic cross-clamping, the "clamp and sew" technique, has been used in the past, but it yields higher rates of paraplegia than techniques that use extracorporeal lower body perfusion (**Table 1**).[3] Cross-clamp times greater than 30 minutes have been associated with paraplegia rates of 15% to 30%.[3,76] In the AAST prospective database, only 33% of repairs were accomplished in less than 30 minutes.[3] A meta-analysis by von Oppell and colleagues[76] reported an average cross-clamp time of 41.0 minutes. Although some experienced groups have reported very low paraplegia rates with simple clamping, they still rely on short cross-clamp times (<20–25 minutes), with little margin for difficult cases.[77,78] Their results have not been reproducible across many centers.

Various perfusion techniques and adjuncts have been developed to reduce the incidence of paraplegia resulting from spinal cord ischemia. The spinal cord blood supply is through the anterior and posterior spinal arteries. The anterior two-thirds of the spinal cord is supplied by the anterior spinal artery, which arises from radicular and medullary branches of the paired posterior intercostal arteries coming directly from the aorta. The anterior spinal artery is well developed in the upper thorax and receives collateral flow from the left vertebral artery and the internal mammary artery through

Table 1		
Incidence of postoperative paraplegia in relation to surgical management: AAST Prospective Trial		
Operative Technique	**No. of Patients**	**Paraplegia (%)**
Bypass	134	4.5[a]
Gott shunt	4	0
Full bypass	22	4.5
Partial bypass	39	7.7
Centrifugal pump	69	2.9[b]
Clamp and sew	24	6.4[a,b]

[a] $P<.004$, bypass versus clamp and sew.
[b] $P<.01$, centrifugal pump versus clamp and sew.
   Data from Fabian T, Richardson J, Croce M, et al. Prospective study of blunt aortic injury: multicenter trial of the American Association for the Surgery of Trauma. J Trauma 1997;42(3):374–80.

the intercostals. The anterior spinal artery is less developed in the lower thorax and abdomen, and it is more dependent on collateral flow that it receives from the intercostals and lumbar arteries at these levels. At the level of the first lumbar vertebra (variations T8 to L4), the anterior spinal artery receives the arteria radicularis magna (artery of Adamkiewicz). This artery is essential for the blood supply to the spinal cord in this region in at least 25% of patients.[79,80] Unlike patients with chronic aneurysmal disease, young trauma patients lack well-developed collateral circulation to the spinal cord and are therefore at increased risk of spinal cord ischemia.

Risk factors for postoperative paraplegia include increased cross-clamp time, the length of the aorta excluded, low distal perfusion pressure, systemic hypotension, the number of intercostal arteries ligated, increased body temperature, and increased cerebrospinal fluid pressure. Aortic cross-clamping near the aortic isthmus produces profound hypotension in the lower body and spinal cord, and the risk of spinal cord injury is proportionate to cross-clamp time.[81] Furthermore, the aorta often must be clamped proximal to the origin of the left subclavian artery, which may occlude collateral flow and predispose to cord ischemia. Paraplegia has been reported to occur with as little as 9 minutes of cross-clamp time when lower body perfusion was not used.[82] These factors have influenced many centers to adopt a strategy of routine lower body perfusion with various forms of extracorporeal circulation. However, no factor has been identified as the single most important contributor to paraplegia, and the cause is likely multifactorial.

Distal perfusion with the use of a passive shunt was first described by Gott in 1972.[81] Of predominantly historical interest, this shunt consisted of a tapered, heparin-coated polyvinyl tube that shunted blood from the proximal aorta (ascending aorta, aortic arch, or left subclavian artery) to the distal aorta (descending thoracic aorta or femoral artery). The diameter of the tube is fixed, and flow is therefore passive, unmonitored, and dependent on a pressure gradient. Experimental data later indicated that this shunt was inadequate to prevent paraplegia.[82] Although the AAST database reported no cases of paraplegia with use of the Gott shunt, it was used in only four patients in this study.[3]

Use of a centrifugal pump with heparin-bonded tubing and active partial left-heart bypass is an option that does not require systemic heparinization.[83,84] Full heparinization should be avoided in cases of brain injury or severe pulmonary contusion. The addition of a heat exchanger allows active warming in these patients who frequently present hypothermic. A venous reservoir can also be included in the circuit to allow capture of shed blood and to allow rapid volume control. However, the stasis that occurs with a reservoir and the surface area added by incorporating these components necessitate full systemic heparinization to decrease thrombotic risks. Despite concerns with heparinization in trauma patients, many groups that use active partial left-heart bypass with full heparinization have not reported increased bleeding complications.[3,85] Partial left-heart bypass set up in this manner serves several purposes: (1) to maintain lower body perfusion, (2) to unload the left heart and control proximal hypertension at the time of aortic cross-clamping, (3) to control intravascular volume (rapid infusion or removal), and (4) to allow active warming in cases of associated hypothermia. The circuit for left-heart bypass entails blood outflow through the left atrium and arterial inflow by way of cannulation of the distal descending thoracic aorta or the femoral artery. Radial and femoral arterial pressure monitoring are required. The lower body is perfused at a rate of 2 to 3 L/min to maintain a lower body mean arterial pressure (MAP) of 60 to 70 mm Hg. The upper body MAP is maintained at 70 to 80 mm Hg. All shed blood can be returned to the circuit through pump reservoir or is collected and returned by way of cell saver.

Full cardiopulmonary bypass can be achieved by venous cannulation at the inferior vena cava-right atrial (RA) junction by way of a left thoracotomy by opening the pericardium posterior to the phrenic nerve. Alternatively, RA drainage can be accomplished through the common femoral vein with use of a long venous drainage catheter. The catheter is threaded over a guidewire and TEE is used to confirm its placement at the level of the RA. RA venous drainage through the femoral vein to femoral arterial bypass has the added advantage of allowing cardiopulmonary bypass support before left thoracotomy in patients who may not otherwise tolerate single-lung ventilation. Full cardiopulmonary bypass also allows for active cooling and facilitates a period of hypothermic circulatory arrest, which may be necessary to repair complex aortic arch injuries. Ascending aorta and arch injuries proximal to the left common carotid artery are better approached with anterior exposure through a sternotomy or thoracosternotomy.

In addition to lower-body perfusion, several adjunctive measures can be used to reduce the risk of spinal cord ischemia during thoracic aortic surgery, such as monitoring motor or somatosensory evoked potentials, lumbar cerebrospinal fluid drainage, and hypothermia;[86–88] however, these modalities are often impractical in emergent settings. The use of theoretical neuroprotective pharmaceuticals, such as steroids, lidocaine, or magnesium, has also been described.[89] These adjuncts have not been well studied in the trauma population.

The standard approach to open repair is through a left posterolateral thoracotomy in the fourth intercostal space, providing excellent exposure to the aortic isthmus. The incision should be large enough to allow exposure of the aorta from the left common carotid artery for proximal control to the distal descending thoracic aorta for arterial inflow cannulation. Notching the fifth rib posteriorly may help with this exposure. Emergency department thoracotomies are commonly done in haste and are often placed too inferiorly to allow for adequate exposure and repair of an aortic transection. Given this situation, it is best to make a second thoracotomy in the fourth interspace, using the same skin incision if possible. Patients with a history of previous thoracotomy likely have significant left-pleural adhesions. Although the adhesions may be beneficial in preventing free rupture of the aorta, the dissection can be cumbersome. Optimally, heparinization should be held until the lung is fully mobilized. If the patient will not tolerate single-lung ventilation during thoracotomy, full cardiopulmonary bypass may be required. The left groin should be prepped after the patient is placed in the right lateral decubitus position to allow access to the left femoral vessels.

As with any other vascular repair, proximal and distal control is accomplished before dissecting near the injury. The distal descending aorta is exposed first because it is the least likely to precipitate free rupture of the contained hematoma. The paired intercostal arteries are preserved as the aorta is encircled with an umbilical tape. The left subclavian artery is then isolated and encircled. Next, proximal control is obtained by encircling the aorta between the left common carotid and left subclavian arteries. Because the injury most often occurs just distal to the origin of the left subclavian artery, it is usually not possible to expose the aorta distal to the subclavian without disrupting the contained hematoma surrounding the injury. Furthermore, the proximity of the injury to the subclavian artery usually precludes adequate debridement with a technically sound repair if the clamp is placed distal to the subclavian. If left-heart bypass is to be used, the descending aorta can be cannulated for arterial inflow. Venous drainage is then established by cannulation at the left superior pulmonary vein-left atrial junction. If heparin is to be used, it is given just before cannulation. A reservoir in the left-heart bypass circuit allows drainage of blood to unload the left ventricle and prevent proximal hypertension just before placing the proximal aortic cross clamp. Flow and pressures are maintained as describedearlier. The mediastinal pleura is now opened to expose the injury. Care is taken to avoid injury to the phrenic, vagus, or left recurrent laryngeal nerves during the dissection. The edges of the aorta are debrided, and the transection is repaired with an appropriately sized interposition graft. The distal clamp is removed first as the graft is deaired. Partial left-heart bypass is weaned after removal of the cross clamps. After ensuring a technically sound repair, the cannulas are removed, and the heparin is reversed with protamine. Chest tubes are placed and the thoracotomy closed. Ongoing resuscitation is continued, and non–life-threatening injuries are addressed as dictated by the patient's clinical status.

Thoracic endovascular aortic repair

There are now many reports of the efficacy of thoracic endovascular aortic repair (TEVAR) for acute traumatic aortic disruption.[90–92] TEVAR has been used selectively based on a predicted higher risk with conventional open repair in patients with significant comorbidities, for example, preexisting illness, advanced age, or severe associated injuries. Given that severe associated injuries are so common and experience with the technique has increased, TEVAR has become the preferred management for BAI in many institutions. Although the long-term durability of these grafts in young trauma patients is not yet known, many have accepted the risk of possible chronic complications in favor of the benefits afforded by a less-invasive, less time-consuming technique where the added potential morbidity of an open repair is avoided. It should be made clear to the patient and family that thoracic aortic stent grafting for acute aortic trauma has not been approved by the Food and Drug Administration (FDA). The lack of long-term follow-up should be discussed in the context of the efficacy of open repair, and a clear rationale as to why an endovascular approach is preferred should be explained and documented as part of the informed consent process.There are three commercially available stent grafts that are FDA approved in the United States for aneurysmal disease: the Gore Thoracic Aortic Graft (W. L. Gore and Associates, Flagstaff, Arizona), the Cook-Zenith TX2 (Cook, Bloomington, Indiana), and the Medtronic Talent (Medtronic, Santa Rosa, California).

When performing TEVAR for aortic injury, the priorities of initial evaluation, resuscitation and antiimpulse therapy are the same as with open repair. TEVAR should be performed in a hybrid operating room/angiography suite with a dedicated fluoroscopy unit designed for endovascular surgery, when possible. A portable C-arm fluoroscopy unit can be used in a conventional operating room when necessary, but it does not allow optimal angling of the fluoroscopy image to visualize the aortic arch. The rate of conversion from TEVAR to open repair is higher with management of aortic disruption than aneurysms, and the operative team must be capable of making the conversion immediately.[93] TEVAR is usually performed under general anesthesia with a single-lumen endotracheal tube.

Aortic access is retrograde through the femoral or iliac arteries. Bilateral access is often obtained, one for angiography and the other for delivery of the stent graft. Percutaneous femoral, direct femoral, and iliac arterial puncture and iliac access by way of a silo graft sewn to the iliac artery have all been used. After establishing arterial access, 5000 units of heparin is routinely given intravenously, although it is possible to avoid heparin altogether in cases where there is concern for bleeding complications at remote sites.[94] A floppy J-tipped wire is advanced to the ascending aorta under fluoroscopic and/or TEE guidance. A marked catheter is subsequently passed over the wire. An aortogram is performed using a steep anterior oblique projection (~60°) to accurately assess and measure the aortic arch anatomy relative to the site of transection. **Fig. 2** demonstrates an intraoperative aortogram performed during

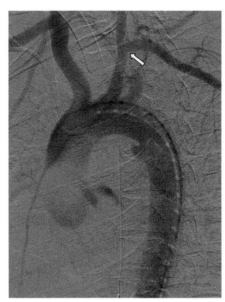

Fig. 2. CTA just before TEVAR with marked catheter in place. Note the left subclavian artery–to–carotid artery transposition (*white arrow*). Transposition was performed just before TEVAR in this 80-year-old patient because of concerns of vertebrobasilar insufficiency.

TEVAR. The diameter of the prosthesis should be based on aortic measurements obtained preoperatively by CT angiography or by intravascular ultrasound (IVUS). Length of graft coverage should be based on intraoperative angiographic or IVUS measurements. A stiff wire is advanced from the side of device delivery. The device delivery sheath is advanced over the stiff wire under continuous fluoroscopy. The device is brought into position. The image intensifier is rotated to the ideal angle, and angiography is performed with respirations suspended (20 mL of contrast per second for 2 seconds). A roadmap is obtained, or the landmarks are marked on the fluoroscopy screen with a felt pen. The pigtail used for the angiogram is now withdrawn, and the stent graft is deployed under fluoroscopy. A completion angiogram is performed. Completion angiograms of the grafted injury and of the pelvis are performed. Follow-up is based on guidelines to evaluate thoracic endografting for atherosclerotic aneurysms with CT angiography performed at 48 hours; at time of discharge; and at 1, 6, and 12 months.

Complications occurring after TEVAR include endoleak, stent-graft collapse, stroke, embolization, bronchial obstruction, migration, paralysis, dissection, or rupture. Endoleaks are categorized as type I (leak around the proximal [A] or distal ends [B] of the graft); type II (leak from an artery excluded by the graft that perfuses the vessel in a retrograde fashion between the wall of the aorta and the graft); type III (leak between modular components); and type IV (failure of graft integrity). Ballooning can be done if a type I endoleak is noted or if there is a lip of the graft not in apposition to the inner curve of the aorta. The predominant mechanism of endograft leak in trauma patients is the combination of a short landing zone and lack of apposition along the inner curvature of the arch.Ballooning of the graft should be avoided in trauma cases to prevent proximal hypertension and graft displacement. Extending the graft with placement of a proximal modular cuff may be necessary if this fails to resolve the endoleak.

Based on the proximity to the aortic injury, the left subclavian artery will need to be covered in many patients to adequately exclude the injury. A type II endoleak can develop from retrograde flow in the left subclavian artery. This can be resolved with coil embolization of the takeoff of the left subclavian by way of a left brachial arterial approach or by transposing the subclavian artery to the left common carotid artery. Transposition has the added benefit of avoiding problems of ischemia to the left arm or vertebrobasilar system. However, coverage of the left subclavian artery without revascularization is well tolerated in young trauma patients.[95,96] **Fig. 3** shows the final result of TEVAR for BAI followed by a left subclavian artery-to-carotid artery transposition, which was performed in a delayed fashion for persistent symptoms of subclavian steal. Type II endoleaks can also be secondary to patent bronchial or intercostal arteries. Most endoleaks found on follow-up can be managed with repeat intervention or even observed in some cases.

Stent-graft collapse is a catastrophic complication that usually leads to immediate aortic occlusion and possibly rupture. It can occur immediately or in a delayed fashion and has been seen up to 3 months post procedure.[97] It likely results from graft oversizing and lack of apposition along the inner curve of the aorta. In young hyperdynamic aortas, with their degree of pliability, the force of the cardiac ejection that hits the underside of the graft can cause collapse of the graft. If this occurs post implantation, the patient can develop signs of acute coarctation, and the rapid onset of paralysis and renal failure can occur. This can be treated by extending the graft proximally, by repeat ballooning, or by conventional open repair. Uncovered bare metal stents have also been used in this situation, but late aortic perforation has been reported.[98] Cuff extenders, which may be deployed sequentially and fit the curvature of the aorta better, may prove to perform better than longer thoracic stent grafts in patients with aortic diameters less than 24 mm.

Stroke occurs at a rate of 3% to 5% with thoracic endografting. The incidence is reported to be lower in the trauma population at 0% to 2%.[99] Possible causes may include occlusion of the left vertebral artery, embolization of arch thrombus in older patients, inadvertent guidewire advancement into the carotid, or air embolism. Distal

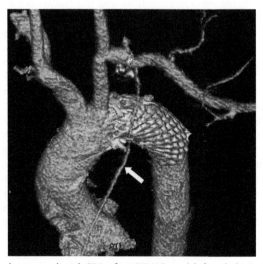

Fig. 3. Follow-up volume rendered CTA after TEVAR and left subclavian artery–to–carotid artery transposition. Note intact left internal mammary artery (*white arrow*).

embolization can occur in older patients with diffuse atheromata or from thrombus at the site of injury. If distal embolization is possible, angiography should be performed. Peripheral pulses should be recorded at the start and completion of the procedure.

Table 2 summarizes the mortality and paraplegia rates for open repair and TEVAR. Paraplegia rates vary widely depending on the operative technique used, with a range of 0% to 20%. The preponderance of data suggests that the combination of partial left-heart bypass for lower-body perfusion with short (<30 min) cross-clamp time affords the lowest rate of paraplegia. The early results of TEVAR suggest that this technique may reduce the risk of paraplegia further.

Unpublished data on the 2-year follow-up of a European experience with the Medtronic Talent thoracic graft in 41 trauma patients was presented at the 45th Annual Society of Thoracic Surgeons meeting. This is a retrospective registry of 457 consecutive TEVARs from 1996 to 2004, where 41 patients underwent endovascular repair of a traumatic aortic injury.[104] Stent-graft implantation was technically successful in all 41 cases. There was 1 hospital mortality (2.4%) and 100% survival in the remaining 40 patients, with a median follow-up of 13 months (1–69 mo). There were no cases of paraplegia reported. A single stent graft was required in 40 of the 41 patients (98%). A proximal extension graft was placed in 1 patient (2%) for a primary endoleak at the time of the initial procedure. Despite covering the left subclavian artery in only 8% of cases, no secondary endoleaks have been discovered in follow-up. Long-term follow-up data are necessary.

Chronic pseudoaneurysms

Chronic traumatic pseudoaneurysms of the aorta are seen infrequently in clinical practice and likely evade detection because of the lack of symptoms. Therefore, the true incidence is not known. Once discovered, these injuries are followed with serial CT angiography. Traumatic pseudoaneurysms have been treated similar to true thoracic aneurysms, with intervention for increase in size or the development of symptoms. Open repair yields very low mortality rates.[105]

Nonaortic Great Vessel Injury

Most injuries of the great venous structures and the pulmonary arteries are due to penetrating trauma. Blunt trauma to these vessels is rare, presumably because of their distensibility and low pressure. The overall incidence of great vessel injury in penetrating trauma is approximately 5% with gunshot wounds and 2% with stab wounds.[106] Wounds penetrating the thoracic "box" bordered by the midclavicular lines, the thoracic outlet, and the xiphoid process should be explored operatively. Chest tubes should be inserted as a diagnostic and therapeutic measure, and an echocardiogram or a subxiphoid pericardial window should be performed to rule out hemopericardium. Patients with a high index of suspicion of mediastinal great vessel injury or with a confirmed hemopericardium should undergo sternotomy. Patients with central venous or pulmonary arterial rupture decompensate from pericardial tamponade. Expeditious pericardial decompression often provides enough stability to facilitate definitive repair. Exsanguination from a venous or pulmonary arterial injury into one of the hemithoraces requires immediate massive volume resuscitation and transfer to the operating room. Choice of incision should be made based on clinical suspicion of site of injury or objective data (arteriography, chest radiograph, or bleeding site). When the site of injury is not clear, median sternotomy provides excellent access to the heart and great vessels, and it can be extended across a hemithorax or up the neck along either sternocleidomastoid to facilitate exposure of any vascular structure in the chest. Most venous injuries and pulmonary arterial injuries, when

Table 2
Operative results of open repair or TEVAR for aortic transection

Authors, Year	Study Period (Years)	No. of Cases		Mortality		Paraplegia	
		Open Repair	TEVAR	Open Repair (%)	TEVAR (%)	Open Repair (%)	TEVAR (%)
Cook et al, 2006[12]	20	79	19	24.1	21.1	4	0
Pacini et al, 2005[100]	23	51	15	7.8	0	5.9	0
Rousseau et al, 2005[92]	18	35	29	17	0	5.7	0
Andrassy et al, 2006[101]	14	16	15	18.8	13.3	12.5	0
Ott et al, 2004[102]	11	12	6	17	0	17	0
Morishita et al, 2004[93]	3	11	18	9	17	0	5.6
Reed et al, 2006[18]	5	9	13	11	23	0	0
Lachat et al, 2002[103]	n/a	n/a	12	n/a	0	n/a	0
Peterson et al, 2005[91]	4	n/a	11	n/a	0	n/a	0
Ehrlich et al, 2009[104]	8	n/a	41	n/a	0	n/a	0
Pooled data	—	214	179	16.8%	4.5%	5.6%	0.6%

Abbreviation: n/a, not applicable.

localized and simple, can be repaired without cardiopulmonary bypass. Large or complex venous, and particularly pulmonary arterial, injuries are often more easily repaired on full cardiopulmonary bypass with a decompressed heart. When repairing pulmonary venous injuries, it is important to safeguard against air embolus, the result of which can be devastating. Therefore, complex pulmonary venous injury may require aortic cross-clamping with cardioplegia to prevent emboli to the brain.

CARDIAC TRAUMA
Blunt Cardiac Trauma

Cardiac rupture resulting from blunt trauma was observed and described by Senac in 1778. Today, motor vehicle crashes cause the majority of blunt cardiac injuries, with other causes including falls, crush or blast injuries, and street violence.

The compression and deceleration forces that yield blunt aortic injuries are similar to those that result in cardiac injuries. Abruptly occurring high pressures within and around the heart can cause disruption of the fairly static components of the heart. Subsequent high intraventricular pressure may cause injury to the cardiac free wall, the ventricular septum, coronary arteries, the tensor apparatus of the mitral and tricuspid valves, or the cusps of the aortic valve. Less dramatically, these forces can cause myocardial contusion, and the right ventricle has been shown to be the most susceptible because of its anterior position.

Rarely, sudden cardiac death can occur as a result of a direct blow to the anterior chest, *commotio cordis*. A blow to the precordium during the vulnerable period of repolarization (just before the T-wave peak) results in ventricular fibrillation or asystole. Most injuries occur in males (95%), and most are children or adolescents (78%).[107] Survival is only 13% and is predicated on immediate recognition and rapid defibrillation.

Screening for cardiac injury begins with a chest radiograph and electrocardiogram (ECG). These have been shown to have sufficient negative predictive value for blunt cardiac injury in young patients. Thus, stable patients with normal ECG and chest radiograph generally require no further cardiac imaging. A normal serum troponin I level increases the negative predictive value, and an elevated troponin significantly increases the specificity for blunt cardiac injury.[108]

Although evidence does not support echocardiography as a screening tool, patients with positive findings on physical examination or screening with ECG, chest radiograph, and serum troponin require a morphologic assessment of the heart and pericardium. Because of its portability, TEE is ideal for detection of pericardial effusion, valvular heart dysfunction, and wall motion abnormalities. In patients with suboptimal transthoracic studies, TEE improves resolution and also allows for identification of aortic trauma. Given the advances in echocardiographic imaging, pericardiocentesis and pericardial window are rarely used for diagnosis, but they may be useful as therapeutic maneuvers when tamponade exists.

Cardiac injuries have been graded according to their lethal potential (**Table 3**). The management of patients with blunt cardiac trauma is most often dictated by the presence of structural injury and hemodynamic compromise. Stable patients with grades I and II injuries require close monitoring but no immediate surgical intervention. Distal coronary artery thrombosis may be managed conservatively or with percutaneous coronary intervention. Patients with heart failure and no structural damage may require immediate or delayed surgical repair based on the presence of heart failure, hemodynamic compromise, and other associated injuries. Disruptions of the right atrium or right ventricle may be tolerated for a brief period allowing patients to survive transport

Table 3
American Association for the Surgery of Trauma cardiac injury scale

Grade	Description of Injury
I	Blunt injury with minor electrocardiographic abnormalities Blunt or penetrating pericardial wound without cardiac injury, tamponade, or herniation
II	Blunt cardiac injury with heart block or ischemic changes without heart failure Penetrating tangential myocardial wound up to, but not extending through, endocardium, without tamponade
III	Blunt cardiac injury with sustained (>5 beats/min) or multifocal ventricular contractions Blunt or penetrating injury with septal rupture, pulmonary or tricuspid valvular incompetence, papillary muscle dysfunction, or distal coronary arterial occlusion without cardiac failure Blunt pericardial laceration with cardiac herniation Blunt cardiac injury with cardiac failure Penetrating tangential myocardial wound up to, but not extending through, endocardium, with tamponade
IV	Blunt or penetrating injury with septal rupture, pulmonary or tricuspid valvular incompetence, papillary muscle dysfunction, or distal coronary arterial occlusion with cardiac failure Blunt or penetrating injury with aortic or mitral valve incompetence Blunt or penetration injury of the right ventricle, right atrium, or left atrium
V	Blunt or penetrating injury with proximal coronary artery occlusion Blunt or penetrating perforation of the left ventricle Stellate wound with <50% tissue loss of the right ventricle, right atrium, or left atrium
VI	Blunt avulsion of the heart Penetrating wound producing >50% tissue loss of a chamber

to the operating room. Traumatic cardiac tamponade always warrants immediate sternotomy. For limited cardiac ruptures, digital control and repair may often be accomplished without the use of cardiopulmonary bypass. For more complicated disruptions, cardiopulmonary bypass is necessary to facilitate hemodynamic stability and cardiac repair. Traumatic left-sided valvular lesions typically require immediate intervention, whereas tricuspid valvular injuries or small septal injuries can often be managed medically or in a delayed fashion.

Penetrating Cardiac Trauma

In 1897, Rehn[109] reported the first successful repair of a right ventricular stab wound using interrupted sutures. Ten years later, he reported on 124 penetrating cardiac injury patients with a 40% survival rate. Since that time period, the results of penetrating cardiac trauma have continued to improve. Among patients with stab wounds who reach the hospital, approximately 35% have an isolated right ventricular injury.[110] The left ventricle is involved in 25%, and in 30%, more than one chamber is involved.[111] Other injuries include coronary artery lacerations (most often the left anterior descending and diagonal branches), valve injury, and ventricular septal defects. Missile injuries often produce through-and-through injury resulting in hemorrhage, tamponade, and shock.

Although prehospital emergency care continues to improve, the most important factor determining survival is the character of the offending penetrating agent. Large penetrating low-velocity wounds and high-velocity missile injuries are frequently fatal. Patients with penetrating cardiac injuries who survive transport are often intoxicated or combative, and classic signs of cardiac tamponade (Beck triad of hypotension, distended neck veins, and muffled heart sounds) may be difficult to assess.

Management of an unstable patient with penetrating cardiac trauma begins with fluid resuscitation and immediate transfer to the operating room. Pericardial decompression may be required to achieve enough stability to allow transfer. A 3 to 4 cm skin incision can be made just to the left side of the xiphoid process facilitating passage of a blunt-tipped clamp into the pericardium for immediate decompression. Emergency department thoracotomy can occasionally salvage unstable penetrating cardiac trauma patients. However, emergency department thoracotomy has significant limitations with respect to injury exposure and surgeon experience. It may be reasonable to perform emergency department thoracotomy in patients who arrive with vital signs, but then arrest in the emergency department.

Identifying penetrating cardiac injuries in hemodynamically stable patients can be more difficult. A retrospective analysis from the Kings County Hospital in New York demonstrated excellent negative predictive value using a combination of transthoracic echocardiography and chest CT to screen stable patients with suspected injury.[112] If identified by noninvasive means, penetrating cardiac injury in a hemodynamically stable patient warrants sternotomy and exploration.

Once in the operating room, median sternotomy should be performed without delay. Simultaneous TEE is useful for assessing function and intracardiac pathology. Immediate digital control of bleeding injuries can facilitate resuscitation and hemodynamic stability. Most lacerations can be repaired with pledgeted polypropylene sutures. Occasionally, more complex wounds may require patch-grafting with autologous or bovine pericardium. Except for distal coronary artery injuries, most coronary artery injuries warrant bypass grafting. Coronary bypass grafting for trauma can usually be accomplished without the use of cardiopulmonary bypass, unless ventricular function is markedly compromised. In the rare instance where myocardial laceration is directly adjacent to, but not involving, a coronary artery, a horizontal mattress suture can be passed under the coronary to completely close the defect without incorporating the artery in the repair. After cardiac repair, a thorough exploration of the rest of the mediastinum should be performed, including visualization of the pleural spaces, posterior pericardium, and, specifically, the mammary arteries, which are often injured but are in spasm and may not be actively bleeding.

During the past 30 years, the reported outcomes after treatment of penetrating cardiac injuries have been variable.[112–116] Multiple factors account for this variability, including differing transport systems, extent and mechanism of injury, and the presence of other associated injuries. A report suggests that physiologic indexes in the field, on transport and on arrival, and the mechanism of injury in correlation with the AAST cardiac injury scale (see **Table 3**) were the strongest predictors of outcome.[117] Specifically, mechanism of injury revealed mortality of 84% for gunshot wounds compared with 35% for stab wounds. Grades IV, V, and VI injuries had a mortality of 56%, 76%, and 91%, respectively. Penetrating left atrial and ventricular injuries had a higher mortality rate between 77% and 80%, whereas RA and right ventricular injuries had mortality rates of 63% and 49%, respectively. Additional predictors of mortality were failure to restore a normal sinus rhythm and the requirement of aortic cross-clamping. In contradistinction to previous retrospective analyses, pericardial tamponade on presentation was not predictive of outcome.

SUMMARY

The diagnosis and management of thoracic aortic and cardiac trauma has continued to evolve with advancement in diagnostic and interventional technologies. The ability to manage blunt aortic injuries safely and effectively has been significantly improved with the use of antiimpulse therapy preoperatively, the use of left-heart bypass for open reconstructions, and the development of thoracic aortic stent grafts for endovascular repair. Operative timing is based on hemodynamic status and the presence of other immediately life-threatening injuries. Morbidity and mortality remain significant because these injuries are often seen in the face of severe associated injuries. Traumatic cardiac injuries remain highly lethal. Cardiac injuries that result in bleeding, tamponade, myocardial ischemia, or structural intracardiac injury require immediate surgical intervention. Collectively, it is imperative that a multidisciplinary team approach be used in managing these thoracic injuries in multitrauma patients to capitalize on the expertise of trauma surgeons, cardiovascular surgeons, and radiologists. The management should be streamlined and disease-driven rather than specialty- or technology-driven, and the operative strategies used should be tailored to each individual patient.

REFERENCES

1. Mattox K, Feliciano D, Beal A. Five thousand seven hundred and sixty cardiovascular injuries in 4459 patients: epidemiologic evolution 1958–1988. Ann Surg 1989;209:698–705.
2. Fitzharris M, Frankly M, Frampton R, et al. Thoracic aortic injury in motor vehicle crashes: the effect of impact direction, side of body struck, and seat belt use. J Trauma 2004;57:582–90.
3. Fabian T, Richardson J, Croce M, et al. Prospective study of blunt aortic injury: multicenter trial of the American Association for the Surgery of Trauma. J Trauma 1997;42(3):374–80.
4. McGwin G Jr, Reiff DA, Morgan SG, et al. Incidence and characteristics of motor vehicle collision-related blunt thoracic aortic injury according to age. J Trauma 2002;52:859–65.
5. Dischinger P, Cowley R, Shankar B. The incidence of ruptured aorta among vehicle fatalities. Proc Assoc Adv Automot Med Conf 1988;32:15.
6. Greendyke R. Traumatic rupture of aorta: special reference to automobile accidents. JAMA 1966;195(7):527–30.
7. Richens D, Kotidis K, Neale M, et al. Rupture of the aorta following road traffic accidents in the United Kingdom 1992–1999: the results of the cooperative crash injury study. Eur J Cardiothorac Surg 2003;23(2):143–8.
8. Brasel K, Quickel R, Yoganandan N, et al. Seat belts are more effective than airbags in reducing thoracic aortic injury in frontal motor vehicle crashes. J Trauma 2002;53:309 [discussion: 313].
9. Pillgram-Larsen J, Geiran O. Airbags influence the pattern of injury in severe thoracic trauma. Tidsskr Nor Laegeforen 1997;117:2437–9.
10. Dunn J, Williams M. Occult ascending aortic rupture in the presence of an air bag. Ann Thorac Surg 1996;62:577.
11. deGuzman B, Morgan A, Pharr W. Aortic transection following airbag deployment. N Engl J Med 1997;337:573–4.
12. Cook J, Salerno C, Krishnadasan B, et al. The effect of changing presentation and management on the outcome of blunt rupture of the thoracic aorta. J Thorac Cardiovasc Surg 2006;131:594–600.

13. Arajarvi E, Santavirta S. Chest injuries sustained in severe traffic accidents by seatbelt wearers. J Trauma 1989;29:37–41.
14. Demetriades D, Gomez H, Velmahos G, et al. Routine helical computed tomographic evaluation of the mediastinum in high-risk blunt trauma patients. Arch Surg 1998;133:1084.
15. Duhaylongsod F, Glower D, Wolfe W. Acute traumatic aortic aneurysm: The Duke experience from 1970 to 1990. J Vasc Surg 1992;15:331–42 [discussion: 342].
16. Pezzella A. Blunt traumatic injury of the thoracic aorta following commercial airline crashes. Tex Heart Inst J 1996;23:65–7.
17. Parmley L, Mattingly T, Manion W, et al. Nonpenetrating traumatic injury of the aorta. Circulation 1958;17:1086–101.
18. Reed A, Thompson J, Crafton C, et al. Timing of endovascular repair of blunt traumatic thoracic aortic transections. J Vasc Surg 2006;43:684–8.
19. Bennett D, Cherry J. The natural history of traumatic aneurysms of the aorta. J Trauma 1967;61:516–23.
20. Albuquerque F, Krasna M, McLaughlin J. Chronic, traumatic pseudoaneurysm of the ascending aorta. Ann Thorac Surg 1992;54:980–2.
21. McCollum C, Graham J, Noon G, et al. Chronic traumatic aneurysms of the thoracic aorta: an analysis of 50 patients. J Trauma 1979;19:248–52.
22. Prat A, Warembourg H Jr, Watel A, et al. Chronic traumatic aneurysms of the descending thoracic aorta (19 cases). J Cardiovasc Surg 1986;27:268–72.
23. Feczko J, Lynch L, Pless J, et al. An autopsy case review of 142 nonpenetrating (blunt) injuries of the aorta. J Trauma 1992;33:845–9.
24. Rabinsly I, Sidhu G, Wagner R. Mid-descending aortic traumatic aneurysms. Ann Thorac Surg 1990;50:155–60.
25. Brundage S, Harruff R, Jurkovich G, et al. The epidemiology of thoracic aortic injuries in pedestrians. J Trauma 1998;45:1010–4.
26. Lundevall J. Traumatic rupture of the aorta, with special reference to road accidents. Acta Pathol Microbiol Scand 1964;62:29–33.
27. Finkelmeier B, Mentzer R Jr, Kaiser D, et al. Chronic traumatic thoracic aneurysm. Influence of operative treatment on natural history: An analysis of reported cases, 1950–1980. J Thorac Cardiovasc Surg 1982;84:257–66.
28. John L, Hornick P, Edmondson S. Chronic traumatic aneurysm of the aorta: To resect or not. The role of exploration operation. J Cardiovasc Surg 1992;33:106–8.
29. Hirose H, Svensson L. Chronic posttraumatic aneurysm of descending aorta with fistulous communication into pulmonary artery. J Vasc Surg 2004;40(3):564–6.
30. Pantaleo P, Prothero T, Banning A, et al. Aorto-bronchial fistula resulting from an accidental fall one year earlier. Int J Cardiol 1999;68(2):239–40.
31. Fernandez-Gonzalez A, Montero J, Luna D, et al. Aortobronchial fistula secondary to chronic post-traumatic thoracic aneurysm. Tex Heart Inst J 1996; 23(2):174–7.
32. Baba M, Yashamita A, Sugimoto S, et al. [A case of a chronic post-traumatic thoracic aneurysm with compression of left main bronchus at the isthmus]. Koybu Geka 1998;51(10):860–3 [In Japanese].
33. Sevitt S. The mechanisms of traumatic rupture of the thoracic aorta. Br J Surg 1977;64:166–73.
34. Marsh C, Moore R. Deceleration trauma. Am J Surg 1957;93:623–31.
35. Stapp J. Human tolerance to deceleration. Am J Surg 1957;93:734–40.
36. Voigt G, Wilfort K. Mechanisms of injuries to unrestrained drivers in head-on collisions. Proceedings 30th Strapp Car Crash Conference. New York. Society of Automotive Engineers, 1969;295.

37. Mohan D, Melvin J. Failure properties of passive human aortic tissue. J Biomech 1982;15(11):887–902.
38. Zehnder M. Delayed post-traumatic rupture of the aorta in a young healthy individual after closed injury mechanical-etiologoical considerations. Angiology 1956;7:252–67.
39. Ray G, Liu Y, ND. Wall stress in curved aorta in blunt chest trauma. 28th Annual Conference on Engineering in Medicine and Biology. Alliance for Engineering in Medicine and Biology, New Orleans; September 20–24, 1975.
40. Symbas P. Fundamentals of clinical cardiology: great vessel injury. Am Heart J 1977;93:518–22.
41. Crass J, Cohen A, Motta A, et al. A proposed new mechanism of traumatic aortic rupture: the osseous pinch. Radiology 1990;176:645–9.
42. Cohen A, Crass J, Thomas H, et al. CT evidence for the "osseous pinch" mechanism of traumatic aortic injury. AJR Am J Roentgenol 1992;159:271–4.
43. Cohen A, Crass J. Traumatic aortic injuries: current concepts. Semin Ultrasound CT MR 1993;14:71–84.
44. Javadpour H, O'Toole J, McEniff J, et al. Traumatic aortic transection: evidence for the osseous pinch mechanism. Ann Thorac Surg 2002;73:951–3.
45. Richens D, Field M, Neale M, et al. The mechanism of injury in blunt traumatic rupture of the aorta. Eur J Cardiothorac Surg 2002;21:288–93.
46. Smith R, Chang F. Traumatic rupture of the aorta: still a lethal injury. Am J Surg 1986;152:660–3.
47. Clark D, Zeiger M, Wallace K, et al. Blunt aortic trauma: signs of high risk. J Trauma 1990;30:701–5.
48. Gundry S, Williams S, Burney R, et al. Indications for aortography in blunt thoracic trauma: a reassessment. J Trauma 1982;22:664–71.
49. Kram H, Appel P, Wohlmuth D, et al. Diagnosis of traumatic thoracic aortic rupture: a 10-year retrospective analysis. Ann Thorac Surg 1989;47:282–6.
50. Sturm J, Perry J Jr, Olson F, et al. Significance of symptoms and signs in patients with traumatic aortic rupture. Ann Emerg Med 1984;13:876–8.
51. Cook A, Klein J, Rogers F, et al. Chest radiographs of limited utility in the diagnosis of blunt traumatic aortic laceration. J Trauma 2001;50:843–7.
52. Mirvis S, Bidwll J, Buddenmeyer E, et al. Value of chest radiography in excluding traumatic aortic rupture. Radiology 1987;163:487–93.
53. Ho R, Blackmore C, Bloch R. Can we rely on mediastinal widening on chest radiography to identify subjects with aortic injury? Emerg Radiol 2002;9:183–7.
54. Sturm J, Hankins D, Young G. Thoracic aortography following blunt chest trauma. Am J Emerg Med 1990;8:92–6.
55. Kram H, Wohlmuth D, Appel P, et al. Clinical and radiographic indications for aortography in blunt chest trauma. J Vasc Surg 1987;6:168–76.
56. Richardson P, Mirvis S, Scorpio R, et al. Value of CT in determining the need for angiography when findings of mediastinal hemorrhage on chest radiographs are equivocal. Am J Roentgenol 1991;156:273–9.
57. Eddy A, Nance D, Goldman M, et al. Rapid diagnosis of thoracic transection using intravenous digital subtraction angiography. Am J Surg 1990;159:500–3.
58. Bruckner B, DiBardino D, Cumbie T, et al. Critical evaluation of chest computed tomography scans for blunt descending thoracic aortic injury. Ann Thorac Surg 2006;81:1339–46.
59. Dyer D, Moore E, Ilke D, et al. Thoracic aortic injury: how predictive is mechanism and is chest computed tomography a reliable screening tool? A prospective study of 1561 patients. J Trauma 2000;48:673–82.

60. Gavant M. Helical CT grading of traumatic aortic injuries, impact on clinical guidelines for medical and surgical management. Radiol Clin North Am 1999; 37:553–74.
61. Rivas L, Munera F, Fishman J. Multidetector-row computerized tomography of aortic injury. Semin Roentgenol 2006;41(3):226–36.
62. Fishman J, Nunez D, Kane A. Direct versus indirect signs of traumatic aortic injury revealed by helical CT: performance characteristics and interobserver agreement. Am J Roentgenol 1999;172(4):1027–31.
63. Smith M, Cassidy J, Souther S, et al. Transesophageal echocardiography in the diagnosis of traumatic rupture of the aorta. N Engl J Med 1995;332:356–62.
64. Vignon P, Boncoeur M, Francois B, et al. comparison of multiplane transesophageal echocardiography and contrast-enhanced helical CT in the diagnosis of blunt traumatic cardiovascular injuries. Anesthesiology 2001;94:615–22 [discussion: 615A].
65. Fattori R, Celletti F, Bertacinni P. Delayed surgery of traumatic aortic rupture: role of magnetic resonance imaging. Circulation 1996;94:2865–70.
66. Gavelli G, Canini R, Bertaccini P, et al. Traumatic injuries: imaging of thoracic injuries. Eur Radiol 2002;12:1273–94.
67. Kepros J, Angood P, Jaffe C, et al. Aortic intimal injuries from blunt trauma: resolution profile in nonoperative management. J Trauma 2002;52:475–8.
68. Mattox K, Wall M Jr. Historical review of blunt injury to the thoracic aorta. Chest Surg Clin N Am 2000;10:167–82.
69. Fabian T, Davis K, Gavant M, et al. Prospective study of blunt aortic injury: helical CT is diagnostic and antihypertensive therapy reduces rupture. Ann Surg 1998;227:666–76.
70. Pate J, Gavant M, Weiman D, et al. Traumatic rupture of the aortic isthmus: program of selective management. World J Surg 1999;23:59–63.
71. Nzewi O, Slight R, Zamvar V. Management of blunt thoracic aortic injury. Eur J Vasc Endovasc Surg 2006;31:18–27.
72. Camp P, Shackford S. The Western Trauma Association Multicenter Group. Outcome after blunt traumatic aortic laceration: identification of a high-risk cohort. J Trauma 1997;43:413–22.
73. Maggisano R, Nathens A, Alexandrova N, et al. Traumatic rupture of the thoracic aorta: should one always operate immediately? Ann Vasc Surg 1995;9:44–52.
74. Holmes J, Bloch R, Hall R, et al. Natural history of traumatic rupture of the thoracic aorta managed nonoperatively: a longitudinal analysis. Ann Thorac Surg 2002;73:1149–54.
75. Simon B, Leslie C. Factors predicting early hospital death in blunt thoracic aortic injury. J Trauma 2001;51:906–11.
76. von Oppell U, Dunne T, DeGroot M, et al. Traumatic aortic rupture: twenty-year meta analysis of mortality and risk of paraplegia. Ann Thorac Surg 1994;58: 585–93.
77. Razzouk A, Gundry S, Wang N, et al. Repair of traumatic aortic rupture: a 25-year experience. Arch Surg 2000;135:913–8 [discussion: 919].
78. Sweeney M, Young D, Frazier O, et al. Traumatic aortic transections: Eight-year experience with the "clamp-sew" technique. Ann Thorac Surg 1997;64:384–7 [discussion: 387].
79. Gillilan L. The arterial blood supply of the human spinal cord. J Comp Neurol 1958;110:75–103.
80. Adams H, Van Geertruyden H. Neurologic complications of aortic surgery. Ann Surg 1956;144:574–610.

81. Gott V. Heparinized shunts for thoracic vascular operation. Ann Thorac Surg 1972;14:219–20.
82. Molina J, Cogordan J, Einzig S, et al. Adequacy of ascending aortic descending aortic shunt during cross-clamping of the thoracic aorta from prevention of spinal cord injury. J Thorac Cardiovasc Surg 1985;90:126–36.
83. Szwerc M, Benckart D, Lin J, et al. Recent clinical experience with left heart bypass using a centrifugal pump for repair of traumatic aortic transection. Ann Surg 1999;230:484–90 [discussion: 490].
84. Hess P, Howe H Jr, Robicsek F, et al. Traumatic tears of the thoracic aorta: improved results using the Bio-Medicus pump. Ann Thorac Surg 1989;48:6–9.
85. Santaniello J, Miller P, Croce M, et al. Blunt aortic injury with concomitant intra-abdominal solid organ injury: treatment priorities revisited. J Trauma 2002;53:442–5 [discussion: 445].
86. von Oppell U, Dunne T, De Groot M, et al. Spinal cord protection in the absence of collateral circulation: meta-analysis of mortality and paraplegia. J Cardiovasc Surg 1994;9:685–91.
87. Laschinger J, Cunningham J Jr, Catinella F, et al. Detection and prevention of intraoperative spinal cord ischemia after cross-clamping of the thoracic aorta: use of somatosensory evoked potentials. Surgery 1982;92:1109–17.
88. Kouchoukos N, Masetti P, Rokkas C, et al. Safety and efficacy of hypothermic cardiopulmonary bypass and circulatory arrest for operations on the descending thoracic and thoracoabdominal aorta. Ann Thorac Surg 2001;72:699 [discussion: 707].
89. Laschinger J, Cunningham J Jr, Cooper M, et al. Prevention of ischemic spinal cord injury following aortic cross-clamping: Use of corticosteroids. Ann Thorac Surg 1984;38:500.
90. Karmy-Jones R, Hoffer E, Meissner M, et al. Endovascular stent grafts and aortic rupture: a case series. J Trauma 2003;55:805–10.
91. Peterson B, Matsumura J, Morasch M, et al. Percutaneous endovascular repair of blunt thoracic aortic transection. J Trauma 2005;59:1062–5.
92. Rousseau H, Dambrin C, Marcheix B, et al. Acute traumatic aortic rupture: a comparison of surgical and stent graft repair. J Thorac Cardiovasc Surg 2005;129:1050–5.
93. Morishita K, Kurimoto Y, Kawaharada N, et al. Descending thoracic aortic rupture: role of endovascular stent grafting. Ann Thorac Surg 2004;78:1630–4.
94. Tehrani H, Peterson B, Katariya K, et al. Endovascular repair of thoracic aortic tears. Ann Thorac Surg 2006;82:873–7 [discussion: 887–8].
95. Peterson B, Eskandari M, Gleason T, et al. Utility of left subclavian artery revascularization in association with endoluminal repair of acute and chronic thoracic aortic pathology. J Vasc Surg 2006;43:433–9.
96. Riesenman P, Farber M, Mendes R, et al. Coverage of the left subclavian artery during thoracic endovascular aortic repair. J Vasc Surg 2007;45:90–4 [discussion: 94–5].
97. Idu M, Reekers J, Balm R, et al. Collapse of a stent-graft following treatment of a traumatic thoracic aortic rupture. J Endovasc Ther 2005;12:503–7.
98. Malina M, Brunkwall J, Ivancev K, et al. Late aortic arch perforation by graft-anchoring stent: complication of endovascular thoracic aneurysm exclusion. J Endovasc Surg 1998;5:274–7.
99. Dunham M, Zygun D, Petrasek P, et al. Endovascular stent grafts for acute blunt aortic injury. J Trauma 2004;56:1173–8.

100. Pacini D, Angeli E, Fattori R, et al. Traumatic rupture of the thoracic aorta: ten years of delayed management. J Thorac Cardiovasc Surg 2005;129:880–4.
101. Andrassy J, Weidenhagen R, Meimarakis G, et al. Stent versus open surgery for acute and chronic traumatic injury of the thoracic aorta: a single-center experience. J Trauma 2006;60:765–71.
102. Ott M, Stewart T, Lawlor D, et al. Management of blunt thoracic aortic injuries: endovascular stents versus open repair. J Trauma 2004;56:565–70.
103. Lachat M, Pfammatter T, Witzke H, et al. Acute traumatic aortic rupture: early stent-graft repair. Eur J Cardiothorac Surg 2002;21:959–63.
104. Ehrlich M, Rouseau H, Heijmen R, et al. Endovascular treatment of acute traumatic aortic injuries: the Talent Thoracic Retrospective Registry (TTR) [abstract 83]. In: Programs and abstracts of the 45th Annual Society of Thoracic Surgeons Meeting, San Francisco; January 26, 2009. p. 248.
105. Katsumata T, Shinfield A, Westaby S, et al. Operation for chronic traumatic aortic aneurysm: when and how? Ann Thorac Surg 1998;66(3):774–8.
106. Demetriades D. Penetrating injuries to the thoracic great vessels. J Cardiovasc Surg 1997;12:173 [discussion: 179].
107. Maron B, Gohman T, Kyle S, et al. Clinical profile and spectrum of commotio cordis. JAMA 2002;287(9):1142–6.
108. Velmahos G, Karaiskakis M, Salim A, et al. Normal electrocardiography and serum troponin I levels preclude the presence of clinically significant blunt cardiac injury. J Trauma 2003;54:45–50.
109. Rehn L. [Zur chirurgie des herzens und des herzbeutels]. Arch Klin Chir 1907; 83:723.
110. Demetriades D. Cardiac penetrating injuries: personal experience of 45 cases. Br J Surg 1984;71:95–7.
111. Symbas P, Harlaftis N, Waldo W. Penetrating cardiac wounds: a comparison of different therapeutic methods. Ann Surg 1976;83:377–81.
112. Burack J, Kandil E, Sawas A, et al. Triage and outcome of patients with mediastinal penetrating trauma. Ann Thorac Surg 2007;83:377–82.
113. Attar S, Suter C, Hankins J, et al. Penetrating cardiac injuries. Ann Thorac Surg 1991;51:711–5 [discussion: 715–6].
114. Beall A Jr, Patrick T, Okies J, et al. Penetrating wounds of the heart: changing patterns of surgical management. J Trauma 1972;12:468–73.
115. Feliciano D, Bitondo C, Mattox K, et al. Civilian trauma in the 1980s. A 1-year experience with 456 vascular and cardiac injuries. Ann Surg 1984;199:717–24.
116. Sugg W, Rea W, Ecker R, et al. Penetrating wounds of the heart. An analysis of 459 cases. J Thorac Cardiovasc Surg 1968;56:531–45.
117. Asensio J, Petrone P, Karsidag T, et al. Penetrating cardiac injuries. Complex injuries and difficult challenges. Ulus Travma Acil Cerrahi Derg 2003;9:1–16.

Surgical Treatment of Great Vessel Occlusive Disease

Margaret C. Tracci, MD, JD, Kenneth J. Cherry, MD*

KEYWORDS

- Innominate • Brachiocephalic • Subclavian
- Common carotid • Great vessel

Since the early descriptions of symptomatic occlusive disease of the supra-aortic trunks (SATs) by Savory[1] and Broadbent,[2] such lesions have remained a challenge to the clinician in terms of diagnosis and treatment. Takayasu,[3] in 1908, reported the case of a young woman whose ocular findings were observed by his contemporary, Onishi,[4] to be associated with absent radial pulses. Spanish cardiologist Martorell went on, with Fabre, to describe the syndrome of progressive obliteration of the SAT that has subsequently become known as Martorell syndrome, "pulseless disease," or, most commonly, Takayasu arteritis.[5] Subsequently, proximal subclavian disease associated with retrograde vertebral flow was described by Contorni[6] and was later associated with the symptom complex now known as "subclavian steal syndrome," described by Reivich and colleagues[7] and Fisher.[8]

As the surgical treatment of occlusive disease of the SAT has progressed, it has become evident, as discussed later, that the cause of this condition may be arteritic, as in these early descriptions, or atherosclerotic, as is predominant in the United States.[9] Modern surgical therapy of these conditions blossomed in the 1950s and 1960s, marked by the early publications of Bahnson,[10] who described the first great vessel reconstruction using homograft, Davis and colleagues,[11] who described innominate artery endarterectomy by right anterior thoracotomy, and DeBakey and colleagues[12] and Ehrenfeld and colleagues,[13] who described the use of endarterectomy or aortic-origin grafts. The subsequent decade saw remarkable progress in the surgical reconstruction of the SAT, as Parrot[14] described subclavian artery transposition and Diethrich and colleagues[15] described carotid-subclavian bypass, and several groups began to amass enviable series of transthoracic and extrathoracic reconstructions.[16,17] Multiple investigators have added, on the foundation laid by Dotter and Judkins[18] in 1964, to a growing body of literature supporting the use of

Department of Surgery, Division of Vascular Surgery, University of Virginia, PO Box 800709, Charlottesville, VA 22908-0709, USA
* Corresponding author.
E-mail address: kjc5kh@virginia.edu (K.J. Cherry).

Surg Clin N Am 89 (2009) 821–836
doi:10.1016/j.suc.2009.06.002
0039-6109/09/$ – see front matter © 2009 Published by Elsevier Inc.

endovascular techniques in the primary or adjunctive treatment of occlusive SAT disease.

ANATOMY AND ETIOLOGY

The SATs comprise the innominate artery, subclavian arteries, and common carotid arteries. In the standard configuration, the innominate artery, which in turn gives rise to the right subclavian and right common carotid arteries, arises most proximally on the aortic arch, followed by the left common carotid and left subclavian arteries. Anatomic variations are, however, relatively common. Less frequently, embryologic variations, usually associated with a right-sided aortic arch, may be encountered. Occlusive disease of the SATs is predominantly of atherosclerotic etiology, although it is seen far less commonly than atherosclerotic carotid bifurcation disease. Theories and observations regarding the pathophysiology of atherogenesis abound in the literature and are beyond the scope of this article. Typically, these lesions are believed to evolve from fatty streaks containing intracellular lipid deposits in macrophages and smooth muscle cells to atheromas composed of a fibrous plaque of smooth muscle and connective tissue overlying an inner cholesterol-rich core, frequently accompanied by periarterial inflammatory changes.

The localization of atherosclerotic disease is believed to be intimately related to local hemodynamics, with factors such as shear stress, flow separation and stasis, oscillation of flow, turbulence, and hypertension affecting the distribution of plaques.[19] This process may involve more than one of the supra-aortic arteries, with an incidence of multivessel involvement ranging in the literature from 24% in the series reported by Crawford and colleagues[17] to 84% in other contemporary series (**Table 1**). The carotid bifurcation is particularly susceptible to plaque formation, hence the natural history and treatment of bifurcation disease are well described and familiar to the surgeon. Among the supra-aortic vessels, the frequency with which lesions are encountered is the reason that, at present, far less is known about stenosis of the common carotid artery than stenosis of the subclavian, or even innominate arteries.

Takayasu arteritis is a female-predominant large vessel vasculitis that is the second leading cause of great vessel occlusive disease requiring surgical treatment in the

Table 1
Distribution of atherosclerotic lesions

Authors (Year)	No. of Patients	Total Number of Lesions					Multiple (%)
		IA	LC	RC	LS	RS	
Crawford et al (1969)	299	66 (26)*	61 (37)*	24 (19)*	202 (133)*	59 (29)*	24
Kieffer et al (1995)	148	148	47	27	60	52	84
Azakie et al (1998)[a]	94	94	26	29	20	30	68
Berguer et al (1999)	173	—	—	—	—	—	27
Takach et al (I) (2005)[b]	157	150	38	48	26	48	—
Takach et al (II) (2005)[c]	391	—	17 (left + right)		374 (left + right)		—

Abbreviations: IA, Innominate artery; LC, Left common carotid artery; LS, Left subclavian artery; RC, Right common carotid artery; RS, Right subclavian artery.
   [a] Series of patients being treated for innominate artery disease.
   [b] Patients with innominate artery of multivessel disease.
   [c] Patients with single vessel disease. Authors did not distinguish between left- and right-sided lesions.
   * Numbers in parentheses represent complete occlusions.

United States. Its initial, inflammatory phase is frequently characterized by diffuse systemic symptoms, such as fever, arthralgias, weight loss, and fatigue. Hemodynamically significant stenoses of central arteries are present in the later stages of disease. Typical presenting signs and symptoms referable to progressive vascular disease may include effort-induced cramping of the upper extremity, dizziness, headache, focal tenderness over the affected artery, stroke, renovascular hypertension, visual impairment, angina, myocardial infarction, or pulmonary hypertension.[20] The American College of Rheumatology has established six classification criteria, of which patients should fulfill at least three: (1) age at disease onset of 40 years or less; (2) claudication of the extremities; (3) decreased brachial artery pressure; (4) a blood pressure difference of more than 10 mm Hg; (5) a bruit over the subclavian arteries or the aorta; (6) an arteriogram showing occlusion or narrowing of large arteries that is not the result of arteriosclerosis, fibromuscular dysplasia, or a similar cause.[21]

Although serum markers of inflammation, such as erythrocyte sedimentation rate and C-reactive protein, are typically elevated in active arteritis, these tests are not specific to the disease, and the diagnosis is driven by history, clinical examination, and typical imaging findings. Pathologically, the lesion is characteristically a mixture of active inflammation, originating in the vasa vasorum and demonstrating T cell infiltration of the outer media and adventitia, and intimal and adventitial fibrosis. With time, changes typical of atherosclerosis may arise and may be accompanied by aneurysmal degeneration.[22]

Angiography, magnetic resonance imaging (MRI)/magnetic resonance angiography (MRA), computed tomography (CT)/computed tomography angiography (CTA), and ultrasonography have all been studied in the context of Takayasu arteritis. As discussed later, these modalities differ in their ability to demonstrate such characteristics as pressure and pressure gradients, inflammation, arterial wall anatomy, calcification, and distal vessels. They are typically smooth, long-segment proximal stenoses of the arch and descending portions of the aorta and of its primary branches. Of the great vessels, angiographic studies have demonstrated that the subclavian artery is most commonly affected (93%, 42% bilateral), followed by the common carotid (58%, 28% bilateral), the vertebral (35%, 5% bilateral), and the innominate arteries (27%). However, there appear to be ethnic differences in disease distribution among East Asian, South Asian, and Caucasian populations.[20,23] Investigators have used [^{18}F]fluorodeoxyglucose positron emission tomography to demonstrate evidence of central vascular inflammation in patients in whom Takayasu arteritis was suspected.[24,25]

Less frequently, large vessel arteritis resulting in hemodynamically significant or symptomatic occlusive disease may be attributable to radiotherapy of the chest wall, head and neck, or mediastinum. In the multicenter series reported by Hassen-Khodja and Kieffer,[26] head and neck malignancies (50%) were the most commonly encountered indication for radiotherapy, followed by breast cancer (30%) and lymphoma (19%). The distribution of radiation-induced arterial lesions is clearly related to therapy. Pathologic changes associated with radiotherapy-induced arteritis include subintimal fibrosis, degeneration of the endothelial and elastic layers and, particularly in large muscular arteries, myointimal proliferation.[27]

In the previously cited series,[26] the mean interval between therapy and revascularization was 15.2 years, with most patients presenting with symptomatic disease (80%). Clinically, symptomatic patients presented with embolic (transient ischemic attack [TIA], stroke, amaurosis fugax) and global ischemic (claudication, vertebrobasilar insufficiency) patterns. Surgical treatment of radiation-induced arterial disease may be complicated by postsurgical or radiation-related tissue changes and disrupted lymphatic drainage, not only of the artery in question but also of the adjacent structures, such as the neck musculature and esophagus.

DIAGNOSIS

Great vessel occlusive disease, regardless of the cause, may present with either thromboembolic events to the brain, eye, or upper extremity, or symptoms referable to low-flow states, such as claudication, global ischemic symptoms, or vertebrobasilar insufficiency. However, the incidence of each presentation does vary based on the cause of the disease and on the location and extent of occlusive lesions. In general, the irregular lesions and intimal disruption of atherosclerotic disease more frequently give rise to thromboembolic events, whereas the smooth, tapering lesions of Takayasu disease more typically present with low-flow symptoms. In the University Association for Research in Vascular Surgery[26] series of patients who underwent arterial SAT revascularization for radiation arteritis, 13 of 64 patients (20%) were asymptomatic but demonstrated high-grade carotid stenosis. Most patients (51, 80%) were symptomatic, presenting with TIA (26), minor stroke (37), amaurosis fugax (18), upper extremity ischemia (15), or vertebrobasilar insufficiency (10).

In the 10-year Mayo Clinic series[28] of patients treated with direct transsternal aortic-origin reconstruction for great vessel occlusive disease, 63% of patients with an atherosclerotic cause presented with embolic events, predominantly cerebrovascular (53% vs 10% pure upper extremity and 5% mixed). A second large, contemporary series[29] of patients treated surgically for occlusive disease of the SATs was primarily composed of patients with atherosclerotic disease (85%) and demonstrated a similar distribution of clinical presentations. In this population, 44% presented with cerebrovascular embolic events and 9% with upper extremity emboli.

In addition to eliciting patient history, clinicians must be attentive to physical examination, which, in contrast to disease of the carotid bifurcation, may be revealing in patients suffering from occlusive disease of the SAT. Examination of the hands may demonstrate lesions typical of upper extremity thromboemboli, and palpable pulse differentials may lead to the quantification of differences in upper extremity blood pressure. In addition, significant SAT lesions frequently produce audible bruits above the clavicle.

Arch aortography has been considered the gold standard study for arterial lesions and is well studied in the context of each of the disease entities discussed here. This technique permits imaging of the vessel lumen with high resolution that is maintained through the small vessels of the distal circulation. In addition, angiography permits measurement of central aortic pressure and gradients across stenoses. Perhaps most importantly, it permits interventions such as percutaneous angioplasty or stent placement at the time of the initial study. The use of angiography is limited by its invasiveness and associated rate of vascular complications at and remote from the access site, by complications associated with the administration of iodinated contrast agent, and by radiation exposure. Arterial access is associated with the risk for hematoma, pseudoaneurysm, retroperitoneal hemorrhage, dissection, or distal embolization. In the cerebral and upper extremity circulation, despite the advent and broader use of distal protection devices, distal embolization carries significant clinical consequences.[30] In addition, catheter angiography is unable to provide detailed information on arterial wall anatomy, including the presence of ulceration or wall thickness and surrounding inflammation, afforded by the other imaging techniques.

Ultrasonography is favored in many settings as it is noninvasive, widely available, radiation-free, and relatively inexpensive. It provides high-resolution imaging of vessel wall, flow characteristics, and occlusive lesions of the carotid, axillary, vertebral, and subclavian arteries. Because of these advantages, many centers consider duplex ultrasonography to be an appropriate first-line study. However, because of limitations of the technique, imaging may be compromised in more proximal or central locations, where it is affected by overlying bony structures, and by the patient's body habitus. In addition, the precision of measurements of degree of stenosis may be compromised because ultrasonography yields estimates based on flow velocities rather than direct measurements of luminal diameter within the area of stenosis.

CTA is able not only to visualize the vessel lumen with increasing accuracy, but also to characterize the arterial wall with regard to thickness, calcification, and surrounding inflammation. This additional information may prove invaluable by yielding, in the case of atherosclerotic disease, information crucial to selecting clamp sites and other matters of operative planning or, in Takayasu arteritis, evidence of inflammation important in formulating the patient's prognosis for restenosis at the operative site or of progression of disease in remote locations.[31] The performance of this modality has been examined most closely in the context of carotid imaging. Two meta-analyses reported a pooled sensitivity of 85% to 95% and specificity of 93% to 98% for detecting a greater than 70% carotid stenosis.[32,33] These investigators primarily examined studies using single-slice CT scanners, suggesting that current results obtained with state-of-the-art multidetector CT scanners and improved software for reconstructions may be superior. The newer scanners are thought to address the traditional limitation on the ability of CTA to accurately assess residual lumen in the setting of heavy calcification.[34] Additional drawbacks of CTA are the need for iodinated contrast, with its attendant risks of renal dysfunction and allergic reactions, and substantial radiation doses.

MRA has also found wide acceptance in the imaging evaluation of arterial occlusive disease. A 2003 meta-analysis[35] of 21 studies using MRA or contrast-enhanced (CE-) or gadolinium-enhanced (GE-) MRA yielded a pooled sensitivity of 95% and a pooled specificity of 90% for the diagnosis of a 70% to 99% carotid stenosis. For the diagnosis of occlusion, the sensitivity and specificity were 98% and 100%, respectively. This review did not demonstrate a clear difference in performance between CE-MRA and non-CE-MRA (two-dimensional and three-dimensional time-of-flight [TOF]). CE-MRA may be more accurate in some aspects than TOF-MRA, which relies on flow-related enhancement rather than direct vessel filling, particularly with regard to minimizing motion artifact and signal loss in tortuous arteries and visualizing ulcers and other subtleties.[34] In their comparison of CE-MRA with digital subtraction angiography for the detection of ostial stenosis of the proximal great vessels, Randoux and colleagues[36] found MRA to be quite sensitive and specific (100% and 98%, respectively) in the nonvertebral craniocervical vessels for the detection of stenosis greater than 50%. However, in the vertebral artery, the specificity dropped to 85%, correlating with the findings of others that MR angiography may tend to overestimate the degree of stenosis.

In addition, similar to CT, MR provides imaging of the vessel wall to permit assessment of inflammation in vasculitides and, potentially, plaque vulnerability in atherosclerotic disease. It must be noted that recent findings regarding gadolinium-associated nephrogenic systemic fibrosis appear to negate the previously perceived advantage, in patients with renal insufficiency, of substituting GE-MRI for the iodinated contrast agents used in CT and conventional angiography.[37]

INDICATIONS FOR RECONSTRUCTION

Most reconstructions continue to be performed for symptomatic disease with typical occlusive or embolic presentation or for global ischemic syndromes. However, several circumstances may warrant treatment of asymptomatic disease, although these indications remain more controversial. Asymptomatic common carotid or innominate disease may be treated on the basis of the degree of stenosis, as determined either by direct imaging or angiographic pressure gradients, based on criteria adopted from the better-studied clinical course of carotid bifurcation disease.[38]

In addition, subclavian or innominate reconstruction may be indicated for the treatment of coronary-subclavian steal in the setting of patent mammary grafts or in anticipation of coronary revascularization.[39,40] If sternotomy is to be performed, it is certainly preferable to perform great vessel reconstruction at this time rather than later through a reoperative field. Similarly, asymptomatic carotid stenoses of more than 80% may be addressed at the time of planned SAT reconstruction. In addition, SAT lesions may also be addressed by either surgical or endovascular means to either facilitate the establishment of hemodialysis access using distal vessels or to treat occlusive disease that compromises the efficacy of existing access. Other indications include anticipation or salvage of axillary-origin grafts and facilitation of brachial blood pressure monitoring (**Box 1**).[41,42]

The etiology of disease and planned mode of intervention should be thoroughly considered in planning the evaluation of a patient presenting with occlusive disease of the SAT. Patients presenting with atherosclerotic lesions must be thoroughly evaluated for coexisting coronary disease. Those with Takayasu arteritis should undergo echocardiography for the detection of valvular heart disease resulting from hypertension or involvement of aortic valve leaflets, pulmonary hypertension, or left ventricular hypertrophy, and a thorough evaluation for coronary artery disease. In addition, conduction system abnormalities, including complete heart block, have been reported arising from scarring and lymphocytic infiltration.[43] Statistically significant predictors of left ventricular dysfunction (ejection fraction <50%) in these patients include arch involvement and the number of involved segments, with nonstatistically significant trends toward increased dysfunction in patients presenting with aortic insufficiency and hypertension.[44] Finally, the diagnosis of SAT occlusive disease attributed to radiation arteritis should trigger an evaluation for associated cardiomyopathy or coronary artery disease.

RECONSTRUCTION: TECHNIQUES AND OUTCOMES
Direct Transsternal Reconstruction

In appropriately selected patients, innominate endarterectomy is an important part of the surgeon's armamentarium. A thorough preoperative assessment is necessary to ensure that the aorta is not significantly calcified at the innominate origin, to ensure that there is sufficient distance between the innominate and the left common carotid origin (approximately 1.5 cm) to permit clamp placement, and to identify any relevant anatomic anomalies, such as a common brachiocephalic trunk, which would mandate graft reconstruction.[45] Where these criteria are met, the innominate origin may be excluded using a partially occluding aortic clamp, with subsequent longitudinal arteriotomy of the innominate and distal-to-proximal endarterectomy ending at this clamp.[13,45] In the University of California, San Francisco series,[16] endarterectomy performed in this manner yielded patency rates superior to those achieved with synthetic bypass graft. Most of these patients also underwent additional concurrent distal endarterectomy or, in a small number of cases, bypass grafting. The most common complication was compromise of the adventitia during endarterectomy, necessitating conversion to either an interposition or bypass graft in 4 of 72 patients. This technique, as Kieffer and colleagues[46] note, may be of particular use when coronary grafting is anticipated, to preserve the ascending aorta for coronary inflow. The Texas Heart Institute group's finding that 24% of patients treated for innominate or multivessel

---

Box 1
Indications for reconstruction

Symptomatic disease

Occlusive

    Upper extremity effort-related ischemia

    Wounds/tissue loss

    Vertebrobasilar insufficiency: ataxia, diplopia, vertigo, syncope, dizziness, nausea/vomiting

    Global ischemia

Embolic

    Distal embolization

        Amaurosis fugax, TIA/cerebral vascular accident (CVA): carotid, innominate (rare)

        Hand/digital embolization: subclavian, innominate

Asymptomatic disease

"Critical" stenosis

Special circumstances

Coronary artery disease

    Postoperative angina (patent internal mammary artery [IMA] graft)

    Preoperative

Hemodialysis access

    Subclavian and innominate stenoses

        Established access

        Anticipated access

Axillary-origin graft

    Salvage

    Anticipation

Blood pressure monitoring

SAT occlusive disease had concurrent, symptomatic coronary artery disease[47] under-scores the prevalence of the combination and the ongoing role of innominate endar-terectomy in the therapy of this patient population.

When the selection criteria for innominate endarterectomy are not met, or in the setting of multiple vessel disease, aortic-origin bypass reconstruction may be accomplished using either a simple prosthetic bypass graft to the innominate or a bifurcated graft. Exposure may be gained through median sternotomy or, as has been described, through a minimally invasive ministernotomy to the level of the third intercostal space with transaction of the sternum.[48] The sternotomy incision can be extended onto the right neck if appropriate, or separate cervical incisions may be made to expose more distal carotid targets (**Fig. 1**).

Care must be taken to avoid kinking of the grafts upon closure of the sternotomy, which may be facilitated by locating the proximal anastomosis laterally on the ascending aorta, mobilizing or even dividing the left brachiocephalic vein, or resection of the diseased innominate. The authors prefer a single limb 8- or 10-mm graft with

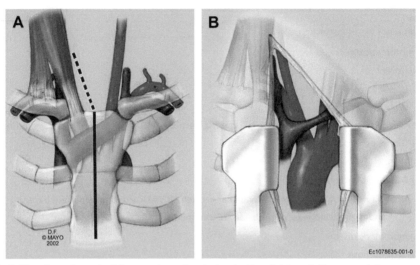

Fig. 1. The sternotomy incision can be extended onto the right neck if appropriate, or separate cervical incisions may be made to expose more distal carotid targets. (*From* Mayo Foundation for Medical Education and Research, copyrighted and all rights reserved; with permission.)

additional side arms placed as indicated (**Fig. 2**). However, if a bifurcated graft is used, the proximal trunk should be left relatively long to avoid high flow lesions in the proximal limbs (**Fig. 3**).[45]

Continuous electroencephalographic monitoring or cerebral oximetry may assist in assessing the need for shunt placement in situations in which this decision has not previously been dictated by preoperative assessment of the occlusive lesions. With regard to staging elements of the reconstruction, the Mayo Clinic group advocated that arteries with complete proximal occlusions be generally addressed first, and they found in their series that reconstruction of the left subclavian may be deferred without negative consequences (**Fig. 4**).[28] Much has been made of the morbidity and mortality associated with transsternal repair. However, the role of experience in achieving acceptable mortality rates is clearly noted in the series most frequently cited in this regard. Crawford and colleagues[17] noted that experience and improved technique reduced the operative mortality rate for transthoracic repair from 22.2% during the 1957 to 1960 period to 5.6% from 1960 to 1967, a rate well in keeping with other large modern series.[16,28,46,47,49,50] When considering options in the treatment of innominate artery occlusive disease, it is also worth noting that in four major series,[28,46,49,51] the average age of patients treated surgically for innominate disease ranged from 54 to 61 years, rendering transsternal reconstruction attractive because of the overall youth of these patients and the effectiveness and durability of the repair.

Extrathoracic Reconstruction

Short-segment single vessel disease is amenable to reconstruction either by transposition or short-segment bypass cervical reconstruction. Berguer and colleagues[29] advocate for the preferential use of transpositions, where possible, and their series does demonstrate excellent long-term patency. Arterial transpositions may be performed through a transverse supraclavicular incision. There are several excellent technical descriptions of this procedure available in the literature;[52] key elements of this

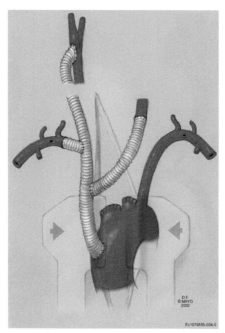

Fig. 2. Single limb 8- or 10-mm graft with additional side arms placed as indicated. (Copyrighted and used with permission of Mayo Foundation for Medical Education and Research. All rights reserved.)

procedure include careful identification, ligation, and division of cervical lymphatics including, on the left side, the thoracic duct. Particular care must be taken in identifying and controlling the origins of the vertebral and internal mammary arteries, and in configuring the anastomosis to avoid excessive tortuosity of the proximal vertebral artery, which arises in a somewhat awkward posteromedial orientation. In addition, transposition is precluded in the event of a proximal origin of the vertebral artery, atheromatous involvement distal to the origin of the vertebral artery, or a patent mammary artery graft.[53] Complications, as with cervical bypass, include stroke or TIA, lymphatic leak, Horner syndrome, postoperative hemorrhage, laryngeal or phrenic nerve palsy, brachial plexus injury, and entry of the pleural space with resultant pneumo-, hemo-, or chylothorax.

In patients presenting a prohibitive risk for transsternal repair, reconstruction may be through remote bypasses, including axillo-axillary, carotid-carotid, contralateral carotid-subclavian, and femoral-axillary bypasses. The axillary approach in these reconstructions uses a subclavicular incision at the level of the deltopectoral groove. The pectoralis major can then be retracted and the pectoralis minor either sectioned or retracted to facilitate exposure of the axillary artery. A subcutaneous tunnel is then used to access either the contralateral axillary artery or a femoral graft origin. The graft itself may be an externally supported expanded polytetrafluoroethylene membrane, Dacron, or autogenous vein.[54] Carotid-carotid bypasses may be tunneled either subcutaneously in a pretracheal position or in a retropharyngeal position, as advocated by Berguer and Kieffer.[55] Pretracheal carotid-carotid bypasses and extrathoracic bypasses that cross the anterior chest may interfere significantly with subsequent procedures such as sternotomy and tracheostomy. However, dysphagia associated with retropharyngeal carotid-carotid bypass has also been observed.

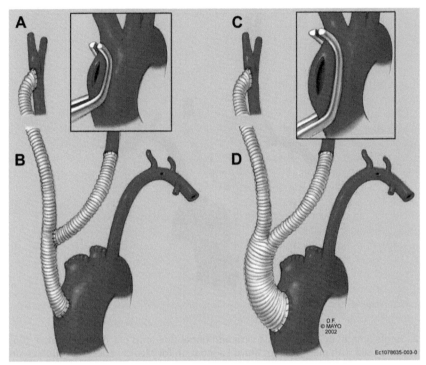

Fig. 3. If a bifurcated graft is used, the proximal trunk should be left relatively long to avoid high flow lesions in the proximal limbs. (Copyrighted and used with permission of Mayo Foundation for Medical Education and Research. All rights reserved.)

Endovascular Treatment

Although the transluminal treatment of SAT lesions was described by Dotter and Judkins[18] in 1964, and isolated reports accumulated throughout the literature of the 1980s, the broad adoption of endovascular techniques in the treatment of SAT disease has occurred during the past two decades.[42,56–58] Early therapy (pre-1990) relied on angioplasty alone, which yielded relatively high rates of complications and restenosis.[58] Whereas newer wires, smaller sheaths and balloon catheters, distal protection devices, and experience have improved the complication rate, restenosis and long-term patency has remained a significant limitation of endovascular interventions.[53,58] In addition, this approach proved suitable only for focal stenoses, with inferior results in patients with more advanced disease presenting with long stenoses or occlusions.[56] However, endovascular treatment of restenosis can provide good results after either primary endovascular[41] or surgical therapy.[59]

The advent of self-expanding nitinol and balloon-expandable stainless steel stents has improved technical success and patency rates.[42] This improvement in results has tipped the balance at most institutions in favor of primary stenting of most lesions addressed with endovascular therapy and has driven the broader use of endovascular treatment. The location and characteristics of a lesion should dictate the choice of stent. Self-expanding nitinol stents are appropriate where precision of deployment is not critical and where surrounding structures may expose the deployed stent to external compressive forces. Balloon-expandable stents are preferable where

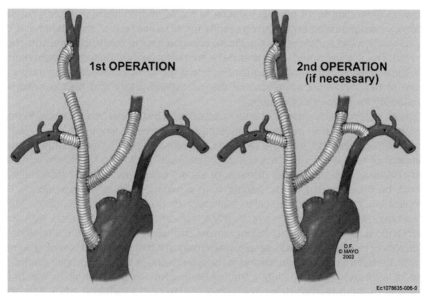

Fig. 4. With regard to staging elements of the reconstruction, the Mayo Clinic group advocated that arteries with complete proximal occlusions be generally addressed first, and found in their series that reconstruction of the left subclavian may be deferred without negative consequences. (Copyrighted and used with permission of Mayo Foundation for Medical Education and Research. All rights reserved.)

deployment must be exact, in locations such as the very proximal or ostial segments of the SAT.[58,60]

As the bulk of the literature regarding the endovascular treatment of SAT disease pertains primarily to atherosclerotic disease, patients who present with symptomatic occlusive disease due to arteritis remain exceptionally challenging. In the setting of symptomatic Takayasu arteritis, percutaneous treatment of occlusive great vessel lesions has demonstrated encouraging early and midterm results in a number of case reports, although the transmural nature of this disease may mitigate its use. Tyagi and colleagues,[61] compared early and long-term outcomes of subclavian artery angioplasty (PTA) alone in patients with Takayasu arteritis and atherosclerotic occlusive disease, and found good technical success rates in both groups (88.2 vs 100%) but a statistically significantly higher rate of restenosis in Takayasu patients and a trend toward higher restenosis rates at both treated and remote sites in this group. Reports suggest that stent placement may improve restenosis rates, even in patients with active disease.[62]

Similarly, Hassen-Khodja and Kieffer,[26] evaluating surgical and endovascular therapies for radiotherapy-induced disease found that the cause of disease does, indeed, affect therapy. Their multicenter, 10-year study of 64 patients with radiation arteritis demonstrated acceptable life-table primary and secondary patency rates of 79% and 88%, respectively, at the 48 to 60 month interval. Important caveats included reminders of the difficulty of dissection in an irradiated field and the subsequent greater risk of postoperative infection or lymphatic leak. In addition, though vein grafts were found to have a lower complication rate, the authors noted that saphenous vein, even when available, may not provide adequate resistance to compression in the setting of dense, sclerotic, irradiated tissue. Endovascular therapy, with a mean follow-up extending to 18 months (relative to the 42-month average among surgical patients), demonstrated encouraging results for the treatment of short lesions. It did not, however, yield a statistically significant improvement in periprocedural complication rate. The authors noted, parenthetically, that the apparent underrepresentation of subclavian lesions in the endovascular treatment group likely reflected the extensive nature of radiation-induced lesions of the subclavian artery and their consequent unsuitability for endovascular therapy.

Overall, potential advantages of endovascular over traditional open surgical therapy may include avoidance of general anesthesia, decreased length of stay, relative appeal to patients, and, in some analyses, decreased cost.[63] The patients meriting treatment of SAT lesions for "special circumstances" including significant coronary artery disease, end-stage renal disease, or severe peripheral vascular disease may, indeed, be those most likely to benefit from a minimally invasive approach.[64] The complication rate for endovascular treatment is not, however, negligible. Major complications include embolic events (CVA, TIA, extremity embolization, IMA graft embolization), dissection, renal failure, vessel occlusion due to stent malposition or migration, or injuries to access vessels, which may result in significant bleeding, symptomatic hematoma or pseudoaneurysm, or arteriovenous fistula. Embolic complications of subclavian lesions only infrequently involve thromboemboli to the brain, likely due to the observed delay in reversal of retrograde vertebral artery flow after subclavian angioplasty,[65] and the overall rate of embolic complications of SAT interventions has, presumably, by inference from carotid stent experience, been improved by the introduction of embolic protection devices.[66] As with all new advances, however, the introduction of embolic protection has its own new complications.[67]

SUMMARY

Occlusive disease of the SAT remains a diagnostic and therapeutic challenge to the surgeon. Although most cases in Western series are attributable to atherosclerotic disease, other entities such as Takayasu arteritis and radiation arteritis account for a substantial subset of patients in whom choice of therapy and clinical response may be significantly affected by the peculiarities of the disease process involved. Presenting symptoms may be related to distal thromboembolic phenomena or low-flow states producing local or global ischemic conditions, such as upper extremity exertional discomfort or vertebrobasilar insufficiency.

With regard to the surgical management of SAT disease, although direct transsternal repair carries a somewhat greater perioperative morbidity and mortality than short-segment anatomic or remote extraanatomic bypass, it subsequently provides excellent long-term patency and freedom from reintervention. In patients with relatively focal, single vessel lesions amenable to direct reconstruction by arterial transposition, this approach is technically elegant, carries relatively low associated morbidity and mortality, and yields superior patency. In single vessel lesions not suited to this approach, short-segment extraanatomic bypass is well tolerated and provides acceptable, although slightly lower, primary patency. Successful endovascular treatment of restenosis has been described, and although long-term follow-up is not yet available, it may improve the overall long-term durability of these reconstructions. Remote bypass yields somewhat lower patency rates, but may be an acceptable alternative in patients who are poor candidates for transsternal reconstruction. Broader application of endovascular therapy continues, as in all areas, to be driven by the favorable morbidity and mortality profile. Although early results of angioplasty alone yielded somewhat disappointing results with regard to restenosis, more recent midterm results of combined angioplasty and stent placement are more encouraging and seem to be driving the growing use of endovascular therapy as first-line treatment for SAT lesions.

REFERENCES

1. Savory WS. Case of a young woman in whom the main arteries of both upper extremities and of the left side of the neck were throughout completely obliterated. Med Chir Trans 1856;39:205.
2. Broadbent WH. Absence of pulsations on both radial arteries, vessels being full of blood. Trans Clin Soc London 1875;8:165–8.
3. Takayasu M. [A case with peculiar changes of the retinal central vessels] [in Japanese]. Acta Soc Ophthal Jpn 1908;12:554–5.
4. Numano F. The story of Takayasu arteritis. Rheumatology 2002;41:103–6.
5. Martorell F, Fabre J. [The syndrome of obliteration of the supra-aortic trunks] [in Spanish]. Med Clin 1944;2:26–30.
6. Contorni L. Il circulo collaterale vertebro-vertebrale obliterazione dell'arteria succlavia alla origine. [The vertebro-vertebral collateral circulation in obliteration of the subclavian artery at its origin] [in Italian]. Minerva Chir 1960;15:268–71.
7. Reivich M, Holling E, Roberts B, et al. Reversal of blood flow through the vertebral artery and its effect on cerebral circulation. N Engl J Med 1961;265:878–85.
8. Fisher CM. A new vascular syndrome: "the subclavian steal". N Engl J Med 1961; 265:912–3.
9. Ochsner JL, Hewitt RL. Aortic arch syndrome (brachiocephalic ischemia). Dis Chest 1967;52:69–82.
10. Bahnson HT. Consideration in the excision of aortic aneurysms. Ann Surg 1953; 138:377–86.
11. Davis JV, Grove WJ, Julian OC. Thrombic occlusion of branches of aortic arch. Martorell's syndrome: report of a case treated surgically. Ann Surg 1956;144: 124–6.
12. DeBakey ME, Crawford ES, Cooley DA. Surgical considerations of occlusive disease of innominate, carotid, subclavian and vertebral arteries. Ann Surg 1959;149:690–710.
13. Ehrenfeld WK, Chapman RD, Wylie EJ. Management of occlusive lesions of the branches of the aortic arch. Am J Surg 1969;118:236–43.
14. Parrot JD. The subclavian steal syndrome. Arch Surg 1969;88:661–5.
15. Diethrich EB, Garret H, Ameriso J, et al. Occlusive disease of the common carotid and subclavian arteries treated by carotid-subclavian bypass. Analysis of 125 cases. Am J Surg 1967;114(5):800–8.
16. Carlson RE, Ehrenfeld WK, Stoney RJ, et al. Innominate artery endarterectomy. A 16-year experience. Arch Surg 1977;12:1389–93.
17. Crawford SE, DeBakey ME, Morris GE Jr, et al. Surgical treatment of occlusion of the innominate, common carotid, and subclavian arteries: a 10-year experience. Surgery 1969;65(1):17–31.
18. Dotter ET, Judkins MR. Transluminal treatment of arteriosclerotic obstructions: description of new technique and preliminary report of its application. Circulation 1964;30:654–70.
19. Zarins CK, Xu C, Glagov S. Arterial wall pathology in atherosclerosis. In: Vascular surgery. 6th edition. Philadelphia: Elsevier Saunders; 2005. p. 123–48.
20. Schmidt WA, Gromnica-Ihle E. What is the best approach to diagnosing large-vessel vasculitis? Best Pract Res Clin Rheumatol 2005;19(2):223–42.

21. Arend WP, Michel BA, Bloch DA, et al. The American College of Rheumatology 1990 criteria for the classification of Takayasu arteritis. Arthritis Rheum 1990;33: 1129–34.

22. Ogino H, Matsuda H, Minatoya K, et al. Overview of late outcome of medical and surgical treatment for Takayasu arteritis. Circulation 2008;118:2738–47.

23. Kerr GS, Hallahan CW, Giordano J, et al. Takayasu arteritis. Ann Intern Med 1994; 120:919–29.

24. Meave A, Soto ME, Reyes PA, et al. Pre-pulseless Takayasu's arteritis evaluated with ¹⁸F-FDG positron emission tomography and gadolinium-enhanced magnetic resonance angiography. Tex Heart Inst J 2007;34(4):466–9.

25. Kobayashi Y, Ishii K, Oda K, et al. Aortic wall inflammation due to Takayasu arteritis imaged with 18F-FDG PET coregistered with enhanced CT. J Nucl Med 2005; 46:917–22.

26. Hassen-Khodja R, Kieffer E. Radiotherapy-induced supra-aortic trunk disease: early and long-term results of surgical and endovascular reconstruction. J Vasc Surg 2004;40(2):254–61.

27. Conomy JP, Kellermeyer RW. Delayed cerebrovascular consequences of therapeutic radiation. Cancer 1975;36:1702–8.

28. Rhodes JM, Cherry KJ Jr, Clark R, et al. Aortic-origin reconstruction of the great vesels: risk factors of early and late complications. J Vasc Surg 2000;31(2):260–9.

29. Berguer R, Morasch M, Kline R, et al. Cervical reconstruction of the supra-aortic trunks: a 16-year experience. J Vasc Surg 1999;29(2):239–48.

30. Willinsky RA, Taylor SM, TerBrugge K, et al. Neurologic complications of cerebral angiography: prospective analysis of 2,899 procedures and review of the literature. Radiology 2003;227(2):522–8.

31. Fields CF, Bower TC, Cooper LT, et al. Takayasu's arteritis: operative results and influence of disease activity. J Vasc Surg 2006;43:64–71.

32. Koelemay MJ, Nederkoorn PJ, Reitsma JB, et al. Systematic review of computed tomographic angiography for assessment of carotid artery disease. Stroke 2004; 35:2306–12.

33. Hollingworth W, Nathens AB, Kanne JP, et al. The diagnostic accuracy of computed tomography angiography for traumatic or atherosclerotic lesions of the carotid and vertebral arteries: a systematic review. Eur J Radiol 2003;48:88–102.

34. Kaufmann TJ, Kallmes DF. Utility of MRI and CTA in the evaluation of carotid occlusive disease. Semin Vasc Surg 2005;18:75–82.

35. Nederkoorn PJ, van der Graaf Y, Hunink MGM. Duplex ultrasound and magnetic resonance angiography compared with digital subtraction angiography in carotid artery stenosis: a systematic review. Stroke 2003;34:1324–31.

36. Randoux B, Marro B, Koskas F, et al. Proximal great vessels of aortic arch: comparison of three-dimensional gadolinium-enhanced MR angiography and digital subtraction angiography. Radiology 2003;229:697–702.

37. Thomsen HJ. Nephrogenic systemic fibrosis: a serious late adverse reaction to gadodiamide. Eur Radiol 2006;16:2619–21. FDA alert Available at: http://www.fda.gov/cder/drug/InfoSheets/HCP/gcca_200705.htm. Accessed May 23, 2007.

38. Peterson BG, Resnick SA, Morasch MD, et al. Aortic arch vessel stenting. A single-center experience using cerebral protection. Arch Surg 2006;141:560–4.

39. Takach TJ, Reul GJ, Cooley DA, et al. Myocardial thievery: the coronary-subclavian steal syndrome. Ann Thorac Surg 2006;81:386–92.

40. Takach TJ, Reul GJ, Duncan MD, et al. Concomitant brachiocephalic and coronary artery disease: outcome and decision analysis. Ann Thorac Surg 2005;80: 564–9.

41. Brountzos EN, Petersen B, Binkert C, et al. Primary stenting of subclavian and innominate artery occlusive disease: a single center's experience. Cardiovasc Intervent Radiol 2004;27:616–23.
42. Sullivan TM, Gray BH, Bacharach JM, et al. Angioplasty and primary stenting of the subclavian, innominate, and common carotid arteries in 83 patients. J Vasc Surg 1998;28:1059–65.
43. Longo MJ, Remetz MS. Cardiovascular manifestations of severe systemic auto-immune diseases. Clin Chest Med 1998;19:793–808.
44. Pfizenmeier DH. Predictors of left ventricular dysfunction in patients with Takaya-su's or giant cell aortitis. Clin Exp Rheumatol 2004;22(6 Suppl 36):S41–5.
45. Cherry KJ Jr, McCullough JL, Hallett JW Jr, et al. Technical principles of direct innominate artery revascularization: a comparison of endarterectomy and bypass grafts. J Vasc Surg 1989;9:718–24.
46. Kieffer E, Sabatier J, Koskas F, et al. Atherosclerotic innominate artery occlusive disease: early and long-term results of surgical reconstruction. J Vasc Surg 1995; 21:326–7.
47. Takach TJ, Reul GJ, Cooley DA, et al. Brachiocephalic reconstruction I: operative and long-term results for complex disease. J Vasc Surg 2005;42:47–54.
48. Sakapoulos AG, Ballard JL, Gundry SR. Minimally invasive approach for aortic arch branch vessel reconstruction. J Vasc Surg 2000;31:200–2.
49. Berguer R, Morasch MD, Kline RA, et al. Transthoracic repair of innominate and common carotid artery disease: immediate and long-term outcome for 100 consecutive surgical reconstructions. J Vasc Surg 1998;27(1):34–42.
50. Azakie A, McElhinney DB, Higashima R, et al. Innominate artery reconstruction: over 3 decades of experience. Ann Surg 1998;228(3):402–10.
51. Uurto IT, Lautamatti V, Zeitlin R, et al. Long-term outcome of surgical revascular-ization of supraaortic vessels. World J Surg 2002;26(12):1503–6.
52. Morasch MM. Technique for subclavian to carotid transposition, tips, and tricks. J Vasc Surg 2008;49(1):251–4.
53. Brountzos EN, Malagari K, Kelekis DA. Endovascular treatment of occlusive lesions of the subclavian and innominate arteries. Cardiovasc Intervent Radiol 2006;29:503–10.
54. Mingoli A, Sapienza P, Feldhaus RJ, et al. Long-term results and outcomes of crossover axilloaxillary bypass grafting: a 24-year experience. J Vasc Surg 1999;29(5):894–901.
55. Berguer R, Kieffer E. Surgery of the arteries to the head. New York: Springer-Verlag; 1992.
56. Motarjeme A. Percutaneous transluminal angioplasty of supra-aortic vessels. J Endovasc Surg 1996;3:171–81.
57. Hadjipetrou P, Cox S, Piemonte T. Percutaneous revascularization of atheroscle-rotic obstruction of aortic arch vessels. J Am Coll Cardiol 1999;33:1238–45.
58. Wholey MH, Wholey MH. The supraaortic and vertebral endovascular interven-tions. Tech Vasc Interv Radiol 2005;7(4):215–25.
59. Anziuni A, Chiesa R, Vivekanathan K, et al. Endovascular stenting for stenoses in surgically reconstructed brachiocephalic bypass grafts: immediate and midterm outcomes. J Endovasc Ther 2004;11(3):263–8.
60. Criado FJ, Abul-Khoudoud O. Interventional techniques to facilitate supraaortic angioplasty and stenting. Vasc Endovascular Surg 2006;40:141–7.
61. Tyagi S, Verma PK, Gambhir DS, et al. Early and long-term results of subclavian angioplasty in aortoarteritis (Takayasu disease): comparison with atherosclerosis. Cardiovasc Intervent Radiol 1998;21:219–24.

62. Takahashi JC, Sakai N, Manaka H, et al. Multiple supra-aortic stenting for Takayasu arteritis: extensive revascularization and two-year follow-up. AJNR Am J Neuroradiol 2002;23:790–3.

63. Takach TJ, Duncan JM, Livesay JJ, et al. Brachiocephalic reconstruction II: operative and endovascular management of single-vessel disease. J Vasc Surg 2005; 42:55–61.

64. Angle JF, Matsumoto AH, McGraw K, et al. Percutaneous angioplasty and stenting of left subclavian artery stenosis in patients with left internal mammary-coronary bypass grafts: clinical experience and long-term followup. Vasc Endovascular Surg 2003;37:89–97.

65. Ringelstein EF, Zeumer H. Delayed reversal of vertebral artery blood flow following percutaneous transluminal angioplasty for subclavian steal syndrome. Neuroradiology 1984;26:189–98.

66. Kastrup A, Groschel K, Krapf H, et al. Early outcome of carotid angioplasty and stenting with and without cerebral protection devices. A systematic review of the literature. Stroke 2003;34:813–9.

67. Shilling K, Uretsky BF, Hunter GC. Entrapment of a cerebral embolic protection device. A case report. Vasc Endovascular Surg 2006;40(3):229–33.

Valve-Sparing Aortic Root Reconstruction

Robert L. Smith, MD[a],*, Irving L. Kron, MD[b]

KEYWORDS

- Aorta • Valve • Conserving • Sparing • Reconstruction
- Root • Remodeling • Cardiac surgery

Aortic valve–sparing root reconstructive techniques are generally applied to treat aortic root pathology that spares the leaflets but may lead to aortic insufficiency as a result of distracting the leaflets from their point of coaptation. The classic example is Marfan syndrome, where pathologic cystic medial necrosis leads to dilation of the sinuses, sinotubular junction, and aortic annulus. The leaflets tend to be spared from a pathologic standpoint in these disease states, but they are distracted by the progressive dilation of all the root components. This leads to aortic insufficiency. This can occur in other disease states, such as aortic root and ascending aortic dissection, annuloaortic ectasia, and aortic root dilation secondary to an ascending aortic aneurysm.

The standard operation for aortic root aneurysm is the composite of a conduit containing a mechanical or tissue valve. Aortic valve–sparing operations have evolved during the past few decades to address various aortic root aneurysms, where the leaflets are spared in an effort to preserve the hemodynamics and durability of the native valve leaflets, to avoid the need for anticoagulation therapy, and to reduce the incidence of artificial valve–related thromboembolism. However, there are only a few centers that perform a significant number of these operations, despite the growing interest in patients for valve-sparing surgical options. The success of this approach is predicated on identifying the correct patients for these techniques, understanding the functional anatomy of the aortic valve and aortic root complex, and choosing the appropriate operation for the situation. The goal of this article is to review the development of these operations, to clarify some of their key differences, and to assess their outcomes.

EVOLUTION OF THE AORTIC VALVE–SPARING ROOT RECONSTRUCTION

In 1968, Bentall and De Bono[1] reported on a single patient, who was treated with a composite graft-valve procedure with implantation of the coronaries into the graft

a Division of Thoracic and Cardiovascular Surgery, Department of Surgery, University of Virginia Health System, PO Box 800709, Charlottesville, VA 22908-0709, USA
b Division of Thoracic and Cardiovascular Surgery, Department of Surgery, University of Virginia Health System, PO Box 800679, Charlottesville, VA 22908-0679, USA
* Corresponding author.
E-mail address: rls9t@virginia.edu (R.L. Smith).

Surg Clin N Am 89 (2009) 837–844
doi:10.1016/j.suc.2009.05.004
0039-6109/09/$ – see front matter

for replacement of the aortic root. This procedure became the gold standard repair, and studies by Gott and others[2,3] have underscored the success of this repair, especially when done in an early, elective setting. However, as aortic root deformation is often found in the setting of morphologically normal valve leaflets, the potential exists for realigning the leaflets to reform the native valve coaptation, thus preventing complications related to chronic anticoagulation, hemodynamic mismatch, hydraulic dysfunction, and bacterial endocarditis. The putative advantages of using the native valve led to the concept of the valve-sparing root replacement. In general, these procedures fall into 2 categories: "remodeling" procedures and "reimplantation" procedures.

Remodeling

The remodeling procedure was described by Sir Magdi Yacoub and colleagues[4] in 1983, and a more collective experience was reported in 1993 by Sarsam and Yacoub.[5] This technique emphasizes the replacement of all 3 sinuses, which are trimmed down to 4 to 5 mm of the annulus. Horizontal mattress sutures are then placed just above the apex of each commissure. With the commissures suspended, the valve is positioned to coapt without prolapse. Coaptation is tested with a blunt instrument. The graft size selected is based on the intercommissural distance where the valve demonstrates maximal nonprolapsing coaptation. A Dacron graft is cut into a tripartite, scallop-shaped tube on the proximal end to be sewn to the residual annular tissue. The coronary buttons are then reimplanted into the graft. The height of the commissural pillars is increased by the incisions in the graft. The result is a cylinder, but as the graft fills, the neosinuses billow. The action of this repair is considered fairly natural because it preserves the independent mobility of the sinuses and recreates the normal opening and closing action of the valve leaflets.[6] Also, by not placing subannular sutures to secure the annulus, the dynamic properties of the ventriculo-aortic junction are conserved, and this, along with improved leaflet action, may enhance long-term valve durability.

Besides the technique describedearlier, there are other remodeling techniques.[7–10] In general, this technique is considered faster and is technically less complicated than the reimplantation techniques described later because it only requires 2 suture lines. The disadvantage of this technique is that it does not reinforce the annular base of the root, and it does not recreate the sinotubular junction, though these deficiencies are addressed by other remodeling techniques.[7,8,10] Additionally, because the suture lines are all exposed, there is a greater risk for surgical bleeding. In the end, it may be easier to teach and get reliable results across a broader group of surgeons, but there may be significant limits to its broad applicability. There are also questions regarding its durability, which are discussed later.

Reimplantation

The concept of aortic root repair with a valve-sparing reimplantation technique was first described by David and Feindel in 1992.[11] Their report included 10 patients treated with what has commonly become known as the Tirone David I repair. The technique involves excising the aortic root aneurysm and leaving the coronary buttons as Carrel patches, the leaflets attached to 5 mm aortic wall remnants, and the intact annulus. A conduit composed of Dacron is then selected based on the measurement of the aortic base (annulus). Pledgeted sutures are placed from underneath the leaflets through the base of the aortic outflow tract and secured to the Dacron graft. This move stabilizes the ventriculo-aortic junction to prevent further dilation. Next, the commissures are resuspended within the tube graft, and the leaflets are secured to the graft wall. The coronary buttons are then sutured to the area of the neosinuses. A distal anastamosis is then created in a standard end-to-end fashion to the normal diameter aorta, which completes the repair.

The key concept to any reimplantation technique is securing a replacement graft to the aorto-ventricular junction below the leaflets and resuspending the commissures within the conduit. The obvious advantage of the reimplantation technique is that the annulus is reinforced to stabilize the repair and prevent further dilation, which is a concern for patients with annuloaortic ectacic diseases, such as Marfan syndrome. However, with the straight Dacron tube graft secured to the annulus with the interiorized valve leaflets, there was concern that the natural leaflet mobility provided by the Yacoub repair technique was not being accomplished. In 1995, Cochran and colleagues[12] reported on a technique that used a modified conduit to create pseudosinuses in an aortic valve–sparing procedure. The reason for the modification was concern that the absence of sinuses did not allow for appropriate DaVinci eddy currents in the supravalvular region. These currents are important in initiating and coordinating trileaflet valve closure and promoting coronary artery blood flow.[13] Without these currents, the valve leaflets would theoretically contact the graft surface, and this would potentially affect load sharing by the leaflets on closure. The ultimate concern is that the leaflets would fatigue at an advanced rate resulting in decreased valve durability. In the modification described earlier, the pseudosinuses are created by scalloping the proximal graft (the "annular" end) and securing this end to the subannular horizontal mattress sutures of the Tirone David I repair. The commissures are suspended as in the Tirone David I repair, and the coronary buttons are placed in the neosinuses. By scalloping the graft, a significant increase in free edge graft length is created, which is also increased by increasing the height of the scallops. When pressurized blood fills the graft, the extra material in the scalloped margin pushes upward and outward bowing at the sinuses. In their study, the effect was confirmed by transesophageal echocardiography and was not seen in the original Tirone David I repair, the single case control for their series.

The next step in the evolution of the reimplantation technique was to specifically address the sinotubular junction, which the previously noted procedure failed to do. This is addressed by the Tirone David IV and Tirone David V operations, which preselect a larger Dacron graft size (diameter + 4–8 mm) that requires tapering down proximally and distally. The result was the creation of pseudosinuses and circumferential tapering distally to recreate the sinotubular junction.[8] The Miller modification of the David V operation uses 2 grafts of different sizes.[14] The proximal graft is the diameter + 8 mm and is plicated around a valve sizer to even the tapering circumferentially. The tapered proximal end is then secured to the ventriculo-aortic junction, and the commissures are suspended within the graft. A separate graft is sized to the distal native aorta for a size match. The distal end of the proximal graft is then tapered when sewing the anastamosis between the 2 grafts. A benefit of the 2-graft technique is that it provides significant flexibility in creating the proximal graft to match different annulus sizes and commisural heights and still taper down to a more normal sinotubular junction while matching the distal native aorta. The Valsalva graft (Sulzer Vascutek, Renfrewshire, Scotland) is a modified Dacron graft introduced by DePaulis and colleagues[15] that incorporates sinuses of Valsalva and tapered proximal and distal ends as part of a single graft. Although useful for select patients, this graft is limited by the sizes that are commercially available. In patients with tall commissures or annulus diameters larger than the commercially available ends, the Valsalva graft is not an option for the reimplantation technique (but may be used in a remodeling technique).

As the procedures for reimplantation have evolved, the techniques have become more complicated with time, which has likely prevented its more universal acceptance by surgeons as a viable option for appropriate patients. To simplify the process, Hess and colleagues[16] from the University of Florida developed the Florida Sleeve as an approach to aortic valve–sparing root repair. The conduit size is determined by the degree of dilatation of the sinus of Valsalva. The goal is to achieve a normal annulus to sinotubular junction with a large-enough graft to allow for sinus expansion, yet maintain adequate leaflet coaptation. To place the graft, the aorta is transected just above the sinotubular junction. The proximal coronary arteries are mobilized to allow the graft to slip down over the root and fit into the "coronary keyholes" created on the graft. Subannular pledgeted sutures are placed that secure the graft below the annulus and are tied down with a Hegar dilator of appropriate size through the valve. This assures a secure but not overly reduced annuloplasty. The leaflets are then checked for coaptation. The sleeve is cut at the sinotubular junction and secured to the sinotubular junction with a running Prolene suture. (A Hegar dilator can also be used here to help assure a reduction in size of the sinotubular junction as appropriate for smaller aortas.) The distal anastamosis is then completed.

The Florida Sleeve operation is similar to a repair described earlier by van Son and colleagues.[17] In their repair, the coronaries were removed as buttons for reimplanting, and the dilated sinuses were reduced in size. The repair was then sleeved with the conduit as earlier, with correction of the annuloaortic ectasia, if present. The edge of the sinotubular junction is sewn to the conduit. A second conduit is used to replace the remainder of the ascending aorta, and the coronaries are reimplanted into this graft. In this repair and the Florida Sleeve, leaving the natural sinus tissue in place prevents the leaflets from interfacing with the Dacron and potentially reduces their deterioration. Additionally, there is some preservation of the sinus billowing, which may reduce closing tension on the leaflets. By reducing the needed excision steps, the Florida Sleeve definitely simplifies the technique of aortic valve–sparing reimplantation. Additionally, there is theoretical reduced risk of bleeding because there are fewer suture lines. For both techniques, though, concern remains regarding all the remaining diseased tissue and its ability to dissect or continue to dilate.

It is clear that aortic valve–sparing root repair is feasible. The continual developments make it hard to track the data well regarding how efficacious these repairs are. Additionally, there are few comparative studies that shed light on true outcome differences between the varied techniques. Until good data become available, it is understandable why the procedures have not been easily accepted.

REASONS FOR FAILURE

Aortic valve–sparing root reconstruction is still in its relative infancy. The techniques are constantly being evaluated to address new concerns that were not addressed by previous iterations. As the patient population treated by these operations ages, observations are made regarding the reasons for valve failure after repair. Three primary reasons for failure deserve discussion: late annular dilation, early or accelerated valve degeneration, and failure of the repair itself by placing the leaflet coaptation point too low in the annulus.

One of the primary causes of failure of valve-sparing operations is failing to secure the aortic annulus. Patients with aortic root aneurysm often have annuloaortic ectasia, and in patients with Marfan syndrome, the expression may be temporal. Therefore, procedures that only remodel the root but do not stabilize the annular base are prone to permitting annular dilation later. In David and colleagues' direct comparison of reimplantation versus remodeling, the reimplantation technique demonstrated better valve durability that was statistically significant as determined by decreased incidence of moderate or severe aortic insufficiency. This difference was attributed to a dilating annulus associated with the remodeling repair.[18]

The reimplantation technique secures the annulus and prevents dilatation by containing the valve apparatus within the cylindrical confines of a Dacron conduit. However, there are concerns that the contact between the leaflets on opening with the graft material will eventually lead to early leaflet degeneration. This has been addressed in later iterations of the reimplantation technique with the creation of pseudo-sinuses[8,12,14,15] and by limiting contact of the leaflets to the natural sinuses contained within the graft.[16,17] There is also evidence that this concern may be all theoretical with the good outcomes posted by the Hannover group using the classic Tirone David I repair with a cylindrical graft.[19] Leaflet trauma can also occur with overcrowding the valve components within the graft. This is a particular concern for patients with an annulus size greater than 25 to 27 mm.[10] This potential problem is also addressed by the creation of pseudosinuses and may also be related to not achieving the appropriate height for the commissural pillars.

The level of leaflet coaptation within the annulus plays a role in operative failure as was discovered by Pethig and colleagues[20] using echocardiography. The investigators found that when the point of leaflet coaptation sagged below the annulus, aortic insufficiency developed in all patients. Patients whose coaptation plane sat 2 mm above the plane of the annulus remained free of significant aortic insufficiency. These results emphasized the importance of adequately resuspending the commissural pillars to set the coaptation plane at the normal height to prevent early aortic insufficiency.

OUTCOMES AFTER AORTIC VALVE–SPARING RECONSTRUCTION

In general, the perioperative mortality from aortic valve–sparing root reconstruction is low; it ranges from 1.4% to 4.9% for the valve-sparing aortic root repair surgery, for both the remodeling and the reimplantation techniques, and therefore it is considered to be safe.[18,19,21,22] The perioperative mortality data are similar to the classic Bentall and De Bono composite valve graft root replacement in which perioperative mortality rates range from 3% to 4%.[2,3] Additionally, 10-year survival statistics with valve-sparing operations have also been excellent, ranging from 84% to 88% ± 3%.[18,22] Independent predictors of death are age greater than 65 years, preoperative New York Heart Association functional classes III and IV, emergency operation, absence of β-blockers, and left ventricular ejection fraction less than 40%.[18,22]

The biggest concern about aortic valve–sparing root reconstructions is not the survivability of the operation but durability. Do valve-sparing operations last? In a report from David and colleagues[18] that reviewed their reimplantation and remodeling repairs, freedom from moderate and/or severe aortic insufficiency for all patients was 85 ± 5%: 94 ± 4% after reimplantation repairs and 75 ± 10% after remodeling repairs. For patients with Marfan syndrome, 10-year freedom from moderate and/or severe aortic insufficiency was 87 ± 6%, and for those without Marfan syndrome, it was 84 ± 5%. Lastly, in this series, freedom from aortic-valve replacement in all patients at 10 years was 95 ± 3%: 96 ± 3% for reimplantation repairs and 93 ± 4% for remodeling repairs. In a report chronicling Yacoub's remodeling technique for patients with Marfan sydrome, 22.4% of patients had moderate aortic insufficiency in follow-up from surgery, but there were no patients with severe aortic insufficiency.[22] Freedom from aortic-valve replacement was 82.7% for patients at 10 years. Also, there were only 2 valve-related complications beside recurrent aortic insufficiency during this time period. These 2 patients had bovine pericardial extensions of the valve leaflets and later developed endocarditis, and 1 developed a left-ventricular thrombus. No patient in the series received routine anticoagulation. In both series, trivial to mild aortic insufficiency was common.[18,22] The group from Hannover, Germany, reported on 158 patients who underwent reimplantation repair during an 8-year period; 6 (3.8%) required reoperation for aortic valve–related morbidity and only 3 cases were related to failure of the operation.[19]

The existing follow-up data for aortic valve–sparing root reconstruction are limited. Continual changes in technique, heterogeneity of the populations studied, and the limited number of the operations performed make it difficult to reach any significant conclusions about these operations. Additionally, for all the reasons listed, it is also difficult to directly compare these operations with the classic Bentall and De Bono composite valve graft root replacement operation. There is certainly a considerable amount of selection bias that goes into the decision to choosing an operation for disease of the aortic root.Without a concerted effort by higher volume centers to pool data, to strictly define variables and outcomes, and to avoid institutional/surgeon/patient preferences for the varied types of operations for these disease processes, the best answer for how to treat these aortic root diseases will not be available.

WHAT WE DO

At the University of Virginia, we generally use an aortic valve–sparing reimplantation technique in relative consistency with the Tirone David I technique of aortic valve–sparing reimplantation. We treat a moderate-sized population of patients with annuloaortic ectasia. Therefore, we feel it is important to stabilize the annulus to prevent late dilation. All patients have a transesophageal probe placed in the operating room. Central cannulation is usual, and a left ventricular vent is always used. Cardioplegia is initiated retrograde and followed by hand-held cardioplegia catheter, especially to protect the right ventricle. Patients are systemically cooled to 30°C to 32°C. The aortic root is dissected out to the level of the annulus on all sides. The aneurysm is resected, leaving a less than 5 mm cuff of aorta attached to the leaflets and sparing the coronaries, which are removed as Carrel patches. The distal aorta is transected at the transition to normal diameter aorta. Next, the valve is sized using a valve sizer, and the conduit size is upsized up 2 mm from the valve size. Usually twelve 2-0 Ticron, nonpledgeted, interrupted, horizontal mattress sutures are placed in the subannular position through the aortic outflow tract. The graft is brought to the field, and the commissures are marked for orientation on the graft; then 4 to 5 mm triangular wedges are removed at the commissural sites on the graft, similar to scalloping described earlier (Cochran). The subannular sutures are placed through the graft, and the silk sutures tagging the valve commissures are brought up through the center of the graft, as it is lower and secured in the subannular position. The commissures are then suspended in the graft to an adequate height to provide an approximate 5mm coaptation between the cusps. A double-armed, 4-0 Prolene suture is started at the nadir of the each residual aortic sinus tissue and run to each commissure. The graft is clamped distally and a 16-gauge needle is used to give pressurized volume down the graft to check the valve integrity and hemostasis of the suture line. Next, the eye cautery is used to create a defect in the graft in the left neosinus to implant the left coronary button using a 5-0 Prolene. Cardioplegia is again given, using the 16-gauge needle down the graft, so that we can evaluate the left coronary suture line. Next, the distal anastamosis is completed using a nonpledgeted running 4-0 Prolene suture. Because the graft is slightly upsized, there is usually a slight necking down with the distal anastamosis recreating a sinotubular ridge. A DLP cannula is placed through conduit, and cardioplegia is given now to assess placement of the right coronary button. We also fill the heart to make sure the graft does not kink with filling of the right ventricle at the site chosen for reimplantation. (It is difficult to diagnose poor right ventricular function secondary to kinking of the coronary because it does not happen until after the patient is weaned from cardiopulmonary bypass.) One last check is made with cardioplegia distension of the graft before deairing and removing the cross-clamp.

For years, we have seen little to any effect of early leaflet degeneration secondary to leaflet contact with the graft. The benefits of this technique include excellent survivability, short cardiopulmonary bypass times, and an ability to extend the graft to any needed length distally without having to use a second graft reducing the risk of bleeding at an additional suture line, and this technique is teachable. Because all of our cases use intraoperative transesophageal echocardiography, we can immediately address any residual aortic insufficiency that results from a prolapsing leaflet.

As we expanded the use of this repair, more cardiologists refer their patients specifically for valve-sparing reconstructions. Whether this is the preference of cardiologists or patientsis hard to tell. However, for patients who cannot stand the possibility of a second operation for possible valve failure and who demonstrate a compliant nature, we still offer a standard Bentall aortic root replacement.

SUMMARY

The aortic valve–sparing root reconstruction procedure remains an ideal concept, but it has not yet become an ideal operation. There is still great variation and evolution in techniques, which mirrors the increasing understanding of the aortic root's functional anatomy and the disease processes that affect it. These operations remain complex, and the surgeons who perform them well are often times best armed with an experienced eye for what looks right more than a mathematical model that can predetermine who will do well, with what repair type and with what percentage chance of long-term success. Because of this, it will likely still be a while before these operations are more routinely used by a broader group of surgeons, as compared with the very reproducible Bentall and De Bono repair.

REFERENCES

1. Bentall H, De Bono A. A technique for complete replacement of the ascending aorta. Thorax 1968;23(4):338–9.
2. Gott VL, Greene PS, Alejo DE, et al. Replacement of the aortic root in patients with Marfan's syndrome. N Engl J Med 1999;340(17):1307–13.
3. Zehr KJ, Orszulak TA, Mullany CJ, et al. Surgery for aneurysms of the aortic root: a 30-year experience. Circulation 2004;110(11):1364–71.
4. Yacoub M, Fagan A, Stessano P, et al. Results of valve conserving operations for aortic regurgitation. Circulation 1983;68(Suppl 3):321.
5. Sarsam MA, Yacoub M. Remodeling of the aortic valve anulus. J Thorac Cardiovasc Surg 1993;105(3):435–8.
6. Leyh RG, Schmidtke C, Sievers HH, et al. Opening and closing characteristics of the aortic valve after different types of valve-preserving surgery. Circulation 1999; 100(21):2153–60.

7. de Oliveira NC, David TE, Ivanov J, et al. Results of surgery for aortic root aneurysm in patients with Marfan syndrome. J Thorac Cardiovasc Surg 2003;125(4): 789–96.

8. David TE, Armstrong S, Ivanov J, et al. Results of aortic valve-sparing operations. J Thorac Cardiovasc Surg 2001;122(1):39–46.

9. David TE, Armstrong S, Ivanov J, et al. Aortic valve sparing operations: an update. Ann Thorac Surg 1999;67(6):1840–2 [discussion: 53–6].

10. Hopkins RA. Aortic valve leaflet sparing and salvage surgery: evolution of techniques for aortic root reconstruction. Eur J Cardiothorac Surg 2003;24(6):886–97.

11. David TE, Feindel CM. An aortic valve-sparing operation for patients with aortic incompetence and aneurysm of the ascending aorta. J Thorac Cardiovasc Surg 1992;103(4):617–21 [discussion: 22].

12. Cochran RP, Kunzelman KS, Eddy AC, et al. Modified conduit preparation creates a pseudosinus in an aortic valve-sparing procedure for aneurysm of the ascending aorta. J Thorac Cardiovasc Surg 1995;109(6):1049–57 [discussion: 57–8].

13. Kunzelman KS, Grande KJ, David TE, et al. Aortic root and valve relationships. Impact on surgical repair. J Thorac Cardiovasc Surg 1994;107(1):162–70.

14. Demers P, Miller DC. Simple modification of "T. David-V" valve-sparing aortic root replacement to create graft pseudosinuses. Ann Thorac Surg 2004;78(4): 1479–81.

15. De Paulis R, De Matteis GM, Nardi P, et al. One-year appraisal of a new aortic root conduit with sinuses of Valsalva. J Thorac Cardiovasc Surg 2002;123(1):33–9.

16. Hess PJ Jr, Klodell CT, Beaver TM, et al. The Florida Sleeve: a new technique for aortic root remodeling with preservation of the aortic valve and sinuses. Ann Thorac Surg 2005;80(2):748–50.

17. van Son JA, Battellini R, Mierzwa M, et al. Aortic root reconstruction with preservation of native aortic valve and sinuses in aortic root dilatation with aortic regurgitation. J Thorac Cardiovasc Surg 1999;117(6):1151–6.

18. David TE, Feindel CM, Webb GD, et al. Long-term results of aortic valve-sparing operations for aortic root aneurysm. J Thorac Cardiovasc Surg 2006;132(2): 347–54.

19. Kallenbach K, Hagl C, Walles T, et al. Results of valve-sparing aortic root reconstruction in 158 consecutive patients. Ann Thorac Surg 2002;74(6):2026–32 [discussion: 32–3].

20. Pethig K, Milz A, Hagl C, et al. Aortic valve reimplantation in ascending aortic aneurysm: risk factors for early valve failure. Ann Thorac Surg 2002;73(1):29–33.

21. Reece TB, Singh RR, Stiles BM, et al. Replacement of the proximal aorta adds no further risk to aortic valve procedures. Ann Thorac Surg 2007;84(2):473–8 [discussion: 8].

22. Birks EJ, Webb C, Child A, et al. Early and long-term results of a valve-sparing operation for Marfan syndrome. Circulation 1999;100(19 Suppl):II29–35.

Indications for the Treatment of Thoracic Aortic Aneurysms

John A. Elefteriades, MD*, Donald M. Botta Jr, MD

KEYWORDS

- Thoracic • Aortic • Aneurysm • Dissection
- Rupture • Tamponade

Thoracic aortic aneurysms (TAAs) are serious conditions that result in significant morbidity, with a population-based incidence of mortality comparable to that of human immunodeficiency virus infection.[1–4] As precise thoracic imaging technology has become widespread, the incidence of diagnosis of TAAs before the feared complications of rupture, dissection, or death has increased, and the results of operative repair have improved.[5] With increasing numbers of people presenting to clinicians for evaluation of TAAs, clinicians are more often faced with the difficult decision of determining the correct timing to treat TAAs. More importantly, as operative repair becomes safer, minimally invasive approaches enter the clinician's armamentarium, and the promise of medical therapy for TAAs comes closer to fruition, the choice of which treatment modality to employ becomes even more complex. The indications for treatment of TAAs are moving targets. Some indications are clear-cut, whereby the risk of observation clearly outweighs the risk of treatment (see later discussion). Other indications are subject to change as operative and nonoperative techniques become safer.

The first step in developing a rational approach to this changing clinical environment is to understand the behavior of TAAs as much as possible. In this article, the natural behavior of the aneurysmal thoracic aorta is examined, the currently available diagnostic and therapeutic modalities and the outlook for the future are explored. How best to harness knowledge of the behavior of TAAs to bring about optimal treatment with appropriate timing is discussed.

THE NATURAL BEHAVIOR OF TAAs

Over the last 10 years at the Yale Center for Thoracic Aortic Disease, the authors have made a concerted effort to learn more about the natural history of aortic diseases

Section of Cardiac Surgery, Yale University School of Medicine, 330 Cedar Street, Boardman 204, New Haven, CT 06510, USA
* Corresponding author.
E-mail address: john.elefteriades@yale.edu (J.A. Elefteriades).

Surg Clin N Am 89 (2009) 845–867
doi:10.1016/j.suc.2009.06.005
0039-6109/09/$ – see front matter © 2009 Elsevier Inc. All rights reserved.

surgical.theclinics.com

based on a dataset that includes information on 3000 patients, with 9000 years of patient follow-up and 9000 serial imaging studies. Analysis of this dataset has helped to elucidate the behavior of thoracic aortic diseases.

The feared complications of TAAs are rupture, dissection, and death. Free rupture of the thoracic aorta is almost always fatal. Its close relative, aortic dissection, is one of the most catastrophic acute natural events that can befall a human being. The pain of this disorder is often described by those affected as the most severe pain imaginable, eclipsing that of childbirth and kidney stones. It is interesting that nature perceives the pain of dissection as a splitting or tearing quality, much apropos of the pathologic process itself. Because acute aortic dissection often masquerades as a heart attack, its true incidence is often underestimated. If a middle-aged or elderly person arrives in the emergency room with acute onset of chest pain, clutches his/her chest, and promptly dies, he/she is likely to be signed out as having experienced a myocardial infarction. However, many such presentations represent undiagnosed aortic dissections. It takes autopsy series to document the true incidence of acute aortic dissection. Such series have indicated that aortic dissection is actually the most common lethal condition affecting the human aorta, more common than the better-appreciated ruptured abdominal aortic aneurysm.[6] Furthermore, with the increasing frequency of three-dimensional imaging of the human body; including the so-called drive-in CT scanners, aortic pathology is being diagnosed more thoroughly. For all these reasons, acute aortic dissection is a condition of great importance not only to the surgical specialist but also to the generalist and to other specialists in emergency medicine, radiology, and cardiology, among others. The risks of these feared complications are enumerated in this review. The risks associated with current and emerging treatments for TAAs are discussed, and a rational approach to specifying evidence-based indications for treatment is developed. The findings from the Yale Center for Thoracic Aortic Disease in terms of specific individual questions that have been answered over the last 10 years are also discussed.

How Fast does the Aneurysmal Thoracic Aorta Grow?

When the authors started their investigations, little was known about the natural behavior of the aneurysmal thoracic aorta. Although hundreds of articles had been written about *how* to do aortic operations, little had been written about *when* to do them, or about how the thoracic aorta behaves. The authors began with the fundamental question of how fast the aneurysmal thoracic aorta grows, and found that, although a *virulent* disease, TAA is an *indolent* process. The thoracic aorta grows slowly, at about 0.1 cm/y. The descending aorta grows a bit faster than the ascending aorta (**Fig. 1**). Prior estimates had failed to account for negative observed growth (measurements of any object will vary about a mean) and other statistical complexities, leading to overestimates of actual growth. Dr. John Rizzo developed exponential equations specifically for the purpose of accurately estimating growth rates.[7] Reports of rapid growth of the thoracic aorta are usually reflective of measurement error, specifically, measuring across an oblique portion of the aorta, especially the aortic arch (**Fig. 2**). The only condition in which the thoracic aorta truly grows rapidly in a short time is when there has been an intercurrent aortic dissection; this should be suspected when the diameter of the aorta truly has grown rapidly.

At What Size does the Aorta Dissect or Rupture?

The poor prognosis after dissection indicates how critically important it is to intervene before aortic dissection occurs. Detailed studies of the natural history of the enlarged aorta have defined criteria that predict when dissection and rupture are likely to occur

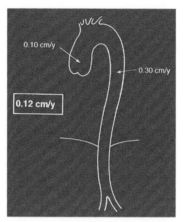

Fig. 1. Annual growth rates of TAAs. TAA, although virulent, is an indolent disease; the aorta grows slowly (about a centimeter per decade). The descending aorta generally grows faster than the ascending aorta.

in an enlarged thoracic aorta. Analysis of the lifetime risk of rupture or dissection revealed sharp hinge points in the aortic size at which rupture or dissection occurs. These hinge points occur at 6 cm in the ascending aorta and 7 cm in the descending aorta (**Fig. 3**). It is important to intervene before the aorta reaches these hinge point dimensions. Specifically, as seen in the figure, an individual with TAA incurs a 34% risk of rupture or dissection by the time that the ascending aorta reaches a diameter of 6 cm. As seen in the figure, the descending aorta, for inexplicable reasons, does not rupture until a larger dimension.

To calculate yearly growth rates required even more robust data, which have now become available in the database. This analysis reveals that the incidence of rupture, dissection, or death increases in a roughly linear fashion as the aorta grows, reaching maximal levels at an aortic dimension of 6 cm (**Fig. 4**). There is something special about the dimension of 6 cm; it is important mechanically as well as clinically.

In addition to sporadically occurring TAAs, several heritable causes of TAAs are known. Patients with Marfan disease are known to rupture or dissect their TAAs at smaller diameters than those described above. Patients with TAAs, and a family history of TAAs, are also at increased risk. Familial patterns have emerged, and this should be taken into account when estimating risk (see later discussion). Patients

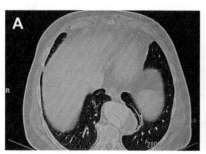
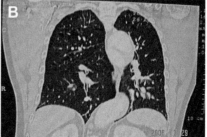

Fig. 2. Two perspectives on the same widespread aneurysm. (*A*) Transverse cross-section. (*B*) Oblique cross-section.

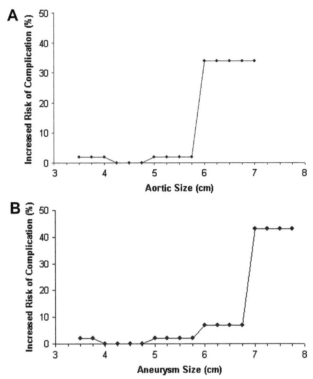

Fig. 3. Lifetime increase in risk of rupture or dissection as the aorta enlarges to specific dimensions. Note the abrupt hinge point at 6 cm for the ascending aorta (*A*) and 7 cm for the descending aorta (*B*).

with bicuspid aortic valves deserve special consideration, as our group and others have shown them to be biologically deficient in terms of the balance of matrix metalloproteinases (MMPs) and their restraining tissue inhibitors, the MMPs or tissue inhibitor of metalloproteinases (TIMPs).[8] Bicuspid aortic valves are a common congenital

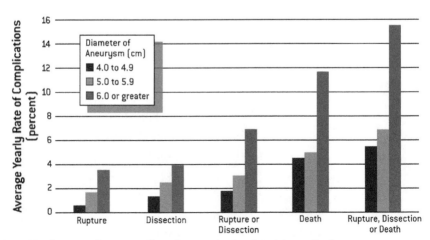

Fig. 4. Yearly rates of rupture, dissection, or death related to aortic size.

condition (1%–2% of the general population) with a predisposition to aortic dissection. One in 20 patients with a bicuspid aortic valve will develop aortic dissection. Dissection usually occurs *before* the onset of symptomatic aortic stenosis or regurgitation in these patients.

The risk of rupture or dissection varies based on the size of the patient. It is appropriate to use body size corrections, especially for very small or very large individuals. The authors have been able to calculate the risk of complications based on an aortic size index, which takes into account aneurysm size and the patient's body surface area (**Fig. 5**).

What Causes TAA? Is this a Genetic Disease?

Marfan syndrome, based on any of a large number of mutations on the fibrillin-1 gene, is a well-known cause of aortic dissection. Patients with Marfan disease, if denied surgical intervention, run a 50% risk of developing aortic dissection during their lifetime. Marfan disease accounts for about 5% of all cases of aortic dissection.

A small number of other collagen vascular diseases (including Ehler-Danlos syndrome) cause an even smaller percentage of aortic dissections. The condition of cystic medial necrosis provides the anatomic backdrop in which the dissecting process can occur. **Figure 6** provides a classic example of this pathologic entity. One can easily picture how a tear in the endothelium can permit blood under pressure to enter one of the intramedial lacunae and how such pressurized entry can split the aortic wall and propagate distally. Cystic medial necrosis is a nonspecific degenerative condition of the media that can occur from one of the collagen vascular syndromes like Marfan disease, from the effects of chronic hypertension, or from the aging process itself. Although the medial degeneration may take decades to develop, the process of dissection itself is literally instantaneous: one moment the aorta is whole, and a split second later, it is dissected. The authors have visualized this process in an animal model of experimental aortic dissection by direct aortic examination and by echocardiography.[9] By the naked eye and by echo, it is possible to see the dissection extend from the proximal descending aorta, where an intimal tear is induced, along the entire length of the aorta. By producing the intimal tear and then inducing severe iatrogenic hypertension

BSA	Aortic Size (cm)									
	3.5	4.0	4.5	5.0	5.5	6.0	6.5	7.0	7.5	8.0
1.30	2.69	3.08	3.46	3.85	4.23	4.62	5.00	5.38	5.77	6.15
1.40	2.50	2.86	3.21	3.57	3.93	4.29	4.64	5.00	5.36	5.71
1.50	2.33	2.67	3.00	3.33	3.67	4.00	4.33	4.67	5.00	5.33
1.60	2.19	2.50	2.80	3.13	3.44	3.75	4.06	4.38	4.69	5.00
1.70	2.05	2.35	2.65	2.94	3.24	3.53	3.82	4.12	4.41	4.71
1.80	1.94	2.22	2.50	2.78	3.06	3.33	3.61	3.89	4.17	4.44
1.90	1.84	2.11	2.37	2.63	2.89	3.16	3.42	3.68	3.95	4.22
2.00	1.75	2.00	2.25	2.50	2.75	3.00	3.25	3.50	3.75	4.00
2.10	1.67	1.90	2.14	2.38	2.62	2.86	3.10	3.33	3.57	3.80
2.20	1.59	1.82	2.05	2.27	2.50	2.72	2.95	3.18	3.41	3.64
2.30	1.52	1.74	1.96	2.17	2.39	2.61	2.83	3.04	3.26	3.48
2.40	1.46	1.67	1.88	2.08	2.29	2.50	2.71	2.92	3.13	3.33
2.50	1.40	1.60	1.80	2.00	2.20	2.40	2.60	2.80	3.00	3.20

□ = low risk (~4% /y)   ▨ = moderate risk (~8% /y)   ■ = severe risk (~20% /y)

Fig. 5. Aortic size index nomogram. (*Reproduced from* Davies RR, Gallo A, Coady MA, et al. Novel measurement of relative aortic size predicts rupture of TAA. Ann Thorac Surg 2006;81:169–77; with permission.)

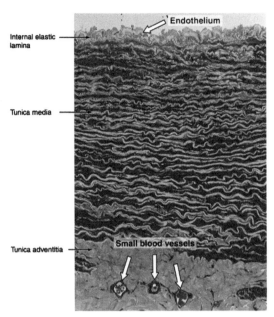

Fig. 6. Classic cystic medial necrosis. The dropout of medial cell bodies and the cystic spaces within the media can be evidenced here.

(blood pressure 300 mm Hg after epinephrine injection), these aortic phenomena can be produced reliably for evaluation of various surgical treatments.

Marfan disease has been elucidated for decades. However, Marfan disease explains only about 5% of known TAAs. The question arises whether genetic abnormalities explain some of the remaining 95% of patients with TAA. The answer is a resounding yes. The Yale database has allowed us to recognize that many patients with aortic dissection do not fit any acknowledged syndrome of collagen vascular disease. Marfan disease and similar disorders account for only the tip of the iceberg of TAA and dissection. Studies have indicated a strong genetic component in patients with TAA and dissection among those patients without Marfan disease.

The construction of nearly 500 family trees of patients with TAA or dissection has indicated that 21% of the probands have at least one family member with a known aneurysm somewhere in the arterial tree.[10,11] The patients with positive family trees showed a higher rate of growth of their aortas and presentation with clinical disease at an earlier age, two findings that strongly support the presence of an inherent genetic defect of the aortic wall. **Figure 7** shows the positive family trees from among the first 100 family pedigrees. The predominant mode of inheritance is autosomal dominant, but other genetic patterns are also expressed. The true rate of inheritance is likely to be much higher than shown, as many family members may harbor aneurysms without being aware of their presence.

Our most recent analysis indicates that the location of the aneurysm in the proband has a strong impact on the site at which family members develop their aneurysms.[11] Specifically, probands with ascending aortic aneurysm have family members with predominantly ascending aortic aneurysms (**Fig. 8**). However, probands with descending thoracic aneurysms most commonly have family members with abdominal aortic aneurysms. This analysis fits a conception that aneurysm disease divides itself into two entities at the ligamentum arteriosum: above the ligament is one disease and

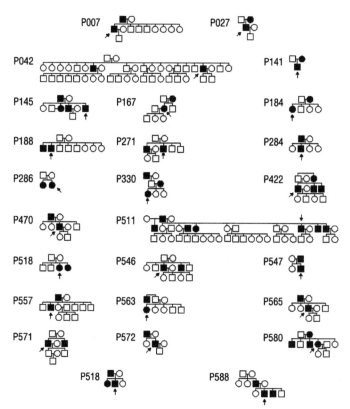

Fig. 7. Among the first 100 family pedigrees constructed, these 21 showed a family pattern for TAA. Autosomal dominant inheritance predominates, but other patterns are also discernable.

below the ligament another. The authors have made intensive efforts aimed to identify the specific genetic aberrations that underlie these family transmissions. RNA expression patterns in the blood of 30,000 patients with TAA have been studied and compared with control patients. A 31-single nucleotide polymorphism (SNP) panel could discriminate quite well between patients with and without aneurysm from a blood test alone (**Fig. 9**).[12] This RNA signature is more than 80% accurate in determining from a blood test alone whether the patient has an aneurysm. This may eventuate in a screening test for family members or even the general public. This level of accuracy far exceeds that of the prostate specific antigen test used so widely for prostate cancer.

In collaboration with colleagues at Celera Diagnostics in California, the authors have also performed genome-wide scans for SNPs associated with TAA and dissection. More than 600 Yale patients and their spousal controls have been studied in this manner. Results are encouraging, with several SNPs strongly predicting the aneurysm disease. Replication studies from European collections sites are currently underway.

How is the Thoracic Aorta Degraded in Aneurysmal Diseases?

To better understand the risks associated with TAAs, and to rationally correlate them with emerging diagnostic and therapeutic methods, the authors have begun to analyze

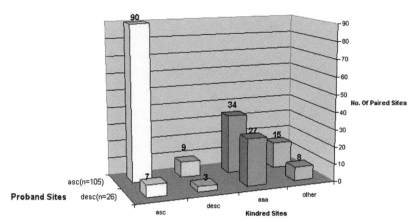

Fig. 8. Distribution of arterial aneurysms and dissection sites in kindred of familial probands. The location of the proband aneurysms influences the location of aneurysms in the family members. Probands with ascending aneurysms have family members with ascending aneurysm, whereas probands with descending thoracic aneurysm are more likely to have family members with abdominal aortic aneurysm.

the process by which thoracic aneurysms form. The pathogenesis of aneurysms is complex, involving, among other factors, inflammation, proteolysis, and disturbed survival and function of smooth muscle cells in the aortic wall.[13] The authors have looked specifically at the profiles of proteolytic enzymes in the aortic wall of aneurysm patients and compared these profiles to those of normal individuals. Work at Yale has implicated the MMP enzymes in the wall of the aorta as a prime agent of deleterious change in aneurysm and dissection disease. Marked elevation of the proteolytic enzymes (MMPs) and a marked depression of the inhibitory enzymes (TIMPs) have been found (**Fig. 10**).[14] Thus, in aneurysm patients, the balance is shifted strongly toward increased proteolysis, indicating an enzymatic attack on the fibrillin and

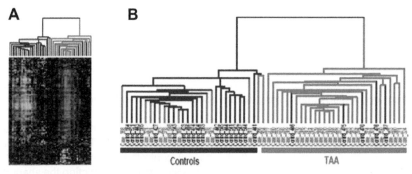

Fig. 9. The RNA signature test for thoracic aortic aneurysm. (*A*) In the hierarchical cluster diagram, each vertical line represents a patient, and each horizontal line represents an RNA. (*B*) In the grid, the lighter gray indicates underexpression and the darker gray indicates overexpression. The diagram on side A displays the overexpression and underexpression cluster, depending on phenotype. On side B, if all the lighter grays were together and all the darker grays were together, the test would have been 100% accurate. As it turns out, the overall accuracy was more than 82%.

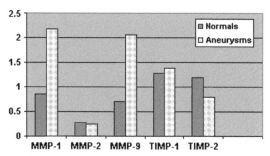

Fig. 10. The elevation of MMP-1and MMP-9 in aneurysm patients.

collagen that form the structural basis of the aortic wall. These lytic enzymes have a hand in destroying the aortic wall, so that, in an extreme case, it can become as thin and translucent as seen in the inset in **Fig. 10**.

What Mechanical Forces Play on the Dilated Aorta?

In addition to the changes in the microchemical environment that occur with TAAs, the mechanical forces at work in the aneurysmal aorta are different from those at play in the normal aorta. To better understand the role that these forces play, and the risks that they pose, a detailed engineering analysis on the aortic wall has been carried out on patients with ascending aortic aneurysms. The analysis was done by epiaortic echocardiography at the time of aortic surgery. The full spectrum of engineering calculations of the mechanical properties of the dilated aorta can be determined by measurement of 6 independent variables: aortic pressure in systole and diastole, aortic diameter in systole and diastole, and aortic wall thickness in systole and diastole. These measurements have shown that as the aorta enlarges, distensibility of the aortic wall falls, so that by about a size of 6 cm, the aorta becomes a rigid tube.[15] The end result is that because the aneurysmal aortic wall cannot stretch in systole, all the force of cardiac contraction is translated into wall stress. The result of this is that the enlarged aorta demonstrates a high wall tension. These findings are shown in **Fig. 11**. The dotted line in **Fig. 11**B represents the ultimate strength of the human aorta. During episodes of moderate hypertension, part of everyday life, an individual with a 6-cm aorta will flirt with the ultimate bursting strength of human aortic tissue (see **Fig. 11**B). The engineering data dovetail well with the clinical data. It is at 6 cm that the mechanical properties of the aneurysmal aorta deteriorate markedly. It is at precisely 6 cm that the malignant behaviors of the dilated human aorta (rupture and dissection) commonly become manifest.

A thinner wall, larger diameter, and increased intraaortic pressure all contribute to increased wall stress, and increased risk of aortic rupture or dissection. The authors have also demonstrated that times of physical or emotional stress tend to be present at the onset of aortic dissection.[16] Let us presume that a patient is rendered susceptible to aortic dissection due to his genetic makeup and then consider what factors or forces might precipitate dissection at one particular moment in time. A few years ago, the authors noticed a cluster of healthy young weight lifters who had presented to Yale with acute ascending aortic dissection and required urgent surgery. The authors reported this cluster in the Journal of the American Medical Association.[17] The authors did a biomechanical study on themselves and found that, during severe weight lifting, blood pressures approaching or exceeding 300 mm Hg were reached (**Fig. 12**). These

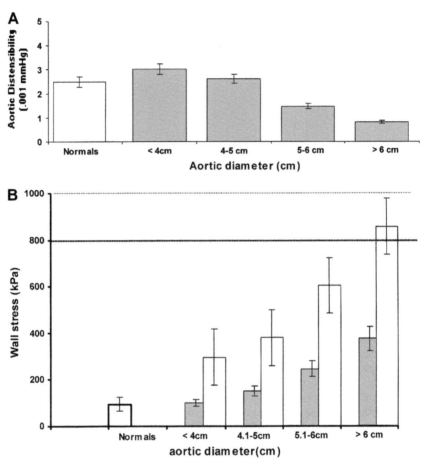

Fig. 11. (*A*) Distensibility values in normal aortas and aortic aneurysms of different diameters. Distensibility of ascending aortic aneurysms decreases rapidly as diameter increases to low values at dimensions greater than 6 cm. (*B*) Exponential relationship between wall stress and aneurysm size in ascending aortic aneurysms. The dark columns represent a blood pressure of 100 mm Hg, and the light columns represent a blood pressure of 200 mm Hg. The lines at 800 to 1000 kPa represent the range of maximum tensile strength of the human aorta.

are levels of hypertension simply not seen in any type of cardiac care, be it in the coronary care unit or in the cardiothoracic surgical unit. The authors hypothesized that extreme elevation of blood pressure during lifting was a factor in the cluster of dissections that had been treated in the weight lifters. After publication of their original report, the authors received details of cases from around the country. A follow-up report enumerated 31 similar cases of acute aortic dissection in the setting of weight lifting or other severe straining activity.[18] All of these dissections occurred in young men with previously unknown moderate aortic enlargement (4–5 cm). The authors recommended routine screening of all athletes embarking on weight lifting or other heavy athletic activity as the only means to protect these young athletes from needless death. The International Olympic Committee now requires an echocardiogram for every athlete competing in the Olympics. Another study was carried out in which

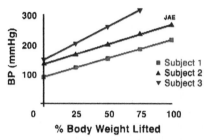

Fig. 12. Relationship of systolic blood pressure to weight lifted. There is marked elevation in blood pressure for these 3 scientists as they lift various percentages of their body weight in the bench press.

each patient or family member who had been treated for acute aortic dissection at Yale University was contacted. This investigation implicated emotion as well as exertion as a causative factor in the acute onset of aortic dissection. Specifically, most of the patients could recall a specific episode of severe emotional upset or extreme exertion at the time of their dissection. Dissection is so painful that most patients can remember the pain (**Fig. 13**). The authors conclude that the extreme increase in blood pressure from the emotion or exertion is the immediate precipitating trigger for dissection in a susceptible individual.

The susceptibilities to aortic aneurysm and dissection are set from birth by genetics. The aorta is destroyed over time, at least in part by excess proteolysis by the MMPs. The aorta enlarges as its wall is damaged. As the aorta enlarges, the mechanical properties deteriorate, with loss of distensibility and imposition of excess wall tension. An acute hypertensive event supervenes, usually emotional or exertional, and exceeds the tensile limit of the aortic wall, producing an acute aortic dissection or rupture.

RISKS OF THE TREATMENTS

Having explored the natural risks of TAA, and the biologic mechanisms of these risks, the risks of the growing number of treatments available are examined. The available treatments for TAA include conventional surgical, endovascular, and emerging

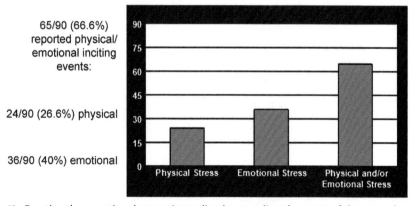

Fig. 13. Emotional or exertional events immediately preceding the onset of the pain of acute aortic dissection.

medical therapies. Unfortunately, there are no level one data to guide the decision making process. However, the observational data that have been collected, at our institution and others, can be reviewed.

Surgical Therapy

For the conventional surgical approach, the risks are well defined. The complications from 500 consecutive aneurysm repairs in the Yale Center have been analyzed. Overall mortality was 8.6%, with mortality for elective operations on the ascending/arch of 3.0% and mortality for elective operations on the descending aorta of 2.9%. Mortality for elective thoracoabdominal operations was 11.9%. Postoperative survival at 1, 3, and 5 years was 84.7%, 78.3%, and 72.5%, respectively. Among patients younger than 55 years of age, those who derived the greatest benefit from elective aneurysm resection, freedom from stroke, paralysis, or death was 98%.[19]

The techniques available for aneurysm repairs are as follows.

Aortic root

The specifics of the morphology of the proximal aortic root dictate the surgical procedure required to encompass the aneurysm pathology. For supracoronary aneurysms, tube graft replacement suffices. Concomitant aortic valve replacement may be necessary, depending on the degree of aortic stenosis or insufficiency. For aneurysms involving the proximal aortic root, with annuloaortic ectasia, composite graft replacement of the aortic root, and the aortic valve with a one-piece, prefabricated unit is required. This complex procedure requires meticulous reimplantation of the coronary arteries, with buttons of the surrounding aortic wall (**Fig. 14**). Recently, Yacoub and David and colleagues[20,21] have advocated techniques for valve-sparing aortic root replacement, which require further follow-up to determine their long-term efficacy compared with the gold standard composite graft replacement.

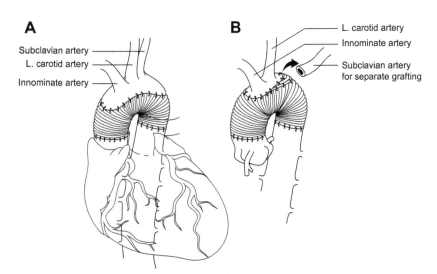

Fig. 14. (A) Methods of re-implantation of head vessels (with or without subclavian artery) using a Carrel patch of aortic tissue. (B) When subclavian artery is not included in the patch (to save time and improve exposure—preferred technique at Yale) it is re-implanted separately after completion of the aortic arch reconstruction.

Aortic arch

Fascinating techniques have evolved for the safe conduct of surgery on the aortic arch. These techniques revolve around (1) methods for reattachment of the great vessels to the brain and arms, and (2) methods for brain preservation during the arch surgery. For reattachment of the great vessels, the authors usually employ Carrel patches (with a rim of aorta carrying the innominate, left carotid, and left subclavian arteries; **Fig. 15**) or prefabricated branched grafts that permit individual anastomosis of each great vessel. To facilitate arch surgery in a still, bloodless field, the fascinating technique of deep hypothermic circulatory arrest (DHCA) is often employed. This technique was originally practiced in Siberia, where infants with holes in the heart were cooled outdoors in the snow, permitting quick open heart surgery without extracorporeal circulation. DHCA was repopularized, in its modern iteration, by Griepp and colleagues[22] in the 1970s and is now in widespread use. This safe and effective technique[23] depends on the exponential decrease in metabolic rate as organs are cooled, a 50% reduction for every 6° to 8° drop in temperature.[24,25] At 18°C, the temperature commonly employed, the metabolic rate is less than 15% of normal, permitting at least 30 to 45 minutes of safe operating time on the aortic arch. The authors have recently documented the safety of DHCA as a sole means of brain protection in aortic arch surgery in nearly 400 patients.[23] DHCA really represents real-life suspended animation, as there is no pulse, blood pressure, ECG activity, electroencephalogram activity, or blood flow during the arrest interval. If longer arrest periods are anticipated, direct cerebral perfusion, by cannulae placed individually in the great vessels, can be employed.

Descending and thoracoabdominal aorta

The key issues in surgery on the thoracoabdominal aorta revolve around (1) protection of the lower body organs during the period of time that the aorta is cross-clamped, and (2) methods for reattachment of the visceral arteries (superior mesenteric artery, celiac axis, and renal arteries). In terms of lower body perfusion, it is the spinal cord that is most vulnerable. The arterial blood supply of the spinal cord is segmental, and viability of the spinal cord cells can be dependent on an artery (arteria magna or artery of

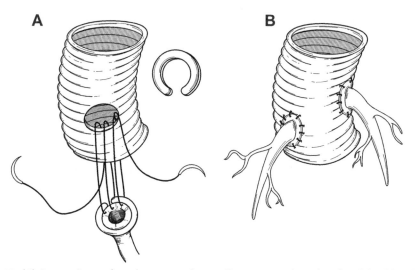

Fig. 15. (A) Composite graft replacement of ascending aorta and aortic valve. (B) With reimplantation of coronary artery "buttons".

Adamkewicz) or arteries arising from the low intercostal or lumbar territory (T8 to L2), which is temporarily or permanently excluded in the process of thoracoabdominal surgery. Intraoperative perfusion of the lower body by blood aspirated from the left atrium seems to be helpful in combating paraplegia.[26] Other techniques believed to be protective include mild systemic hypothermia, cerebrospinal fluid drainage to decrease ambient pressure on the spinal cord, and intercostal artery reimplantation.[27,28] The technical challenges of attaching all the important branch vessels of the abdominal aorta have been met by technical advances (forged by Crawford and continued by Cosellli, Safi, Kouchoukos, and others),[29–31] most specifically by the implementation of reimplantation of the branch arteries on pedicles of surrounding aorta, often by the inclusion technique (in which the pedicle is not mobilized completely from its bed of tissue). Current mortality for these operations runs less than 10%, and paraplegia rates are also equal to or less than 10%, reflecting technical improvements in graft technology, surgical techniques, perfusion, and aftercare.[19,32] Coronary artery disease is the most important risk factor for cardiac events and death in patients undergoing aneurysm surgery.[33–36] No well-designed studies are available that compare the outcome of serial myocardial revascularization and abdominal or TAA repair with aneurysm surgery alone. Efforts should be made to identify those patients at highest cardiac risk preoperatively using noninvasive diagnostic methods.[37,38] Abnormal findings indicating extensive myocardial ischemia may prompt angiography to determine the nature of the coronary artery disease and the level of left ventricular function. Thereafter, decisions regarding coronary revascularization must be based on symptoms, angiographic findings, and other elements of risk. It is reasonable to consider coronary revascularization before aneurysm surgery in patients with left main coronary artery disease, stenosis greater than 70% in each of the three major coronary arteries in the presence of impaired left ventricular function, and in those with active angina pectoris.

For patients with descending and thoracoabdominal aneurysms, the authors usually proceed directly to coronary angiography to determine conclusively whether significant coronary artery disease exists. If severe proximal disease is found in major vessels, the authors revascularize by coronary artery bypass grafting as a first stage; the aneurysm resection is done some weeks later. For patients having ascending aortic aneurysm resection, cardiac catheterization and angiography will have been performed as part of the cardiac assessment; the surgeon will be armed with the knowledge to perform concomitant cardiac surgical corrections, if warranted.

The advent of coronary arteriography by 64-slice CT scanning promises to change the field in terms of preoperative evaluation for coronary artery disease in patients facing aneurysm surgery. The authors are currently experimenting with concomitant 64-slice CT scanning for coronary anatomy, at the time of the CT scan for detailed assessment of the aneurysm morphology.

Endovascular Therapy for Aortic Aneurysms

Parodi and colleagues first reported the technique of transfemoral catheter-based repair of infrarenal abdominal aortic aneurysms in 1991 as an alternative for management of patients at high risk of complications with conventional surgical treatment.[39] Over the ensuing years, a variety of stent grafts and delivery systems have been introduced, many of which commonly require surgical exposure of the common femoral artery for sheath insertion. In addition, extraperitoneal abdominal incisions may be necessary to establish temporary access conduits to the iliac arteries when the size or tortuosity of the external iliac arteries precludes transfemoral cannulation. By avoiding major abdominal/retroperitoneal surgery or thoracic surgery, however, endovascular repair under general anesthesia has become a valuable alternative for patients in whom severe cardiopulmonary disease, advanced age, morbid obesity, or a previously instrumented abdomen present obstacles to safe, direct surgical reconstruction. A virtual frenzy of endograft placement has resulted, with radiologists, cardiologists, and vascular and cardiac surgeons participating in an environment that has often exceeded the valid indications for treatment and resulted in a seemingly endless series of compensatory endograft placements to compensate for shortcomings or complications of the original procedure. The endograft process requires large-bore patency of the iliac arteries (which poses a particular challenge in women, in whom the arteries are generally smaller and more angulated than in men) and suitable landing zones for seating of the proximal and distal limbs of the endograft. Stent therapy seems to have valid roles in ruptured aortic aneurysm (**Fig. 16**),[40,41] in traumatic transaction of the aorta,[42] and in penetrating ulcers.[43] An important study is underway in Europe evaluating whether prophylactic endograft therapy for stable, subacute Type B aortic dissections can improve the long-term natural history of this disease.[44] Initial presentation of data at meetings mandates caution, as multiple complications were noted in endograft treated patients. The role of endograft therapy in typical, fusiform degenerative aneurysms is much less clear. Endograft therapy can be administered safely and has a high rate of early technical success; endograft therapy still produces paraplegia in treating thoracic aneurysms, but this complication seems to occur at a lower rate than in open surgery.[41]

It is important to examine the phenomenon of endoleak, which, despite the euphemistic neologism, really represents a failure of therapy.[45] This new term refers to continued blood flow into the excluded sac of an aneurysm. Type I endoleaks are

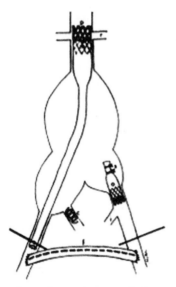

Fig. 16. The Montefiore system for endovascular control of ruptured abdominal aortic aneurysm. An endograft is placed from proximal to the aneurysm into 1 iliac. The other iliac is occluded endovascularly, thus isolating the ruptured aneurysm from the bloodstream. A cross-femoral graft is then performed to provide blood flow to the isolated leg. (The system relies on initial control of bleeding by a transbrachial balloon catheter inflated above the aneurysm, not shown in this diagram.) (*Reproduced from* Veith FJ, Gargiulo NJ, Ohki T. Endovascular treatment of ruptured infrarenal aortic and iliac aneurysms. Acta Chir Belg 2003;103:555–62; with permission.)

caused by incompetent proximal or distal attachments, producing high intrasac pressures that can lead to rupture, and need to be repaired using intraluminal extension cuffs or conversion to open surgery. Type II endoleaks result from retrograde flow from branch vessels (eg, the intercostal, lumbar, or inferior mesenteric arteries) and occur in as many as 40% of patients after endograft implantation. These may be corrected by selective arterial embolization, but more than half seal spontaneously and, when persistent, do not seem to increase the risk for rupture dramatically over a short-term follow-up.[46–55] Type III endoleaks are caused by fabric defects, tears, or disruption of modular graft components. These carry the same potential for delayed aneurysm rupture as Type I endoleaks and should therefore be repaired promptly. Type IV endoleaks, the least common, result from graft porosity and diffuse leakage through interstices and usually occur within 30 days of implantation. These and other complications become increasingly apparent as the follow-up of patients undergoing endograft repair increases and experience is gained. On the other hand, technical improvements in the graft devices and their deployment strategies may lead to improvements in complications as the field advances.

Because of the potential for endoleaks or other complications, follow-up imaging every 6 to 12 months is recommended following endovascular stent graft repair. As open surgical therapy becomes safer and safer, it remains to be seen whether endograft therapy has benefits. It remains to be seen whether endograft therapy is really effective in preventing aneurysm growth, aneurysm rupture, and aneurysm-related death. That endograft therapy is effective in achieving these essential goals is far from clear, and the data available are far from encouraging. It is important for medical science to evaluate endografting of aneurysms with enthusiasm for this new modality, but at the same time, with a grain of skepticism or at least realism. Multiple reasons to be cautious can be cited. Accordingly, one editorial has been titled "Endograft therapy of thoracic aneurysms: wave of the future, or the emperor's new clothes."[45]

Short duration of follow-up of an indolent disease

This line of reasoning leads to another major area of concern: TAA, although ultimately lethal, is an indolent disease. Many years are generally required from the time of diagnosis to the time of aneurysm-related death, especially with small- to moderate-size aneurysms (**Fig. 17**).[56] To have patients alive at 1 or 2 years (as in many abdominal and all thoracic endograft trials) is not at all reassuring. These patients would probably still be alive without any directed therapy whatsoever. As longer-term follow-up becomes available through the EUROSTAR investigation of endografting for abdominal aortic aneurysm, this concern literally comes to life, with mortality and rupture rearing their ugly heads, as the aneurysm disease expresses its natural history, even after successful endografting. The EUROSTAR study of endografting for abdominal aortic aneurysms is much more mature than corresponding studies of TAA. Endoleak becomes increasingly common as the duration of follow-up is extended (**Fig. 18**).[57] It seems that nearly 50% of patients will suffer diagnosed endoleak as follow-up becomes extended toward the 5-year point. It has been demonstrated that endoleak predicts a need for surgical conversion, rupture, and death, which in one EUROSTAR publication affected 14%, 13%, and 27%, respectively, of patients by 5 years postprocedure among patients presenting originally with large aneurysms; sobering statistics after endograft therapy.[58] Also concerning is the emergence of substantial rates of aneurysm-related death after endograft therapy, when follow-up extends to 4 years, especially for large aneurysms.[59] This is shown vividly in **Fig. 19**; the aneurysm is ignoring the endograft and merely expressing its natural tendency to rupture. In recognition of these sobering statistics, several major

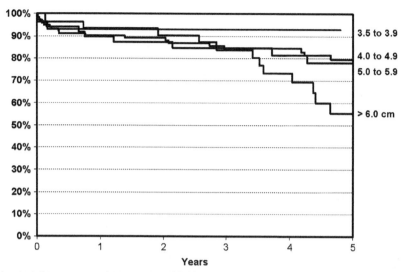

Fig. 17. Indolent nature of TAA. Survival before operative repair is show, for different size classes. Note that years generally pass before the mortality risk expresses itself, even for large aneurysms.

EUROSTAR publications conclude with serious cautionary statements about endograft therapy, calling attention to concerns about its long-term effectiveness and safety.[59–61]

Medical Treatment of Chronic Aneurysms

Patients with aneurysms are often treated with β-blocking medications, to decrease the virulence of the impact of systole on the aortic wall. The effectiveness of this treatment is largely unproven and somewhat controversial, but this has become standard

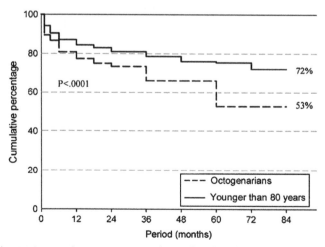

Fig. 18. Kaplan-Meier graph represents cumulative freedom from any endoleak in patients operated for abdominal aortic aneurysm with endovascular aneurysm repair. (*Reprinted from* Lange C, Leurs LJ, Buth J, et al. Endovascular repair of abdominal aortic aneurysm in octogenarians: an analysis based on EUROSTAR data. J Vasc Surg 2005;42:624–30; with permission.)

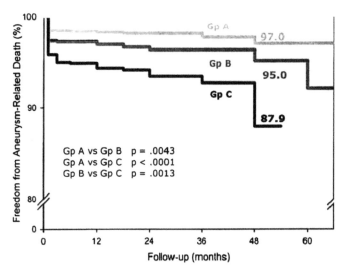

Fig.19. Cumulative freedom from aneurysm-related death after endograft therapy. Note the low attrition of survival in the first 3 years of follow-up and rapid attrition in the fourth year. Gp, Group. Groups represent increasing initial aneurysm size: Gp A = 4.0 to 5.4 cm, Gp B = 5.5 to 6.4, Gp C ≥ 6.5 cm. (*Reprinted from* Peppelenbosch N, Buth J, Harris PL, et al. Diameter of abdominal aortic aneurysm and outcome of endovascular aneurysm repair: does size matter? A report from EUROSTAR. J Vasc Surg 2004;39:288–97; with permission.)

practice. One long-duration study from Johns Hopkins of a moderate-size group (n = 70) of Marfan patients provides support,[62] but there is also reason for doubt regarding this therapy, especially for non-Marfan patients.[63] Concerns revolve around several issues: there is evidence that β-blockers decrease elasticity of the aortic wall, already deficient in aneurysmal aortas. There is concern about the side effects of β-blockers in young people, as treatment is often a lifetime decision. Furthermore, there is concern about a paradoxic adverse impact (increased mortality) in a blinded, randomized, controlled trial of β-blockers for abdominal aneurysm. Nonetheless, the authors do not object to the current standard practice of the prescription of β-blockers for aneurysm disease at the present time, as the negative evidence is not yet overwhelming. Other promising drug treatments are on the horizon (see later discussion). Of course, hypertension must be controlled in aneurysm patients to limit the disruptive forces on the aortic wall. β-Blockers may be important in this regard. Investigation of other medical treatments has also been carried out.[64] The antibiotic doxycycline, an MMP inhibitor, has been tested in large-scale clinical trials in patients with abdominal aneurysm and shows promise. Other drugs that hold theoretical promise and have undergone some animal or clinical testing include antiinflammatory agents (COX-2 inhibitors), statin drugs, immunosuppressants (rapamycin), and angiotensin receptor blockers (losartan).[13] None are of proven clinical benefit at this time. A great deal of excitement was generated by a recent report by Habashi and colleagues[64] showing dramatic suppression of aneurysm disease by the angiotensin receptor blocker, losartan, in an animal model of Marfan syndrome. Clinical trials are underway to investigate this exciting potential avenue of treatment.

PUTTING IT ALL TOGETHER: CRITERIA FOR INTERVENTION

Based on increasing understanding of the pathogenesis of TAAs, their rate of expansion, and their risk of progressing to complications, and based on the current understanding of the risks of various treatment methods, evidence-based guidelines for surgical intervention for TAAs have been formulated and are now widely adopted (**Fig. 20**).

The simple fact is that most ruptures, dissections, and aneurysm-related deaths can be prevented by preemptive extirpation of the aneurysmal ascending thoracic aorta before the critical dimension of 6 cm is reached. It is well known that dissection can occur in patients with Marfan disease whose aortic diameter is small. For this reason, the authors have decreased the intervention criterion for patients with Marfan disease to lower levels, namely 5.0 cm for the ascending aorta and 6.0 cm for the descending aorta. These criteria apply to asymptomatic aneurysms. Symptomatic aneurysms should be resected regardless of size. Symptoms are a harbinger of aortic rupture or dissection and must not be ignored. However, symptoms are rare in this disease; only about 5% of patients are symptomatic before an acute aortic event occurs. For the other 95% of patients, the first symptom is often death. Ascending aneurysms can produce retrosternal pain that is not exertional in nature, and descending aneurysms can produce interscapular back pain. Attention to these symptoms literally can be lifesaving.

Can one set of size criteria for surgical intervention can be applied to all individuals, regardless of body size? It is indeed appropriate to use body size corrections, especially for very small or very large individuals. The authors have been able to determine appropriate criteria for interventions based on an aortic size index, which takes into account aneurysm size and the patient's body surface area (see **Fig. 5**).

The subject of which method to use for repair is an issue of some debate. It is well accepted that ascending aortic aneurysms should be treated using a conventional operative approach. The use of endovascular therapy, with the limitations enumerated earlier, has been extended proximally in the aorta to now involve the aortic arch. Unfortunately, long-term data to support this approach are absent. For arch aneurysms, endovascular therapy should be reserved for those who cannot tolerate open repair, and who are involved in experimental protocols. For descending aneurysms, endovascular therapy should be reserved for those who either cannot tolerate open repair, have a short life expectancy, or have isolated, sacular aneurysms with normal proximal and distal aorta. Endovascular therapy can also be considered appropriate (even as an alternative to conventional surgery) for acute descending aortic transections, and perhaps for localized, single penetrating ulcers.

Greenspan and colleagues have defined conditions of irrational exuberance in the financial world. Irrational exuberance must be avoided in the application of endovascular therapies, despite the push by device manufacturers and the financial incentives to practices and institutions. Specifically, the criteria for intervention must not be made more liberal simply because endovascular therapy is being employed, as the

1. Rupture
2. Acute aortic dissection
   a. Ascending requires urgent operation
   b. Descending requires a "complication-specific approach"
3. Symptomatic states
   a. Pain consistent with rupture and unexplained by other causes
   b. Compression of adjacent organs, especially trachea, esophagus, or left main stem bronchus
   c. Significant aortic insufficiency in con-

junction with ascending aortic aneurysm
4. Documented enlargement
   a. growth ≥1 cm/y or substantial growth and aneurysm is rapidly approaching absolute size criteria
5. Absolute size (cm)

	Marfan	Non-Marfan
Ascending	5.0 cm	5.5 cm
Descending	6.0 cm	6.5 cm

Fig. 20. Surgical intervention guidelines for TAA from the Yale Centre.

long-term efficacy of such therapy for the virulent, but indolent, condition of degenerative thoracic aneurysm is far from secure.

SUMMARY

TAA is a formidable enemy. Once it occurs, the impact on short-term survival in symptomatic patients and on long-term survival in asymptomatic patients is severe. Although advances in imaging techniques and surgical sciences have succeeded to some extent in taming this disorder, it continues to exert a significant impact on the human race. Once the aorta has been rent into 2 layers, despite the most talented surgical efforts, the outlook for that aorta, and, consequently, for the patient, will be irrevocably impaired. The best hope resides in predicting and preventing aortic dissection so that it does not occur. Natural history investigations have clarified criterion levels for preemptive intervention on the basis of aortic size. If the RNA expression studies discussed earlier bear fruit, it may become possible to predict the diathesis for dissection from a simple blood test.[7] Understanding the genetic underpinnings of dissection disease may, in the future, permit conventional therapies aimed at strengthening the abnormal structural proteins coded by those genes. Even specific genetic remedies can be envisioned for the future. As more is learnt about the behavior, monitoring, and management of TAAs, the brighter the future for the increasing number of physicians, colleagues and patients who battle with this disease.

REFERENCES

1. Clouse WD, Hallett JW Jr, Schaff HV, et al. Improved prognosis of thoracic aortic aneurysms: a population-based study. JAMA 1998;280(22):1926–9.
2. Clouse WD, Hallett JW Jr, Schaff HV, et al. Acute aortic dissection: population-based incidence compared with degenerative aortic aneurysm rupture. Mayo Clin Proc 2004;79(2):176–80.
3. Johansson G, Markstrom U, Swedenborg J. Ruptured thoracic aortic aneurysms: a study of incidence and mortality rates. J Vasc Surg 1995;21(6):985–8.
4. Centers for Disease Control and Prevention. National Center for Health Statistics, National Hospital Discharge Survey, 2001. Available at: http://webapp.cdc.gov/cgi-bin/broker.exe.
5. Olsson C, Thelin S, Stahl E, et al. Thoracic aortic aneurysm and dissection: increasing prevalence and improved outcomes reported in a nationwide population-based study of more than 14,000 cases from 1987 to 2002. Circulation 2006; 114:2611–8.
6. Anagnostopoulos CE. Acute aortic dissection. Baltimore (MD): University Park Press; 1975.
7. Rizzo JA, Coady MA, Elefteriades JA. Procedures for estimating growth rates in thoracic aortic aneurysms. J Clin Epidemiol 1998;51(9):747–54.
8. Koullias GJ, Korkolis DP, Ravichandran P, et al. Tissue microarray detection of matrix metalloproteinases, in diseased tricuspid and bicuspid aortic valves with or without pathology of the ascending aorta. Eur J Cardiothorac Surg 2004; 26(6):1098–103.
9. Morales DLS, Quin JA, Braxton JH, et al. Experimental confirmation of effectiveness of fenestration in acute aortic dissection. Ann Thorac Surg 1998;66:1679–83.
10. Coady MA, Davies RB, Roberts M, et al. Familial patterns of thoracic aortic aneurysm. Arch Surg 1999;134:361–7.

11. Albornoz G, Coady MA, Roberts M, et al. Familial thoracic aortic aneurysms and dissections—incidence, modes of inheritance, and phenotypic patterns. Ann Thorac Surg 2006;82(4):1400–5.
12. Wang Y, Barbacioru CC, Shiffman D, et al. Gene expression signature in peripheral blood detects thoracic aortic aneurysm. PLoS ONE 2007;2(10):e1050.
13. Hackman AE, LeMaire SA, Thompson RW. Long term suppressive therapy: clinical reality and future prospects. In: Elefteriades JA, editor. Acute aortic disease. New York: Informa Healthcare; 2007. p. 309–30.
14. Koullias GJ, Ravichandran P, Korkolis DP, et al. Increased tissue microarray MMP expression favors proteolysis in thoracic aortic aneurysms and dissections. Ann Thorac Surg 2004;78(6):2106–10.
15. Koullias G, Modak RK, Korkolis D, et al. Mechanical and elastic properties of the normal and aneurysmal ascending aorta by intraoperative epiaortic echocardiography. J Am Coll Cardiol 2003;41:6(Suppl 2):513a.
16. Hatzaras IS, Bible JE, Kallias GJ, et al. Role of exertion or emotion as inciting events for acute aortic dissection. Am J Cardiol 2007;100:1470–2.
17. Elefteriades AJ, Hatzaras I, Tranquilli M, et al. Weight lifting and rupture of silent aortic aneurysms. JAMA 2003;290:2803.
18. Hatzaras I, Tranquilli M, Coady MA, et al. Weight lifting and aortic dissection: more evidence for a connection. Cardiology 2006;107(2):103–6.
19. Achneck HE, Rizzo JA, Tranquilli M, et al. Safety of thoracic aortic surgery in the present era. Ann Thorac Surg 2007;84(4):1180–5 [discussion: 1185].
20. David TE, Ivanov J, Armstrong S, et al. Aortic valve-sparing operations in patients with aneurysms of the aortic root or ascending aorta. Ann Thorac Surg 2002;74: S1758–61.
21. Yacoub MH, Gehle P, Chandrasekaran V, et al. Late results of a valve-sparing operation in patients with aneurysms of the ascending aorta and root. J Thorac Cardiovasc Surg 1998;115:1080–90.
22. Griepp RB, Stinson EB, Hollinngsworth JF, et al. Prosthetic replacement of the aortic arch. J Thorac Cardiovasc Surg 1975;70:1051–63.
23. Gega A, Rizzo JA, Johnson MH, et al. Straight deep hypothermic arrest: experience in 394 patients supports its effectiveness as a sole means of brain preservation. Ann Thorac Surg 2007;84:759–66.
24. Taylor KM. Cardiac surgery and the brain: an introduction. In: Smith P, Taylor K, editors. Cardiac surgery and the brain. London: Edward Arnold; 1993. p. 1–14.
25. Weir DL. The use of thiopental and propofol. In: Smith P, Taylor K, editors. Cardiac surgery and the brain. London: Edward Arnold; 1993. p. 245–51.
26. Olivier HF Jr, Maher TD, Liebler GA, et al. Use of the BioMedicus centrifugal pump in traumatic tears of the thoracic aorta. Ann Thorac Surg 1984;38: 586–91.
27. Hilgenberg AD. Spinal cord protection for thoracic aortic surgery. In: Elefteriades JA, editor. Diseases of the aorta. Cardiol Clin 1999;17:807–13.
28. Elefteriades JA, Coady MA, Nikas DJ, et al. "Cobrahead" graft for intercostal artery implantation during descending aortic replacement. Ann Thorac Surg 2000;69:1282–4.
29. Coselli JS, LeMaire SA. Surgical techniques: thoracoabdominal aorta. In: Elefteriades JA, editor. Diseases of the aorta. Cardiol Clin 1999;17:751–65.
30. Kouchoukos NT, Masetti P, Murphy S. Hypothermic cardiopulmonary bypass and circulatory arrest in the management of extensive thoracic and thoracoabdominal aortic aneurysms. Semin Thorac Cardiovasc Surg 2003;15:333–9.

31. Jacobs MJ, Meylaerts SA, de Haan P, et al. Assessment of spinal cord ischemia by means of evoked potential monitoring during thoracoabdominal aortic surgery. Semin Vasc Surg 2000;13:299–307.

32. LeMaire SA, Miller CC 3rd, Conklin LD, et al. A new predictive model for adverse outcomes after elective thoracoabdominal aortic aneurysm repair. Ann Thorac Surg 2001;71:1233–8.

33. Gill JB, Ruddy TD, Newell JB, et al. Determination of cardiac risk by dipyrida-mole-thallium imaging before peripheral vascular surgery. N Engl J Med 1985; 312:389–94.

34. Eagle KA, Coley CM, Newell JB, et al. Combining clinical and thallium data optimizes preoperative assessment of cardiac risk before major vascular surgery. Ann Intern Med 1989;110:859–86.

35. Leppo J, Plaja J, Gionet M, et al. Noninvasive evaluation of cardiac risk before elective vascular surgery. J Am Coll Cardiol 1987;9:269–76.

36. Raby KE, Goldman L, Creager MA, et al. Correlation between preoperative ischemia and major cardiac events after peripheral vascular surgery. N Engl J Med 1989;321:1296–300.

37. McCollum CH, Garcia-Rinaldi R, Graham JM, et al. Myocardial revascularization prior to subsequent major surgery in patients with coronary artery disease. Surgery 1977;81:302–4.

38. Fleisher LA, Rosenbaum SH, Nelson AH, et al. The predictive value of preoperative silent ischemia for postoperative ischemic cardiac events in vascular and nonvascular surgery patients. Am Heart J 1991;122:980–6.

39. Parodi JC, Palmaz JC, Barone HD. Transfemoral intraluminal graft implantation for abdominal aortic aneurysms. Ann Vasc Surg 1991;5:491–9.

40. Veith FJ, Gargiulo NJ, Ohki T. Endovascular treatment of ruptured infrarenal aortic and iliac aneurysms. Acta Chir Belg 2003;103:555–62.

41. Brinster DR, Szeto WY, Bavaria JE. Endovascular thoracic aortic stent grafting in acute aortic catastrophes. In: Elefteriades JA, editor. Acute Aortic Disease 1999;17:269–308.

42. Reed AB, Thompson JK, Crafton CJ, et al. Timing of endovascular repair of blunt traumatic thoracic aortic transections. J Vasc Surg 2006;43:684–8.

43. Kaya A, Heijmen RH, Overtoom TT, et al. Thoracic stent grafting for acute aortic pathology. Ann Thorac Surg 2006;82:560–5.

44. Nienaber CA, Zannetti S, Barbieri B, et al. Investigation of stent grafts in patients with type B aortic dissection: design of the INSTEAD trial—a prospective, multicenter European randomized trial. Am Heart J 2005;149:592–9.

45. Elefteriades JA, Percy A. Endovascular stenting for descending aneurysms: wave of the future or the emperor's new clothes? J Thorac Cardiovasc Surg 2007;133:285–8.

46. White RA, Donayre C, Walot I, et al. Abdominal aortic aneurysm rupture following endoluminal graft deployment: report of a predictable event. J Endovasc Ther 2000;7:257–62.

47. Abraham CZ, Chuter TA, Reilly LM, et al. Abdominal aortic aneurysm repair with the Zenith stent graft: short to midterm results. J Vasc Surg 2002;36:217–24 [discussion: 224–5].

48. Zarins CK, White RA, Hodgson KJ, et al. Endoleak as a predictor of outcome after endovascular aneurysm repair: AneuRx multicenter clinical trial. J Vasc Surg 2000;32:90–107.

49. Zarins CK, White RA, Moll FL, et al. The AneuRx stent graft: four-year results and worldwide experience 2000. J Vasc Surg 2001;33:s135–45.

50. Sapirstein W, Chandeysson P, Wentz C. The Food and Drug Administration approval of endovascular grafts for abdominal aortic aneurysm: an 19-month retrospective. J Vasc Surg 2001;34:180–3.
51. Stelter W, Umscheid T, Ziegler P. Three-year experience with modular stent-graft devices for endovascular AAA treatment. J Endovasc Surg 1997;4:362–9.
52. Greenberg RK, Lawrence-Brown M, Bhandari G, et al. An update of the Zenith endovascular graft for abdominal aortic aneurysms: initial implantation and mid-term follow-up data. J Vasc Surg 2001;33:s157–64.
53. Broeders IA, Blankensteijn JD, Wever JJ, et al. Mid-term fixation stability of the EndoVascular Technologies endograft. EVT Investigators. Eur J Vasc Endovasc Surg 1999;18:300–7.
54. Makaroun MS, Deaton DH. Is proximal aortic neck dilatation after endovascular aneurysm exclusion a cause for concern? J Vasc Surg 2001;33:S39–45.
55. Silverberg D, Baril DT, Ellozy SH, et al. An 8-year experience with type II endo-leaks: natural history suggests selective intervention is a safe approach. J Vasc Surg 2006;44:453–9.
56. Coady MA, Rizzo JA, Hammond GL, et al. What is the appropriate size criterion for resection of thoracic aortic aneurysms? J Thorac Cardiovasc Surg 1997;113:476–91.
57. Lange C, Leurs LJ, Buth J, et al. Endovascular repair of abdominal aortic aneu-rysm in octogenarians: an analysis based on EUROSTAR data. J Vasc Surg 2005; 42:624–30.
58. Waasderp EJ, de Vries JP, Hobo R, et al. Aneurysm diameter and proximal aortic neck diameter influence clinical outcome of endovascular abdominal aortic repair: a 4-year EUORSTAR experience. Ann Vasc Surg 2005;19:757–9.
59. Peppelenbosch N, Buth J, Harris PL, et al. Diameter of abdominal aortic aneu-rysm and outcome of endovascular aneurysm repair: does size matter? A report from EUROSTAR. J Vasc Surg 2004;39:288–97.
60. Hobo R, Buth J, and the EUROSTAR investigators. Secondary interventions following endovascular abdominal aortic aneurysm repair using current endog-rafts. A EUROSTAR report. J Vasc Surg 2006;43:896–902.
61. Leurs LJ, Bell R, Degrieck Y, et al. Endovascular treatment of thoracic aortic diseases: combined experience from the EUROSTAR and United Kingdom thoracic endograft registries. J Vasc Surg 2004;40:670–80.
62. Shores J, Berger KR, Murphy EA, et al. Progression of aortic dilatation and the benefit of long-term beta-adrenergic blockade in Marfan's syndrome. N Engl J Med 1994;330(19):1335–41.
63. Sanz J, Einstein J, Fuster V. Acute aortic dissection: anti-impulse therapy. In: Elefteriades JA, editor. Acute aortic disease. New York: Informa Healthcare; 2007. p. 229–49.
64. Habashi JP, Judge DP, Holm TM, et al. Losartan, an AT1 antagonist, prevents aortic aneurysm in a mouse mode syndrome. Science 2006;312:117–21.

Approach to the Treatment of Aortic Dissection

Marc R. Moon, MD

KEYWORDS

- Acute dissection • Chronic dissection
- Diagnosis • Surgical treatment • Medical treatment
- Endovascular treatment

Acute aortic dissection is the most common catastrophic event that involves the aorta, presenting to the emergency room much more often than a ruptured abdominal aortic aneurysm.[1] Timely intervention, whether medical, surgical, or endovascular, is essential to yield the best short-term and long-term results for patients with acute dissection, who are often only a few hours away from death. Unfortunately, the ability of acute aortic dissections to masquerade as a myriad of other pathologic processes can make the diagnosis difficult to pinpoint at times. An aortic dissection essentially represents a pathologic state in which a tear occurs in the intima of the aortic wall, allowing blood to split the aorta in two, like an onion peeling apart. Dissections swirl down the aorta for a variable length, shearing off side branches along the way. Most commonly, the entry tear is short (0.5–3 cm in length or less) and located at the proximal extent of the dissection, with the false lumen extending distally as a consequence of blood shearing off the inner layers in an antegrade fashion. Retrograde dissection can also occur, but it is much less common. **Fig. 1** demonstrates a typical dissection in the ascending aorta on transesophageal echocardiography (TEE). **Fig. 2** demonstrates a typical dissection in the descending aorta on TEE. Side branch involvement occurs in 30%, due to either compression of the branch by the distended false lumen, or by shearing off the side branch as the dissection travels beyond. The most common vessels involved clinically are the renal and iliac arteries, followed by the mesenteric, cerebral, coronary, and spinal arteries.[2–5] Although fenestrations between the true and false lumen are most frequent at branch points, fenestrations can occur anywhere along the aorta, allowing blood to travel between the two lumens in locations beyond the primary tear.

Division of Cardiothoracic Surgery, Center for Diseases of the Thoracic Aorta, Washington University School of Medicine, 660 S. Euclid Avenue, Box 8234, Saint Louis, MO 63110, USA
E-mail address: moonm@wustl.edu

Surg Clin N Am 89 (2009) 869–893
doi:10.1016/j.suc.2009.05.003
0039-6109/09/$ – see front matter

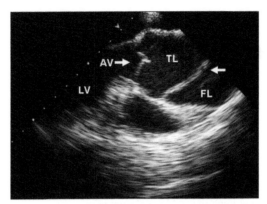

Fig. 1. Transesophageal echocardiogram demonstrating a dissection flap (*unlabeled arrow*) in the ascending aorta. The arrow labeled AV is the aortic valve, LV is left ventricle, TL is true lumen, and FL is false lumen.

NATURAL HISTORY AND CLASSIFICATION OF ACUTE DISSECTION

Acute aortic dissections are lethal if not diagnosed early and treated with aggressive medical or surgical therapy. In a classic natural history study, Hirst and associates demonstrated 30% mortality by 24 hours, 50% mortality by 48 hours, and 90% mortality at 1 year in 505 patients with acute aortic dissection (**Fig. 3**).[6] This study is the source for the commonly referenced "one percent per hour" mortality rate for the first 48 hours following acute dissection. The clinical manifestations of aortic dissection are protean, and some reports suggest that 25% to 50% of aortic dissections are misdiagnosed.[7,8] As for other catastrophic disease processes, a "high-index of suspicion" is important, but it is important to remember that less than 1% of patients with chest or back pain on presentation to the emergency room have an aortic dissection.[9,10]

Numerous classification systems have been proposed, but the 2 that have stood the test of time are the DeBakey classification (3 types: I, II, and III) and the Stanford classification (2 types: A and B).[11,12] The Stanford classification is the most important for determining the need for surgical intervention. **Fig. 4** demonstrates the classification systems.[13] The Stanford system is a functional classification that separates dissections into type A (involving the ascending aorta) (**Fig. 5**) and type B (not involving

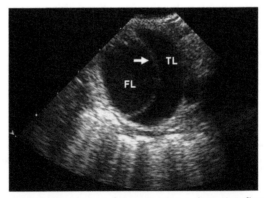

Fig. 2. Transesophageal echocardiogram demonstrating a dissection flap (*arrow*) in the descending aorta. The false lumen (FL) is typically larger and often compresses the true lumen (TL) potentially impacting distal aortic flow.

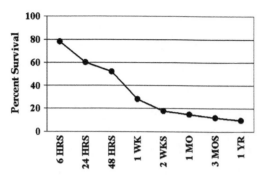

Fig. 3. Mortality rate of untreated acute aortic dissection. (*Data from* Hirst AD, Johns VJ, Kime SW. Dissecting aneurysm of the aorta: a review of 505 cases. Medicine 1958;37:217–79.)

the ascending aorta) (**Figs. 6** and **7**) regardless of the location of the primary tear or the distal extent of the dissection. The DeBakey classification subcategorizes the Stanford type A into either a DeBakey type I or II, depending on its distal extent. DeBakey type I dissections extend beyond the ascending aorta, generally into the descending and possibly abdominal aorta. DeBakey type II dissections do not extend beyond the ascending aorta, the surgical implications of which are that the entire length of the dissection can be replaced without having to deal with the arch (**Fig. 8**). DeBakey type III dissections are equivalent to Stanford type B dissections.

In autopsy series, type A dissections outnumber type B dissection almost 2:1, with isolated arch dissections accounting for only 1% to 2%.[1,8] By far, the most common cause of death in untreated type A dissection is intrapericardial rupture with tamponade (80%–90%) followed by extrapericardial rupture (5%–10%) and obstruction of an aortic tributary causing end-organ failure (5%–10%).[6] The most common causes of death in untreated type B dissection are rupture (60%), which is usually intrathoracic, and obstruction of an aortic tributary causing end-organ failure (40%).

WHEN AND WHY DO DISSECTIONS OCCUR?

Dissections can present at a young age in patients with Marfan syndrome or other connective tissue diseases (Ehlers-Danlos, Loeys-Dietz, Turner syndrome), but they

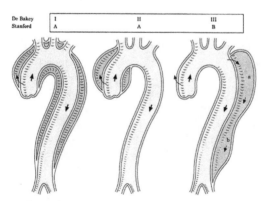

Fig. 4. The Debakey and Stanford classification systems for aortic dissection. (*From* Erbel R, Alfonso F, Boileau C, et al. Diagnosis and management of aortic dissection. Eur Heart J 2001;22:1642–81; with permission.)

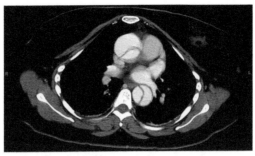

Fig. 5. CT scan demonstrating a Stanford type A dissection that not only involves the ascending aorta but also the descending aorta.

are most common in the 40- to 70-year-old age groups.[5,6] In patients greater than 40 years of age, hypertension is overwhelmingly the most common predisposing factor. In either age group, it is important to consider bicuspid aortic valve disease as a predisposing factor, because dissections are 5 to 10 times more common than in patients with trileaflet valves.[14] The "classic" patient with an acute aortic dissection is a hypertensive man in his 50s, but, unfortunately, this is also the "classic" patient with coronary artery disease. Therefore, although it is interesting to identify subgroups that are most commonly affected, it is not helpful in the diagnosis of an individual patient.

Bicuspid Aortic Disease

Bicuspid aortic valves are often associated with ascending aortic dilation and dissections.[15] At Washington University, the incidence of an ascending aortic aneurysm in patients with bicuspid valves undergoing aortic valve replacement is 22%.[16] The classic teaching that ascending aortic dilation in patients with valvular disease is the consequence of abnormal flow patterns in the root with stenosis or regurgitation does not explain the increased incidence of ascending aortic involvement in patients with bicuspid valves. The authors have identified increased expression of genes associated with cell death and apoptosis (interleukin-1-β, tumor necrosis factor-α) in ascending aortic aneurysms, but not genes associated with atherosclerosis and inflammation (apolipoprotein-E, interleukin-8), as are typically found in descending thoracic and abdominal aortic aneurysms.[17] These findings are consistent with our

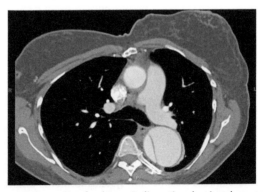

Fig. 6. CT scan demonstrating a Stanford type B dissection (no involvement of the ascending aorta).

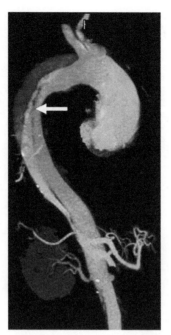

Fig. 7. Three-dimensional CT scan demonstrating a Stanford type B dissection (the *arrow* identifies the dissection flap).

biochemical and histologic analysis demonstrating elastin fragmentation and noninflammatory loss of smooth muscle cells in the ascending aorta of patients with bicuspid valves with a diminution in collagen content strikingly similar to that observed in Marfan syndrome (**Fig. 9**).[18] In contrast to aneurysms associated with Marfan syndrome, however, the genetic predilection to dilation seems mainly to affect the ascending aorta above the sinotubular junction, with relative sparing of the sinuses and arch in many cases. The Stanford group demonstrated recently that the proximal and distal extent of the aortopathy in bicuspid disease represents a spectrum of variable phenotypic expression.[19]

Hypertension and Aortic Wall Stress

In patients with degenerative or atherosclerotic aneurysms, hypertension is the most important factor for instigating a dissection. Elefteriades' group at Yale identified either physical exertion or emotional stress as the direct predecessor of acute pain in two thirds of acute dissections,[20] presumably due to acute blood pressure changes during the event. Ascending aortic tissue was harvested from 35 patients with aneurysms for biomechanical testing.[21] Force transducers were employed for biaxial testing and it was found that, with regard to their respective impact on the determination of aortic wall stress, a 26-mm Hg increase in systolic blood pressure was equivalent to a 1-cm increase in aortic diameter. For example, wall stress in a patient with a 4-cm aorta and a systolic blood pressure of 172 mm Hg is equivalent to a patient with a 6-cm aorta and a systolic blood pressure of 120 mmHg. In addition, the burst strength of intact ascending aortic rings, which identifies the point of stress failure (ie, rupture or dissection), was intimately related to age. Older patients had a greater opening angle, representing stiffer tissue with diminished wall strength (**Fig. 10**). Thus,

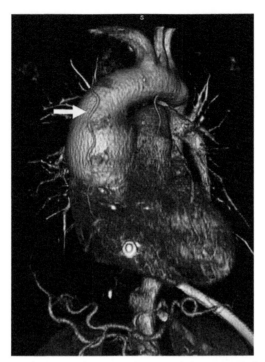

Fig. 8. Three-dimensional CT scan demonstrating a DeBakey type II dissection (the *arrow* identifies the dissection flap).

our biomechanical studies demonstrated that the risk of aortic rupture and dissection is directly related to patient age, aortic size, and blood pressure. Studies examining the cellular and molecular perturbations of ascending aortic disease have also demonstrated an important role for matrix metalloproteinases (specifically MMP-2 and

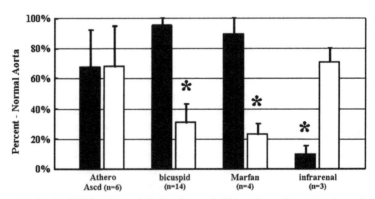

Fig. 9. Aortic elastin (black columns) and collagen (white columns) content in patients with aneurysmal disease of the ascending (atherosclerotic, bicuspid, or Marfan etiology) versus infrarenal aorta. *$P < .01$ versus normal thoracic (n = 8) or abdominal (n = 3) aorta. (*Data from* Curci JA, Thompson RW, Davis CG, et al. Heterogeneity of matrix changes in aneurysms of the thoracic and abdominal aorta. Circulation 2000;102(Suppl II):II-400.)

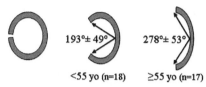

$193° \pm 49°$ $278° \pm 53°$

<55 yo (n=18)   ≥55 yo (n=17)

Fig. 10. Opening angle of intact rings of ascending aortic tissue. After severing rings of ascending aortic tissue, the rings either spring open (large opening angle), demonstrating increased stiffness and wall stress as in the older patients, or they remain intact (small opening angle), demonstrating decreased stiffness and wall stress as in the younger patients. (*Data from* Okamoto RJ, Xu H, Kouchoukos NT, et al. The influence of mechanical properties on wall stress and distensibility of the dilated ascending aorta. J Thorac Cardiovasc Surg 2003;126:842–50.)

MMP-9) and their tissue inhibitors (TIMP-1 and TIMP-2) in the pathophysiology of aneurysms and their progression to dissection.[22–27]

Can Aortic Dissections be Prevented?

Prophylactic oral β-blocker use in patients with Marfan syndrome has been reported to decrease hemodynamic stress and slow aortic growth due to their negative chronotropic and inotropic responses.[28] Prophylactic therapy seems most effective when aortic diameter is less than 40 mm, but although β-blockers may slow aortic growth, they do not prevent growth. Improved results have been suggested with the angiotensin converting enzyme enalapril, and more recently with the angiotension II receptor antagonist losartan in a mouse model of connective tissue disease.[29,30] The use of prophylactic agents in other high-risk groups, specifically patients with bicuspid valves, remains speculative, but as outlined in the discussion of how to manage patients with chronic dissections, it may be appropriate to initiate low-dose β-blocker therapy in patients with bicuspid valves and small aortic aneurysms, as long as there are no contraindications, especially if the patient is borderline hypertension.[31] As outlined in the 36th Bethesda Conference consensus report, exercise limitation is also warranted for patients with known ascending aortic aneurysms between 4.0 cm and 4.5 cm (only noncontact moderate-intensity sports) and for those greater than 4.5 cm (only low-intensity sports, such as bowling or golf).[32,33]

CLINICAL PRESENTATION AND DIAGNOSIS OF ACUTE DISSECTION

Patients with aortic dissection can present with a myriad of symptoms, and although "typical" symptoms are often present, it is not uncommon for patients to arrive in the emergency room following substantial improvement in their presenting complaints. Type A dissection typically presents with sharp, tearing anterior chest pain, often radiating to the neck or through to the back and abdomen, if the descending thoracic or abdominal aorta are involved. Although diaphoresis is common, shortness of breath and other respiratory complaints are less common than with acute coronary syndromes, unless contained rupture with tamponade is present.

Type B dissection typically presents with sharp, tearing pain between the shoulder blades that shoots down to the abdomen. Pain generally abates once blood pressure control is achieved unless there is end-organ compromise. With either type A or B dissection, compromise of the spinal artery or, much more often, one of the iliac arteries, can produce leg pain, parasthesias, or even paralysis. In such circumstances, unlike when treating paralysis or parasthesias that present following thoracoabdominal aneurysm repair,[34] the goal is to lower, rather than raise, systemic blood pressure to diminish pressure within the false lumen, which, with expansion, is generally responsible for obstructing true lumen flow.

It is important to specifically question the patient, rather than to blindly accept the history on the chart or the account of the patient's relatives or friends. Patients can often pinpoint the exact time at which the dissection occurred, which may have been several days before their presentation to the emergency room, yielding more of a subacute than acute presentation. It is not uncommon for a patient with a chronic type B dissection and aneurysmal dilation in the thoracoabdominal region to present to the emergency room with intrascapular, low back, or flank pain that has been present for 3 months following an initial inciting event for which they did not seek medical attention. Although aortic dissection has often been referred to as the "great imitator" in that the presentation can mimic many disease processes depending on the specific aortic tributaries it impacts along its course, with a careful history, its presentation can often be differentiated from a typical myocardial infarction or other catastrophic intrathoracic event. The power to differentiate, for example, an acute type A dissection from an acute coronary syndrome in a patient with a chronic dissection on a computed tomography (CT) scan (a clinical scenario that presents itself at least a couple of times every year in a busy aortic center), depends heavily on the history taken by an experienced aortic surgeon, more so than the physical examination. Nowadays, most trauma centers have rapid CT imaging capabilities, so in a patient with acute, tearing chest pain, following an electrocardiogram that does not show classic signs of acute myocardial infarction, a CT scan of the chest should be performed. Although patients with aortic dissection can present with coronary involvement producing myocardial ischemia and classic ST changes, such a presentation is uncommon.

Patients presenting with an acute coronary syndrome far outnumber those presenting with a type A dissection and myocardial ischemia. Most often, electrocardiographic changes are absent or nonspecific (diffuse ST depression due to pericardial irritation) in patients with an acute dissection.[35] Patients who present with an acute dissection that has sheared off or is obstructing one of the coronary orifices are most often in extremis, and although efforts to save the patient should not be abandoned, prognosis is poor.[36] A patient in extremis with tombstone ST changes is many orders of magnitude more common with myocardial infarction than dissection, and for a patient with a clinical picture and electrocardiogram changes most consistent with an acute coronary syndrome, transfer to the catheterization laboratory should not be delayed to perform a CT scan unless there are other circumstances that question the diagnosis.

Physical Examination

The most important aspects of the patient's evaluation for diagnostic purposes are the history and CT scan. The physical examination becomes important when determining the need (and ultimate approach) for surgical intervention. Important details of the physical examination include:

- *Systemic blood pressure.* Most patients with acute dissection present with severe hypertension, often greater than 200 mmHg systolic. A systemic blood pressure lower than normal (less than 100 mmHg systolic) in a patient with cold and clammy skin should prompt suspicion of a contained rupture with tamponade.

- *Differential blood pressures or pulses in the arms.* Involvement of the innominate artery or subclavian artery is important to identify to avoid maladaptive blood pressure manipulation due to inaccurate monitoring, dissuade use of the axillary artery as a cannulation source, and monitor appropriate flow following surgical reconstruction.
- *Central neurologic changes* (somnolence, coma, hemispheric neglect, or weakness) imply cerebral malperfusion, but not necessarily irreversible stroke. Carotid bruits or an absent carotid pulse, although rare, suggest dissection into the head vessels.
- *Jugular venous distention* suggests contained rupture with tamponade.
- *Cardiac murmurs.* Systolic murmurs are present in patients with underlying aortic stenosis (ie, with a bicuspid valve), and if associated with a transvalvular gradient should prompt valve replacement at the time of ascending aortic repair. Diastolic murmurs are loud along the left sternal border when acute aortic regurgitation is severe, which may alter the intraoperative perfusion and venting strategies. However, in contrast to the prevalent beliefs of the late 1980s, if the aortic valve leaks, it does not necessarily need to be replaced. It is now known that a competent valve is most often the result of a careful reconstruction of the sinotubular junction during ascending aortic repair, without the need to intervene on the valve.
- *Abnormal abdominal findings* (tenderness, distention, absent bowel sounds, flank pain) suggest visceral or renal malperfusion with impending ischemia.
- *Differential femoral pulses or loss of sensation or motor strength in the legs.* Differential femoral pulses in a patient without peripheral vascular disease (ask about chronic leg claudication) suggest iliac obstruction by the false lumen, which may alter the perfusion strategy during cardiopulmonary bypass. Neurologic changes can suggest spinal artery involvement but most often are secondary to iliac malperufsion and often reverse following adequate blood pressure control.

TEE Versus CT Scans

Some units have purported the benefits of TEE over CT scans for its specificity and sensitivity in diagnosing aortic dissection,[13] but at Washington University, although it takes more than 1 or 2 hours to set up for a TEE in the middle of the night, a CT scan can be performed and read by an attending radiologist (who may even be lying in his bed at home) in 20 minutes or less. If a dissection is suspected in the catheterization laboratory following a nondiagnostic coronary examination, a TEE is better than a makeshift low-contrast aortogram, but TEE is generally reserved as a secondary diagnostic tool in equivocal cases following CT imaging. In centers with more ready access to TEE, TEE may be used as a primary diagnostic tool, but it does have limitations depending on the experience of the examiner and his or her ability to visualize the entire ascending aorta and arch.

Transthoracic Echocardiography

Transthoracic echocardiography is most helpful in the acute setting to identify pericardial fluid or tamponade, quantify the degree of aortic regurgitation, and evaluate right and left ventricular function preoperatively. However, a well-performed examination can identify abnormalities in the aortic root and proximal ascending aorta, whereas the arch is difficult, if not impossible, to visualize.

Magnetic Resonance Imaging

Magnetic resonance imaging (MRI) should be reserved for the subacute or chronic evaluation of equivocal cases (ie, to identify the exact location of the initiation point of a dissection in the arch) or to image complex true versus false lumen anatomy in the arch or other branch vessels. In the last few years, MRI has become less important because three-dimensional CT scanning reconstruction techniques can generate beautiful images in patients who do not have a dye allergy or prohibitively elevated creatinine level. Branch vessel three-dimensional reconstructions are ideal when considering a percutaneous interventional approach to treat a peripheral complication (ie, superior mesenteric artery (SMA) stenting for intestinal ischemia or claudication). For acute diagnosis, MRI is not ideal due to prolonged imaging times, inaccessibility of the MRI scanner in most institutions, and its suboptimal environment for monitoring acutely ill patients.

Other (Less Helpful) Tests

Chest radiographs are essentially useless in the diagnosis of aortic dissection, because findings are either absent or so subtle that they cannot be identified on a portable emergency room examination. Furthermore, although mild cardiac enzyme elevation can occur, blood tests are generally unhelpful in the diagnosis. A couple of decades ago, aortography was considered the gold standard for diagnosis of dissection, but today, the only relevant application for aortography is during percutaneous intervention on an aortic tributary (branch vessel stenting) or the thoracic or abdominal aorta (distal fenestration or stent-grafting at the primary tear to improve distal flow).[4,37-41]

GENERAL MANAGEMENT OF ACUTE DISSECTION

With acute type A dissection, operative intervention is performed to prevent the expected sequelae of rupture with cardiac tamponade, acute aortic regurgitation as a consequence of loss of commissural suspension, or myocardial infarction secondary to coronary artery involvement. Operative mortality rates range from 10% to 25% compared with the 90% mortality rate at 3 months for nonoperative management (50% within the first 48 hours).[3,5,42-48] In contrast, acute type B dissections can most often be treated successfully with medical therapy alone as long as complications do not arise. The International Registry of Acute Aortic Dissections (IRAD) has been collecting data prospectively since 1996, and although mortality rates may be underestimated because several patients may have died before they could consent to participate in the study, it provides the best prospective, although unrandomized, contemporary comparison of medical and surgical therapy.[45] The IRAD investigators analyzed hospital mortality in 464 patients with type A (62%) and type B (38%) dissections from 12 centers. For type A dissections, mortality with medical therapy was more than double with surgical therapy (58% versus 26%). However, for type B dissections, mortality with medical therapy was only 11%, compared with 31% with surgical therapy. However, surgery in type B dissections was only performed if complications were present.[49]

With acute type A dissection, surgical intervention should be offered for all patients deemed survivable, including patients with signs of severe cerebrovascular accident (often mental status is impaired due to cerebral malperfusion that can completely reverse following aortic reconstruction),[50] patients in hemodynamic shock (most likely secondary to contained rupture with pericardial tamponade), and patients of all ages. For type B dissections, surgery is reserved for rupture, "impending rupture", malperfusion, persistent pain, and uncontrolled hypertension. Impending rupture is a difficult diagnosis, but the presence of frank blood (not serous or serosanginous fluid) in the pleural space has been used as a criterion to intervene. A reactive, serous, left pleural effusion will develop within 2 to 3 days in almost all patients with dissection in the descending aorta, which should not be interpreted as impending rupture and most often resolves in a few weeks. In addition, persistent pain is most often due to fluctuations in blood pressure, and most patients who return to the hospital with recurrent pain but a CT scan that is unchanged can be managed medically with resolution of symptoms. Occasionally, a patient will return with early dilation of the proximal descending thoracic aorta to 5 cm or greater. These patients may be considered for early surgical intervention, although it is ideal to wait 8 to 12 weeks if possible to allow the aortic wall to thicken and the flap to stabilize to improve surgical risk from a technical standpoint.

SPECIFIC THERAPEUTIC APPROACH FOR TYPE A DISSECTION

The initial goal of therapy in acute aortic dissection is to get the patient out of the operating room and out of the hospital. Issues that need to be addressed during surgical repair of a type A dissection include perfusion strategy, cross-clamping versus circulatory arrest, extent of proximal resection, and extent of distal resection. The specific technical aspects of surgical repair are beyond the scope of this report, but have been described in previous reports from our unit and from others.[8,51–54] The goals of surgical therapy in acute type A dissection are as follows:

- *Obviate the usual causes of death,* which are local phenomena in nearly 90% of cases. The proximal and distal aortic cuffs are reconstructed with a strip of Teflon felt interior and exterior, and occasionally between the intimal and adventitial layers, before insertion of an interposition graft. Reconstruction at both ends eliminates the false lumen proximally and directs flow into the true lumen distally. Reconstruction diminishes direct flow into the false lumen, decreasing the risk of intrapericardial rupture through the previously partial thickness false lumen wall.
- *Reverse hemodynamic shock.* Patients with hemodynamic compromise generally have a contained rupture with pericardial tamponade. Not uncommonly, such patients will sustain a hemodynamic collapse following induction of anesthesia. At that point, the initial surgical move should be to perform immediate sternotomy and open the pericardium to relieve tamponade. This is more important than getting the patient on pump by way of the groin, which may take longer than opening the sternum and does not address the immediate cause of the collapse. Once tamponade has been relieved, shock will reverse and femoral access can be obtained.
- *Extent of proximal resection.* Historically, it was felt that if the aortic valve leaked, it had to be replaced, but this is rarely the case. Patients with Marfan syndrome require total root replacement, and patients with bicuspid aortopathy require aortic valve replacement; however, most patients with aortic dissections have normal trileaflet aortic valves that leak when they are pulled apart consequent to dilation at the sinotubular junction. Following proximal reconstruction, the aortic valve is usually competent, without the need to address the valve itself. At Washington University, although aortic valve replacement was common in the late 1980s (greater than 50% of cases), it is currently rare (less than 10% of cases).[5]
- *Extent of distal resection.* After resecting the region of the aorta containing the primary tear, distal reconstruction can either be performed in the ascending aorta, or to the lesser curve of the arch, a so-called "hemiarch" procedure

with a beveled, open distal aortic anastomosis under profound hypothermic circulatory arrest (**Fig. 11**). The authors do not perform total arch replacement for acute dissection. Total arch replacement increases surgical risk substantially more than any potential benefit in regard to late reoperation. Studies from our center have found that the extent of distal resection does not have an impact on late survival or late reoperation on the distal aorta, although the need for proximal reoperation on the ascending aorta may be lower following hemiarch repair.[3,31] Each surgeon should select an approach with which he or she is most comfortable.

- *Correct compromise of contiguous aortic branches.* As presentation, branch vessel involvement is common; however, redirection of flow in the ascending aorta exclusively into the true lumen at the distal anastomosis is usually adequate to reverse malperfusion without intervention on the branch vessels themselves. The most common site of malperfusion that needs to be addressed following ascending reconstruction is one or both legs. If only one leg is malperfused, a femoral-femoral bypass is sufficient, but if both legs are malperfused, an axillary-femoral bypass may be required. Malperfusion to the renals or viscerals generally requires an interventional radiology approach for branch vessel stenting. Rarely, when there is obstruction to flow at the aortic level, an aortic stent-graft may help restore distal flow, but these types of advanced, experimental procedures should be reserved for centers with extensive endovascular experience.

- *Resect the primary tear.* The authors generally resect the primary tear if practical, but do not perform complete arch replacement during acute dissection unless there is rupture of the arch itself, which is rare. Total arch replacement in this setting is technically hazardous, increases bleeding (which is often troublesome), and doubles circulatory arrest times and mortality rates in most series.[51,55–57] If the primary tear resides in the descending aorta, it is left alone at the time of acute repair. Recent series from centers with extensive endovascular experience have reported initial success in reconstructing the descending aorta with open stent-graft placement at the time of hemiarch repair,[58] but as noted above, these advanced procedures should be reserved for selected centers with defined protocols.

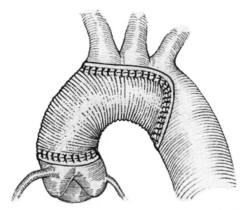

Fig. 11. Hemiarch replacement to the lesser curve of the aortic arch. (*From* Moon MR, Sundt TM: Aortic arch aneurysms. Coron Artery Dis 2002;13:85–92; with permission.)

- *Eliminate flow in the false lumen.* This is seldom accomplished. Studies have shown that the distal false lumen remains patent in most cases (up to 85%) after proximal thoracic aortic repair,[59] and in some cases (especially in chronic dissections), the false channel may be the only source of blood to major organs. At Washington University, the authors found that persistence of the false lumen was associated with a greater chance of aortic growth long-term, but not specifically with the need for late reoperation.[31] In the Mount Sinai series, extending the initial resection into the arch did not necessarily obliterate the false lumen;[48] 23% of patients who underwent partial or total arch replacement for an arch tear had a patent false lumen. Persistence of the false lumen depends more on the presence of distal fenestrations between the true and false lumens rather than complete resection of the primary tear.

Perfusion Strategy

Initial cannulation is generally by way of the femoral artery that has the strongest pulse.[60] After exposing the vessel, an 8-mm Dacron graft is sewn end-to-side to the common femoral artery. The authors prefer the side-graft to direct cannulation because it permits flow down the leg during the period of cardiopulmonary bypass, is immune to the problems associated with atherosclerotic disease of the iliacs or femorals, and at the end of the procedure can be stapled off without having to reconstruct the artery. Venous cannulation is performed following standard sternotomy. If circulatory arrest is planned, then the superior and inferior vena cavae are cannulated separately to allow for retrograde cerebral perfusion if desired. Retrograde cerebral perfusion allows additional cerebral cooling and back flushing of particulate matter during circulatory arrest. Details of retrograde cerebral perfusion can be found in several previous reports.[51,61-63] The axillary artery can also be used for cannulation (with a Dacron side-graft), but is not the initial choice in acute cases, simply because if it turns out to be dissected, manipulation can be troublesome. When cardiopulmonary bypass is initiated, TEE is used to document flow in the true lumen in the ascending aorta, and temperatures are measured above and below the diaphragm to ensure an even distribution of blood flow and cooling. If flow is not adequate, central aortic cannulation can be performed.[64]

Cross-clamping Versus Open Distal with Circulatory Arrest

The distal extent of the dissection repair can be performed either with a cross-clamp on the distal ascending aorta (anastomosis to the mid ascending aorta) or under profound hypothermic circulatory arrest (anastomosis to the mid ascending aorta or lesser curve of the arch). A complete description of the technical aspects of hypothermic circulatory arrest is beyond the scope of this article, but can be found in several excellent previous publications.[8,51-54,65] The potential benefits of using circulatory arrest are that it permits an open distal anastomosis (which may allow a more sound distal anastomosis), facilitates direct inspection of the arch to assess the extent of intimal disruption (if the tear extends into the arch), and avoids clamp injuries to the distal ascending aorta. However, recent studies have failed to demonstrate a difference in operative morbidity or mortality, long-term survival, or the incidence of late aortic growth and reoperation rate between circulatory arrest and cross-clamping,[31,42,66] and bleeding can often be troublesome following circulatory arrest due to extreme perturbations in the coagulation cascade. Our current thinking is that either approach is acceptable, as long as the entire tear is visible within the ascending aorta, and the final choice depends on the experience and preference of the aortic surgeon performing the repair. With either approach, following reconstruction of the distal aorta, the authors generally anastomose a 28-mm Dacron graft with a 10-mm prefabricated side-graft end-to-end. This procedure allows us to reposition the arterial cannula into the side-graft and reconstitute antegrade flow during rewarming, which has been associated with earlier neurologic recovery from circulatory arrest.[46,62] For high-risk patients in whom only a small segment of the aorta had to be removed to resect the primary tear, a primary anastomosis between the two reconstructed ends of the aorta may be possible after freeing up the distal aortic attachments. Such an approach is associated with less bleeding and shorter operative times than standard ascending aortic replacement, but it leaves a significant amount of ascending aorta in situ that may dilate over time.

Operative Results

At Washington University, during a 22-year period ending in 2006, 201 patients underwent acute type A dissection repair by 25 different surgeons. Mean age was 61 years (range 18–88 years) and 64% were men.[5] Operative mortality was 16%, and independent factors predicting death included concomitant aortic valve replacement, preoperative malperfusion, and non-Marfan syndrome patients. Cerebrovascular accident occurred in 5%, but the incidence was not related to the specific surgical technique (circulatory arrest vs cross-clamp, ascending replacement only vs hemiarch, use of retrograde cerebral perfusion). Long-term survival was 75% at 1 year, 63% at 5 years, and 49% at 10 years. Factors associated with diminished long-term survival included advanced age and the presence of coronary artery disease.

Subacute Type A Dissection

With rare exceptions,[67,68] patients who present to the emergency room soon after they develop symptoms should undergo emergent surgical intervention. However, it is not uncommon for the diagnosis of type A dissection to be delayed as a consequence of its complex presentation, such that transfer to a tertiary center does not occur for 48 hours or more following the initial tear. Patients who have survived several days after the onset of symptoms have been fortunate to have passed through the initial, most deadly period of the disease. The timing of surgical intervention under these subacute conditions was recently addressed in two studies from Yale, examining 93 patients over a 20-year period with a delayed presentation or diagnosis.[69,70] In essence, their question was: "If a patient is transferred or presents in the middle of the night with a dissection that occurred more than 48 hours earlier, is it essential to perform emergency surgery at that time, or is it safe to schedule the operation for the following morning?" Their short answer was: "No, it is not necessary to perform nighttime surgery for subacute dissections." Morbidity and mortality rates were similar to those who underwent immediate surgical intervention, leading the Tale group to conclude that patients who present several days after an acute type A dissection can safely be treated with an initial period of medical management, followed by a semi-elective, rather than emergent operation. However, such delays are not recommended within the first 48 hours, as patients can become unstable rapidly during this period. Many centers are simply not experienced enough to perform acute dissection repair, and in such circumstances, the patient's best chance for survival is transfer to a tertiary care hospital. The risks of delayed intervention to allow tertiary transfer are likely far less than immediate surgical intervention by an inexperienced aortic surgeon or surgical team.

Radiologic Versus Surgical Definition of Type A Dissection

The differentiation of aortic dissections into type A and type B represents a surgical definition not a radiologic definition, which is essential to determine the most appropriate initial therapeutic approach for each patient. Occasionally, an attending radiologist, with all good intentions, will dictate that a "type A dissection is present" when the tear resides in the arch, proximal to the left subclavian artery (for example, in the lesser curve across from the left carotid orifice). From a practical therapeutic perspective, if the primary tear extends distally from the arch, these patients should be treated as though they had a type B rather than type A dissection, considering that, with good medical therapy, the dissection will not extend retrograde to involve the ascending aorta. The intent when repairing or replacing the ascending aorta in an acute type A dissection is to eliminate the most common cause of death, that is, intrapericardial rupture with tamponade. Rupture is much more common with type A than type B dissection, potentially due to elevated developed pressure (dP/dt) and flow in the ascending versus descending aorta. With this in mind, emergency surgery by way of sternotomy when the tear resides in the arch is unnecessary. Thus, it is essential for aortic surgeons in busy tertiary centers to have extensive experience reading aortic CT scans (including normal, aneurysmal, and acute and chronic dissections) to allow the surgeon to most appropriately triage the patient from a therapeutic perspective.

SPECIFIC THERAPEUTIC APPROACH FOR TYPE B DISSECTION

Uncomplicated type B dissections are treated medically in most centers, and excellent results can be expected when therapy is continued long-term. Acute operations are performed only when complications are present such as rupture or malperfusion.[71–74] In the classic Stanford-Duke series of patients with acute type B dissection, the 30-day mortality for patients with no compelling indication for emergency operation was 10% with medical therapy versus 19% with surgical therapy.[74] In some centers, there has been a push toward early operation (proximal descending aortic replacement or stent-graft placement over the primary tear) in younger patients in an attempt to prevent the adverse late sequelae of persistent dissection.[58,75–78] Although this type of aggressive surgical approach seems intuitively logical, excellent short-term and long-term results can be expected with aggressive medical therapy, with most patients needing neither an early nor late surgical intervention.[79,80] All new prophylactic-based therapies must be compared with appropriate medical therapy before their widespread use can be advocated.

Estrera and associates in Houston followed 159 patients with a type B dissection who underwent an initial medical management strategy with surgery reserved only for complications.[79] Medical therapy alone was successful in 86% of patients with a mortality rate of 7%. When a surgical or endovascular intervention was necessary (14% of patients), the mortality rate increased to 17%. Overall, 1-year survival was 83% and 5-year survival was 75%. Hsu and colleagues[80] from Taiwan similarly reported excellent results with medical management of type B dissections. Medical therapy alone was successful in 85% of patients, with a 5-year survival rate of 99%. Endovascular options have become popular for complicated dissections, but their use in uncomplicated dissections remains unsupported.

Medical Management

The goals of medical therapy are to first decrease aortic and left ventricular peak dP/dt, then reduce mean, peak, and diastolic recoil aortic pressure. Intravenous β-blockers (typically esmolol) should be initiated to decrease dP/dt, followed by an afterload reducing agent (typically nitroprusside) if additional blood pressure control is needed. Often, decreasing blood pressure from the severely hypertensive levels that are generally present during the initial evaluation of a patient with an acute dissection can reverse malperfusion and stabilize the flap. Pain may wax and wane, possibly due to movement of the flap with blood pressure fluctuations, but severe pain should dissipate. During the initial hospitalization, a complex oral antihypertensive regimen may be necessary to achieve the desired level of blood pressure control, but following hospital discharge, it is often necessary to decrease drug dosages significantly. Blood pressure should be closely monitored (not only by the physician but also the patient) to ensure the most appropriate level of control long-term. Ideally, the patient should become familiar with their disease so that they can play an active role in monitoring changes in therapy.

Endovascular Therapy for Complicated Type B Dissections

Patients who develop ischemic complications due to distal aortic branch compromise should undergo angiographic investigation, potentially with CT or MRI angiography initially to create a three-dimensional roadmap of the aorta and its branches. Bare stenting of branch vessels or covered stent-grafting of the aorta itself can follow to increase distal flow, with or without fenestration of the dissection flap.[37,39–41] The dissection anatomy in these patients is often complex, and these procedures can be challenging. In 2003, the authors published early results for endovascular interventions in type B dissections with malperfusion,[37] and although our initial report was anecdotal in nature, 21 of 23 vascular territories were successfully reperfused with no hospital mortality and no late recurrent ischemia. Dake and associates from Stanford were the first to report their attempts to cover the primary tear with a covered stent-graft in 1999.[38] Using an archaic delivery system, they were able to completely thrombose the false lumen in 79% with a mortality rate of 16%. More recent studies have reported similar results, and studies to compare the endovascular approach to open surgery in complicated type B dissections are being developed.[71–73,76,77]

The goals of endovascular therapy are to reverse malperfusion with either a peripheral or central approach, re-expand the true lumen, exclude or close the primary tear, and obliterate the false lumen. Early experimental work from the Stanford laboratories demonstrated that intravascular stents could restore distal flow in acute type B dissection, but that obliteration of the false lumen required stents to be placed throughout the length of the dissection.[81] Stenting limited to the proximal dissection did not prevent the development of a chronic patent distal false lumen, probably due to branch vessel fenestrations distal to the stents. A study from Vienna evaluated the ability of a stent-graft implanted over the primary tear to thrombose the false lumen.[77] At the level of the stent-graft, they noted a 60% false lumen thrombosis rate immediately postoperatively that increased to 90% at 1 year. In contrast, just distal to the stent-graft, the thrombosis rates fell to 20% and 60% postoperatively and at 1 year, whereas at the celiac artery the rates were 0% and 22% postoperatively and at 1 year.

A meta-analysis of 37 studies was recently published examining the results of endovascular stent-grafting for acute type B dissections in 184 patients.[76] Using the IRAD database, 30-day survival with endovascular therapy compared favorably with medical therapy, both of which were significantly better than open surgical therapy. Also in 2006, the IRAD investigators reviewed 242 patients with acute dissection undergoing either medical (78%), open surgical (11%), or endovascular (11%) therapy with an overall hospital mortality rate of 12%.[82] Survival at 3 years was similar in all groups: 78% ± 7% for medical therapy, 83% ± 19% for open surgical therapy, and 76% ± 25% for endovascular therapy.

The most common indication currently for surgical intervention on the aorta (rather than its branches) in type B dissections is patients who demonstrate early growth (greater than 5 cm diameter) or recurrent refractory pain in the early months following successful initial medical therapy. Subacute dilation is usually isolated to the proximal descending aorta, for which elective proximal descending replacement or placement of a stent-graft over the primary tear should be considered if there are adequate proximal and distal landing zones. The goal is not to remove all dissected aorta, but rather to address the area of maximal dilation. Generally, following replacement of the proximal third of the aorta, the residual dissection will grow in less than 20% of cases with adequate medical therapy.[31,83]

INTRAMURAL HEMATOMA AND PENETRATING ULCER

Intramural hematoma is a variant of aortic dissection in which there is blood present in the aortic wall, but no tear can be identified.[84–88] **Fig. 12** demonstrates an intramural hematoma in the ascending aorta on TEE. Proposed causes include spontaneous bleeding in the wall, but may also simply represent a small entry hole that cannot be identified.[87] Intramural hematomas in the ascending aorta can progress to overt dissection or spontaneous rupture, but the rupture risk is less than with classic dissection. Acceptable results have been reported from a large series employing medical management as first line therapy for patients with type A intramural hematoma;[88] however, this approach requires aggressive monitoring until stabilization (generally for several days), with a watchful eye for progression to overt dissection. In general, it is probably best to perform urgent (not necessarily emergent) surgery in otherwise healthy patients to avoid progression to dissection, which occurs in about one third of patients despite aggressive medical therapy. Penetrating atherosclerotic ulcers in the ascending aorta with surrounding wall hematoma also have a significant risk of rupture and should be considered for urgent surgery if comorbidities do not portend a poor surgical outcome.[84,89,90] Intramural hematomas in the descending aorta should be managed similarly to type B dissection and have been known to resolve over 3 to 6 months with appropriate medical therapy.[91]

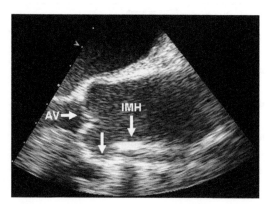

Fig. 12. TEE demonstrating an intramural hematoma of the ascending aorta. The arrow labeled AV is the aortic valve, the arrow labeled IMH is the intima of the intramural hematoma, and the unlabeled arrow is the normal aortic wall proximal to the intramural hematoma.

MANAGEMENT OF CHRONIC DISSECTION

In an attempt to identify important factors that could predict aneurysmal development in a residual dissected aorta, the authors followed 168 operative survivors following acute type A repair.[31] Late reoperation was performed in 15% of patients an average of 5 years postoperatively. Freedom from reoperation among operative survivors was 95% at 1 year, 90% at 5 years, 74% at 10 years, and 65% at 15 years. Risk factors that predicted the need for late reoperation included Marfan syndrome, a nonresected primary tear, absence of postoperative β-blocker therapy, and elevated systolic blood pressure late postoperatively. During long-term follow-up, the incidence of aortic growth between consecutive imaging studies was 18%, with a mean growth rate of 1.3 mm in the abdominal and 1.8 mm in the descending aorta. In several patients, aortic growth was not identified for many years postoperatively (6 years on average and up to 167 months in 1 patient), reinforcing our belief that follow-up for life is essential following successful treatment of an aortic dissection. Independent predictors of aortic growth included (1) increased aortic diameter, (2) patent false lumen, and (3) elevated systolic BP at late follow-up. The incidence of aortic growth increased from 14% to 15% for patients with late systolic BP less than 140 mmHg to 34% when systolic BP was greater than 140 mmHg.

DeBakey and associates were the first to suggest a relationship between poor blood pressure control and dilation in patients with aortic disease, noting that aneurysms subsequently developed in 46% of patients with uncontrolled hypertension, but only in 17% with controlled blood pressure long-term.[83] In our series from Washington University, ideal blood pressure control not only decreased the reoperation rate from 35% to 8%, but the incidence of aortic expansion also fell threefold.[31] **Fig. 13** illustrates the impact of poor blood pressure control on late reoperation, which approaches 50% to 70% at 15 years in those with less than ideal systolic pressures. **Fig. 14** demonstrates the impact of β-blocker therapy to diminish the need for late reoperation from 75% to 25% at 15 years.

To determine the appropriate time interval between which postoperative imaging studies should be obtained, the authors performed a two-way analysis of the impact of aortic diameter and time between scans on the chance of identifying aortic

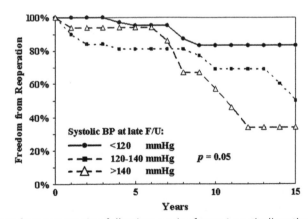

Fig. 13. Freedom from reoperation following repair of type A aortic dissection in relation to the degree of late postoperative systolic blood pressure control. (*From* Zierer A, Voeller RK, Hill KE, et al. Late aortic enlargement and reoperation after repair of acute type A aortic dissection. Ann Thorac Surg 2007;84:479–87; with permission.)

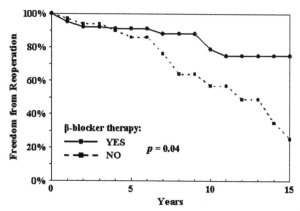

Fig. 14. Freedom from reoperation following repair of type A aortic dissection in relation to late postoperative β-blocker use. (*From* Zierer A, Voeller RK, Hill KE, et al. Late aortic enlargement and reoperation after repair of acute type A aortic dissection. Ann Thorac Surg 2007;84:479–87; with permission.)

growth.[31] **Table 1** demonstrates that when the aortic diameter is small (<35 mm), and the interval between scans is low, it is rare to identify growth. In contrast, when the aorta is large (>50 mm), growth is frequent at all intervals, reaching 83% for intervals greater than 1 year. At the Center for Diseases of the Thoracic Aorta at Washington University, the importance of long-term blood pressure control is reinforced to the patients, with a goal of maintaining systolic BP less than 120 to 140 mmHg, including β-blocker therapy, as long as there are no contraindications to their use. It is often difficult to maintain systolic BP below 120 mmHg, especially in elderly patients with diminished vascular compliance, but when possible, it is an appropriate goal for these patients because of the potential to otherwise need major reoperations as they age. Surveillance of patients with aortic dissection, whether treated medically or surgically, should include a CT scan or MRI before hospital discharge and later studies as follows:

- An initial outpatient scan at 3 to 4 months to identify those who experience rapid early growth (when the aortic wall is most vulnerable).
- If aortic size is stable, a 6-month interval follows.
- Further imaging intervals are based on aortic size; whereas small aneurysms can be followed at 12-month intervals (35–40 mm), large aneurysms (45–50 mm) should be followed at 6-month intervals.

Table 1			
Impact of aortic size and the interval between consecutive imaging studies on the incidence of aortic growth (overall incidence 18%)			
		Incidence (%)	
	<6 mo	6–12 mo	>12 mo
Small (<35 mm)	5	13	21
Moderate (35–49 mm)	12	27	31
Large (≥50 mm)	34	23	83

Data from Zierer A, Voeller RK, Hill KE, et al. Late aortic enlargement and reoperation after repair of acute type A aortic dissection. Ann Thorac Surg 2007;84:479–87.

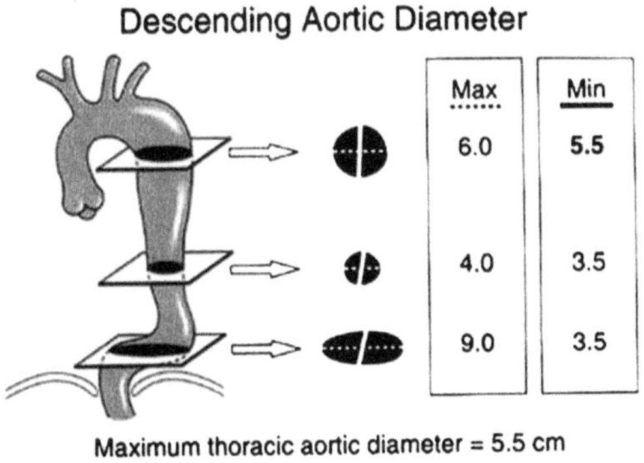

Descending Aortic Diameter

	Max	Min
	6.0	5.5
	4.0	3.5
	9.0	3.5

Maximum thoracic aortic diameter = 5.5 cm

Fig. 15. Inexperienced radiologists often overestimate the size of the aorta due to measurements made on the oblique or as the aorta travels horizontal as demonstrated most obviously at the diaphragm in this schematic. (*From* Juvonen T, Ergin MA, Galla JD, et al. Prospective study of the natural history of thoracic aortic aneurysms. Ann Thorac Surg 1997;63:1533–45; with permission.)

- If aortic expansion is identified, the interval is decreased on subsequent scans until aortic size again becomes stable.
- If diameter measurements are in question, consider three-dimensional CT reconstructions or MRI. It is not uncommon for the aorta to become tortuous following dissection, causing inexperienced radiologists to document inflated aortic sizes **(Fig. 15)**.[92]
- For patients with renal impairment, or for those who require frequent scans, non-contrast images are often satisfactory if the major question regards aortic size.

Our current indications for resection of a chronic residual dissection depend on the region of interest, but in general include: (1) aortic diameter greater than 6 to 6.5 cm (possibly 5.0 cm or 5.5 cm in younger patients with rapid growth); (2) enlargement of more than 7 to 10 mm in 1 year; (3) recurrent persistent pain attributable to the aneurysm that does not respond to medical management (it is important to remember that many patients present with pain during periods of acute hypertension that resolves with blood pressure control); and (4) localized saccular dilation, which might put the patient at a higher risk of rupture. Patients with Marfan syndrome are generally younger and are more prone to rapid dilation, so replacement should be considered when aortic diameter exceeds 5 to 5.5 cm or when expansion exceeds 3 to 5 mm per year in healthy individuals. These criteria need to be individualized by each aortic surgeon after evaluating his own institution-specific morbidity and mortality rates for these often complicated procedures.

SUMMARY

Acute aortic dissection is a fatal disease if not identified and treated appropriately. Even then, there are times when mortality cannot be prevented, despite our greatest efforts. For type A dissections, surgical therapy is essential to offer the patient a reasonable chance at long-term survival; however, it is important to remember that surgical treatment does not cure the generalized disease. For type B dissections, medical therapy is the mainstay of treatment and is associated with excellent survival when continued long-term. With either type A or type B dissections, close medical follow-up is essential after hospital discharge with a mandate for strict blood pressure control, anti-impulse therapy with β-blockers (even if the patient is normotensive), and serial imaging surveillance for the life of the patient. The initial goal of therapy in acute aortic dissection is to get the patient out of the operating room and hospital, whereas the long-term goal is to decrease the risk of late aneurysmal dilation and reoperation.

REFERENCES

1. Coady MA, Rizzo JA, Goldstein LJ, et al. Natural history, pathogenesis, and etiology of thoracic aortic aneurysms and dissections. Cardiol Clin 1999;17: 615–35.
2. Fann JI, Sarris GE, Mitchell RS, et al. Treatment of patients with aortic dissection presenting with peripheral vascular compromise. Ann Surg 1990;212:705–13.
3. Moon MR, Sundt TM 3rd, Pasque MK, et al. Does the extent of proximal or distal resection influence outcome for type A dissections? Ann Thorac Surg 2001;71: 1244–9.
4. Lauterbach SR, Cambria RP, Brewster DC, et al. Contemporary management of aortic branch compromise resulting from acute aortic dissection. J Vasc Surg 2001;33:1185–92.
5. Zierer A, Moon MR, Melby SJ, et al. Impact of perfusion strategy on neurologic recovery for acute type A aortic dissection. Ann Thorac Surg 2007;83:2122–9.
6. Hirst AD, Johns VJ, Kime SW. Dissecting aneurysm of the aorta: a review of 505 cases. Medicine 1958;37:217–79.
7. Beaver TM, Herrbold RN, Hess PJ, et al. Transferring diagnosis versus actual diagnosis at a center for thoracic aortic disease. Ann Thorac Surg 2005;79: 1957–60.
8. Reece TB, Green GR, Kron IL. Aortic dissection. In: Cohn LH, editor. Cardiac surgery in the adult. New York: McGraw-Hill; 2008. p. 1195–222.
9. Elefteriades JA, Barrett PW, Kopf GS. Litigation in nontraumatic aortic diseases: a tempest in the malpractice maelstrom. Cardiology 2008;109:263–72.
10. von Kodolitsch Y, Schwartz AG, Nienaber CA. Clinical prediction of acute aortic dissection. Arch Intern Med 2000;160:2977–82.
11. DeBakey ME, Beall AC, Cooley DA, et al. Dissecting aneurysms of the aorta. Surg Clin North Am 1966;46:1045–55.
12. Daily PO, Trueblood HW, Stinson EB, et al. Management of acute aortic dissections. Ann Thorac Surg 1970;10:237–47.
13. Erbel R, Alfonso F, Boileau C, et al. Diagnosis and management of aortic dissection. Eur Heart J 2001;22:1642–81.
14. Larson EW, Edwards WD. Risk factors for aortic dissection: a necropsy study of 161 cases. Am J Cardiol 1984;53:849–55.
15. Borger MA, Preston M, Ivanov J, et al. Should the ascending aorta be replaced more frequently in patients with bicuspid aortic valve disease? J Thorac Cardiovasc Surg 2004;128:677–83.
16. Braverman AC, Guven H, Beardslee MA, et al. The bicuspid aortic valve. Curr Probl Cardiol 2005;30:470–522.
17. Absi TS, Sundt TM, Tung WS, et al. Altered patterns of gene expression distinguishing ascending aortic aneurysms from abdominal aortic aneurysms. cDNA expression profiling in the molecular characterization of aortic disease. J Thorac Cardiovasc Surg 2003;126:344–57.
18. Curci JA, Thompson RW, Davis CG, et al. Heterogeneity of matrix changes in aneurysms of the thoracic and abdominal aorta. Circulation 2000;102(Suppl II):II-400.

19. Fazel SS, Mallidi HR, Lee RS, et al. The aortopathy of bicuspid aortic valve disease has distinctive patterns and usually involves the transverse aortic arch. J Thorac Cardiovasc Surg 2008;135:901–7.

20. Hartzaras IS, Bible JE, Koullias GJ, et al. Role of exertion or emotion as inciting events for acute aortic dissection. Am J Cardiol 2007;100:1470–2.

21. Okamoto RJ, Xu H, Kouchoukos NT, et al. The influence of mechanical properties on wall stress and distensibility of the dilated ascending aorta. J Thorac Cardiovasc Surg 2003;126:842–50.

22. Koullias GJ, Ravichandran P, Korkolis DP, et al. Increased tissue microarray matrix metalloproteinase expression favors proteolysis in thoracic aortic aneurysms and dissections. Ann Thorac Surg 2004;78:2106–11.

23. Schmoker JD, McPartland KJ, Fellinger EK, et al. Matrix metalloproteinase and tissue inhibitor expression in atherosclerotic and nonatherosclerotic thoracic aortic aneurysms. J Thorac Cardiovasc Surg 2007;133:155–61.

24. Boyum J, Fellinger EK, Schmoker JD, et al. Matrix metalloproteinase activity in thoracic aortic aneurysms associated with bicuspid and tricuspid aortic valves. J Thorac Cardiovasc Surg 2004;127:686–91.

25. Ikonomidis JS, Jones JA, Barbour JR, et al. Expression of matrix metalloproteinases and endogenous inhibitors within ascending aortic aneurysms of patients with Marfan syndrome. Circulation 2006;114(Suppl I):I-365–70.

26. Fedak PWM, de Sa MP, Verma S, et al. Vascular matrix remodeling in patients with bicuspid aortic valve malformations: implications for aortic dilatation. J Thorac Cardiovasc Surg 2003;126:797–806.

27. LeMaire SA, Wang X, Wilks JA, et al. Matrix metalloproteinases in ascending aortic aneurysms: bicuspid versus trileaflet aortic valves. J Surg Res 2005;123: 40–8.

28. Shores J, Berger KR, Murphy EA, et al. Progression of aortic dilatation and the benefit of long-term β-adrenergic blockade in Marfan's syndrome. N Engl J Med 1994;330:1335–41.

29. Yetman AT, Bornemeier RA, McCrindle BW. Usefulness of enalapril versus propranolol or atenolol for prevention of aortic dilation in patients with the Marfan syndrome. Am J Cardiol 2005;95:1125–7.

30. Habashi JP, Judge DP, Holm TM, et al. Losartan, an AT1 antagonist, prevents aortic aneurysm in a mouse model of Marfan syndrome. Science 2006;312:117–21.

31. Zierer A, Voeller RK, Hill KE, et al. Late aortic enlargement and reoperation after repair of acute type A aortic dissection. Ann Thorac Surg 2007;84:479–87.

32. Bonow RO, Cheitlin MD, Crawford MH, et al. Task force 3: valvular heart disease. J Am Coll Cardiol 2005;45:1334–40.

33. Maron BJ, Ackerman MJ, Nishimura RA, et al. Task force 4: HCM and other cardiomyopathies, mitral valve prolapse, myocarditis, and Marfan syndrome. J Am Coll Cardiol 2005;45:1340–5.

34. Maniar HS, Sundt TM, Prasad SM, et al. Delayed paraplegia after thoracic and thoracoabdominal aneurysm repair. A continuing risk. Ann Thorac Surg 2003; 75:113–20.

35. Slater EE, DeSanctis RW. The clinical recognition of dissecting aortic aneurysm. Am J Med 1976;60:625–33.

36. Kawahito K, Adachi H, Murata S, et al. Coronary malperfusion due to type A aortic dissection: mechanism and surgical management. Ann Thorac Surg 2003;76:1471–6.

37. Vedantham S, Picus D, Sanchez LA, et al. Percutaneous management of ischemic complications in patients with type-B aortic dissection. J Vasc Interv Radiol 2003;14:181–94.

38. Dake MD, Kato N, Mitchell RS, et al. Endovascular stent-graft placement for the treatment of acute aortic dissection. N Engl J Med 1999;340:1546–52.
39. Slonim SM, Miller DC, Mitchell RS, et al. Percutaneous balloon fenestration and stenting for life-threatening ischemic complications in patients with acute aortic dissection. J Thorac Cardiovasc Surg 1999;117:1118–26.
40. Pradhan S, Elefteriades JA, Sumpio BE. Utility of the aortic fenestration technique in the management of acute aortic dissections. Ann Thorac Cardiovasc Surg 2007;13:296–300.
41. Sandridge L, Kern JA. Acute descending aortic dissections: management of visceral, spinal cord, and extremity malperfusion. Semin Thorac Cardiovasc Surg 2005;17:256–61.
42. Lai DT, Robbins RC, Mitchell RS, et al. Does profound hypothermic circulatory arrest improve survival in patients with acute type a aortic dissection? Circulation 2002;106(Suppl I):I-218–28.
43. Lai DT, Miller DC, Mitchell RS, et al. Acute type A aortic dissection complicated by aortic regurgitation: composite valve graft versus separate valve graft versus conservative valve repair. J Thorac Cardiovasc Surg 2003;126: 1978–86.
44. Geirsson A, Bavaria JE, Swarr D, et al. Fate of the residual distal and proximal aorta after acute type a dissection repair using a contemporary surgical reconstruction algorithm. Ann Thorac Surg 2007;84:1955–64.
45. Hagan PG, Nienaber CA, Isselbacher EM, et al. The International Registry of Acute Aortic Dissection (IRAD): new insights into an old disease. JAMA 2000; 283:897–903.
46. David TE, Armstrong S, Ivanov J, et al. Surgery for acute type A aortic dissection. Ann Thorac Surg 1999;67:1999–2001.
47. Bavaria JE, Brinster DR, Gorman RC, et al. Advances in the treatment of acute type A dissection: an integrated approach. Ann Thorac Surg 2002;74: S1848–52.
48. Crawford ES, Coselli JS, Safi HJ. Partial cardiopulmonary bypass, hypothermic circulatory arrest, and posterolateral exposure for thoracic aortic aneurysm operation. J Thorac Cardiovasc Surg 1987;94:824–7.
49. Trimarchi S, Nienaber CA, Rampoldi V, et al. Role and results of surgery in acute type B aortic dissection: insights from the International Registry of Acute Aortic Dissection (IRAD). Circulation 2006;114(Suppl I):I-357–64.
50. Estrera AL, Garami Z, Miller CC, et al. Acute type A aortic dissection complicated by stroke: can immediate repair be performed safely? J Thorac Cardiovasc Surg 2006;132:1404–8.
51. Moon MR, Miller DC. Aortic arch replacement for dissection. Op Tech Thorac Cardiovasc Surg 1999;4:33–57.
52. Yun KL, Miller DC. Technique of aortic valve preservation in acute type A aortic dissection. Op Tech Thorac Cardiovasc Surg 1996;1:68–81.
53. David TE. Surgery for acute type A aortic dissection. Op Tech Thorac Cardiovasc Surg 1999;4:2–12.
54. Coselli JS, LeMaire SA, Walkes J. Surgery for acute type A dissection. Op Tech Thorac Cardiovasc Surg 1999;4:13–32.
55. Crawford ES, Kirklin JW, Naftel DC, et al. Surgery for acute dissection of ascending aorta: should the arch be included? J Thorac Cardiovasc Surg 1992;104:46–59.
56. Borst HG, Buhner B, Jurmann M. Tactics and techniques of aortic arch replacement. J Card Surg 1994;9:538–47.

57. Haverich A, Miller DC, Scott WC, et al. Acute and chronic aortic dissections: determinants of long-term outcome for operative survivors. Circulation 1985; 72(Suppl II):II-22–34.

58. Pochettino A, Brinkman WT, Moeller P, et al. Proximal thoracic stent grafting via the open arch during standard repair for acute Debakey I aortic dissection prevents development of dissection thoracoabdominal aortic aneurysms [abstract 24]. In: Program and abstracts of the 55th Annual Meeting of the Southern Thoracic Surgical Association. Austin, TX: November 7, 2008. p. 118–9.

59. Guthaner DF, Miller DC, Silverman JF, et al. Fate of the false lumen following surgical repair of aortic dissections: an angiographic study. Radiology 1979;133:1–8.

60. Fusco DS, Shaw RK, Tranquilli M, et al. Femoral cannulation is safe for type A dissection repair. Ann Thorac Surg 2004;78:1285–9.

61. Moon MR, Sundt TM. Aortic arch aneurysms. Coron Artery Dis 2002;13:85–92.

62. Moon MR, Sundt TM. Influence of retrograde cerebral perfusion during aortic arch procedures. Ann Thorac Surg 2002;74:426–31.

63. Estrera AL, Miller CC, Lee TY, et al. Ascending and transverse aortic arch repair: the impact of retrograde cerebral perfusion. Circulation 2008;118(Suppl 1): S160–6.

64. Reece TB, Tribble CG, Smith RL, et al. Central cannulation is safe in acute aortic dissection repair. J Thorac Cardiovasc Surg 2007;133:428–34.

65. Griepp RB, Stinson EB, Hollingsworth JF, et al. Prosthetic replacement of the aortic arch. J Thorac Cardiovasc Surg 1975;70:1051–63.

66. Kirsch M, Soustelle C, Houel R, et al. Risk factor analysis for proximal and distal reoperations after surgery for acute type A dissection. J Thorac Cardiovasc Surg 2002;123:318–25.

67. Centofanti P, Flocco R, Ceresa F, et al. Is surgery always mandatory for type A aortic dissection? Ann Thorac Surg 2006;82:1658–64.

68. Patel HJ, Williams DM, Dasika NL, et al. Operative delay for peripheral malperfusion syndrome in acute type A aortic dissection: a long-term analysis. J Thorac Cardiovasc Surg 2008;135:1288–95.

69. Scholl FG, Coady MA, Davies R, et al. Interval or permanent nonoperative management of acute type A aortic dissection. Arch Surg 1999;134:402–6.

70. Davies RR, Coe MP, Mandapati D, et al. What is the optimal management of late-presenting survivors of acute type A aortic dissection? Ann Thorac Surg 2007;83: 1593–602.

71. Verhoye JP, Miller DC, Sze D, et al. Complicated acute type B aortic dissection: midterm results of emergency endovascular stent-grafting. J Thorac Cardiovasc Surg 2008;136:424–30.

72. Akin I, Kische S, Ince H, et al. Indication, timing and results of endovascular treatment of type B dissection. Eur J Vasc Endovasc Surg 2009;37:289–96.

73. Szeto WY, McGarvey M, Pochettino A, et al. Results of a new surgical paradigm: endovascular repair for acute complicated type B aortic dissection. Ann Thorac Surg 2008;86:87–94.

74. Glower DD, Fann JI, Speier RH, et al. Comparison of medical and surgical therapy for uncomplicated descending aortic dissection. Circulation 1990; 82(Suppl IV):IV-39–46.

75. Umaña JP, Lai DT, Mitchell RS, et al. Is medical therapy still the optimal treatment strategy for patients with acute type B aortic dissections? J Thorac Cardiovasc Surg 2002;124:896–910.

76. Eggebrecht H, Nienaber CA, Neuhäuser M, et al. Endovascular stent-graft placement in aortic dissection: a meta-analysis. Eur Heart J 2006;27:489–98.

77. Schoder M, Czerny M, Cejna M, et al. Endovascular repair of acute type B aortic dissection: long-term follow-up of true and false lumen diameter changes. Ann Thorac Surg 2007;83:1059–66.

78. Schor JS, Yerlioglu E, Galla JD, et al. Selective management of acute type B aortic dissection: long-term follow-up. Ann Thorac Surg 1996;61:1339–41.

79. Estrera AL, Miler CC, Goodrick J, et al. Update on outcomes of acute type B aortic dissection. Ann Thorac Surg 2007;83:S842–5.

80. Hsu R, Ho Y, Chen RJ, et al. Outcome of medical and surgical treatment in patients with acute type B aortic dissection. Ann Thorac Surg 2005;79:790–5.

81. Moon MR, Dake MD, Pelc L, et al. Intravascular stenting of acute experimental type B dissections. J Surg Res 1993;54:381–8.

82. Tsai TT, Fattori R, Trimarchi S, et al. Long-term survival in patients presenting with type B acute aortic dissection: insights from the International Registry of Acute Aortic Dissection. Circulation 2006;114:2226–31.

83. DeBakey ME, McCollum CH, Crawford ES, et al. Dissection and dissecting aneurysms of the aorta: twenty-year follow-up of five hundred twenty-seven patients treated surgically. Surgery 1982;92:1118–34.

84. Ganaha F, Miller DC, Sugimoto K, et al. Prognosis of aortic intramural hematoma with and without penetrating atherosclerotic ulcer: a clinical and radiological analysis. Circulation 2002;106:342–8.

85. Robbins RC, McManus RP, Mitchell RS, et al. Management of patients with intramural hematoma of the thoracic aorta. Circulation 1993;88(Suppl II):II-1–II-10.

86. Tittle SL, Lynch RJ, Cole PE, et al. Midterm follow-up of penetrating ulcer and intramural hematoma of the aorta. J Thorac Cardiovasc Surg 2002;123:1051–9.

87. Park KH, Lim C, Choi JH, et al. Prevalence of aortic intimal defect in surgically treated acute type A intramural hematoma. Ann Thorac Surg 2008;86:1494–500.

88. Moizumi Y, Komatsu T, Motoyoshi N, et al. Management of patients with intramural hematoma involving the ascending aorta. J Thorac Cardiovasc Surg 2002;124:918–24.

89. Coady MA, Rizzo JA, Hammond GL, et al. Penetrating ulcer of the thoracic aorta: what is it? How do we recognize it? How do we manage it? J Vasc Surg 1998;27:1006–16.

90. Sundt TM. Intramural hematoma and penetrating atherosclerotic ulcer of the aorta. Ann Thorac Surg 2007;83:S835–41.

91. Sueyoshi E, Sakamoto I, Fukuda M, et al. Long-term outcome of type B aortic intramural hematoma: comparison with classic aortic dissection treated by the same therapeutic strategy. Ann Thorac Surg 2004;78:2112–7.

92. Juvonen T, Ergin MA, Galla JD, et al. Prospective study of the natural history of thoracic aortic aneurysms. Ann Thorac Surg 1997;63:1533–45.

Endovascular Repair of the Thoracic Aorta

Joshua D. Adams, MD[a], Lleowell M. Garcia, MD[b], John A. Kern, MD[b],*

KEYWORDS

• Aorta • Endovascular • Stent graft • Aneurysm
• Penetrating ulcer • Aortic dissection

Since first reported more than 50 years ago, surgical repair of the descending thoracic aorta with resection and graft interposition has become the standard treatment strategy for patients with aneurysmal disease.[1] Despite significant clinical advances, which have allowed operative mortality to decrease to as low as 3% in specialized centers,[2] open surgical repair is generally associated with substantial morbidity and mortality in a patient population that is often aged and frail secondary to multiple medical comorbidities.

Endovascular exclusion of aortic aneurysms with covered stent grafts represents a less invasive alternative therapy to patients who might not survive open surgical repair. In addition, either as part of a trial or in an off-label manner, endovascular repair has been applied with increased frequency to other thoracic aortic pathologies such as pseudoaneurysms, type B aortic dissections, traumatic aortic disruptions, intramural hematomas, and treatment of patients with connective tissue disorders. The goals of this review are to: provide information on the 3 commercially available thoracic endografts that have been approved by the US Food and Drug Administration (FDA); detail the preoperative evaluation including imaging, device selection, and sizing; elaborate on certain anatomic considerations that guide therapy; and review the potential complications specific to endovascular repair. The extended use of this evolving technology to treat multiple thoracic aortic pathologies, albeit in an off-label manner, is also discussed.

HISTORY

It was in the early 1990s that treatment of thoracic aortic aneurysms entered the endovascular era. The same guiding principles of complete aneurysm exclusion and subsequent decompression with covered stent grafts used to successfully treat abdominal aortic aneurysms by Parodi[3] were first applied to descending thoracic

[a] Department of Radiology, University of Virginia Health System, PO Box 800170, Charlottesville, VA 22908, USA
[b] Department of Surgery, University of Virginia Health System, PO Box 800679, Charlottesville, VA 22908, USA
* Corresponding author.
E-mail address: jkern@virginia.edu (J.A. Kern).

Surg Clin N Am 89 (2009) 895–912
doi:10.1016/j.suc.2009.06.003
0039-6109/09/$ – see front matter © 2009 Elsevier Inc. All rights reserved.

aneurysms in a high-risk population by Dake and colleagues[4] in 1994. The devices used in these patients consisted of self-expanding stainless steel Z-stents (Cook, Inc, Bloomington, Indiana) covered with woven polyester graft material, which was hand sewn to the stent body with 5-0 polypropylene sutures. Although complication rates were high with this first generation of devices,[5] the development of multiple commercially manufactured endografts with improved flexibility and durability significantly decreased the number of complications.

During the next decade, results steadily improved as device and delivery system designs evolved and as strict inclusion and exclusion criteria were employed to guide patient selection.[6–9] Currently, three devices have been approved by the FDA and are commercially available in the United States for the treatment of thoracic aneurysms, and two of those devices are also approved for treatment of complicated penetrating ulcers of the descending thoracic aorta. With commercial availability, thoracic endovascular aortic repair (TEVAR) of thoracic aortic pathology has significantly increased.[10,11] Many groups have since reported superior short- and mid-term results to those of conventional open surgery, including decreased operative time, shorter intensive care unit (ICU) and hospital stays, and lower perioperative morbidity and mortality rates.[12,13]

AVAILABLE DEVICES

In March of 2005, following publication of the phase 2 multicenter trial with the TAG endoprosthesis (W. L. Gore & Associates, Inc, Flagstaff, Arizona),[6] the first device approved by the FDA became commercially available in the United States to treat descending thoracic aneurysms. More recently, in 2008, the Zenith TX2 TAA Endovascular Graft (Cook, Inc) and the Talent Thoracic Stent Graft System (Medtronic Vascular, Santa Rosa, California) received FDA approval for descending thoracic aneurysms and penetrating aortic ulcers.

TAG Device

The TAG endoprosthesis is a tube composed of expanded polytetrafluoroethylene (ePTFE) externally reinforced with an additional layer of ePTFE and fluorinated ethylene propylene (FEP) and supported by a flexible nitinol exoskeleton available in diameters of 26 to 40 mm and in lengths of 10, 15, and 20 cm (**Fig. 1**). The exoskeleton is commercially bonded to the graft material without sutures and is constrained by an ePTFE-FEP sleeve. EPTFE-covered scalloped flares are present on both ends of the device to aid in fixation. A circumferential ePTFE sealing cuff is located on the external surface of the endoprosthesis at the base of each flared end to enhance sealing of the endoprosthesis to the wall of the aorta. The device profile depends on the size of the graft and requires a 20F to 24F sheath for delivery. Deployment is extremely rapid and occurs with the release of the constraining sleeve in a rip-cord fashion. The TAG expansion initiates from the middle of the endograft and simultaneously extends toward both ends to avoid the "windsock effect" from the high arterial flow that would occur in a standard proximal-to-distal deployment mode (see **Fig. 1**A). The device is then molded with a specially designed trilobed balloon that allows flow to continue during inflation (see **Fig. 1**C).

Multiple clinical trials were conducted leading to FDA approval of the TAG endoprosthesis in March 2005. The pivotal study, which enrolled patients from September 1999 to May 2001, was a nonrandomized multicenter study comparing open surgical repair (n = 94) to endovascular repair (n = 140) in patients with descending thoracic aneurysms. The primary end point compared the incidence of major adverse events

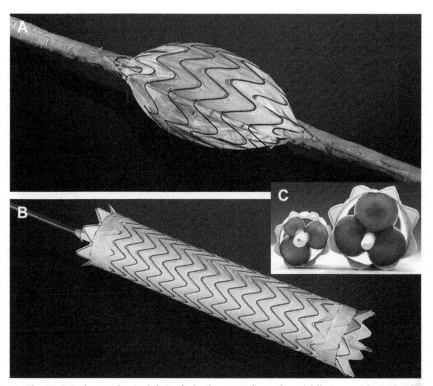

Fig. 1. The TAG Endoprosthesis. (*A*) Graft deployment from the middle to avoid windsocking. (*B*) The fully expanded endoprosthesis. (*C*) The specially designed trilobed balloon that allows flow to continue during inflation. (*Courtesy of* W. L. Gore & Associates, Newark, DE; with permission.)

(MAE) between the two groups for 1 year post-treatment. The study was interrupted secondary to a high rate of fracture of the longitudinal spine. Following a device modification, which included removing the longitudinal spine and adding a low permeability film layer to provide longitudinal stiffness for deployment accuracy and to minimize the potential for aneurysm expansion, a nonrandomized multicenter confirmatory study was conducted from January 2004 to June 2004, which compared 51 patients treated with the TAG device to the original pivotal study control group. From July 2004 to April 2005, while the device was awaiting FDA approval, an additional 80 patients underwent endovascular repair at 13 sites and were enrolled in the treatment investigational device exemption (IDE) study. Enrollment criteria were identical to those used in the pivotal and confirmatory studies, however, the patients were followed according to the investigators' standard of care, which was not defined.

Recently, updated results from the three studies have been released, including follow-up for 5 years for the completed pivotal study, 3 years for the ongoing confirmatory study and 2 years for the ongoing treatment IDE study.[14] At 5 years, patients undergoing endovascular repair reported significantly improved aneurysm-related survival (96% freedom from aneurysm-related death among TEVAR patients versus 88% for open surgical controls) and lower incidence of MAE (37% freedom from MAE among TEVAR patients versus 21% for open surgical controls). At 1 month the difference in freedom from MAE is even more impressive (71% freedom from MAE among TEVAR patients versus 21% for open surgical controls). Pooled data from the three studies demonstrate a rupture incidence of 1.1% (n = 3), a conversion to open incidence of 1.1% (n = 3), and additional implantation incidence of 1.8% (n = 5). Comparison of the pivotal study data with the confirmatory data also validates the previously described device modification as there have been no fractures since the longitudinal spine was removed. Since the additional low permeability film layer was added, the percentage of patients demonstrating a decrease in aneurysm diameter greater than or equal to 5 mm has increased, 64% in the confirmatory patients versus 52.7% in the pivotal study patients; the increase (≥5 mm) in the incidence of aneurysm in the confirmatory and pivotal study patients at 3 years was 6.5%, and 16.4% respectively.

Zenith TX2

The Zenith TX2 is designed as a two-piece modular system with a designated proximal and distal device, although one device or the combination of multiple proximal devices may be used depending on the length and characteristics of the aorta (**Fig. 2**). Both components are constructed from stainless steel modified Gianturco Z-stents, which are sutured to full-thickness woven polyester fabric. The small gaps between the individual Z-stents allow the device to conform to the aorta. The fabric is on the outside of the stents at the proximal and distal ends of the device to maximize fabric-to-aortic

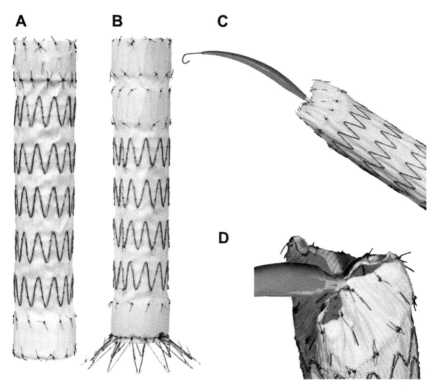

Fig. 2. The Zenith TX2. The proximal (*A*) and distal (*B*) components of the endovascular system. (*C*) The endograft on the H&L-B One-Shot Introduction System. (*D*) The proximal end of the graft in a trifold configuration, thus preventing the "windsock effect" by allowing for blood flow around the graft. (*Courtesy of* Cook Medical Inc., Bloomington, IN; with permission.)

apposition and on the inside of the stents in the midportion to allow fabric-to-fabric overlap zones. A mechanism of active fixation to the aorta is present in both components with multiple 5-mm staggered external barbs oriented in opposing directions at the most proximal and distal ends of the devices designed to prevent migration in either direction (**Fig. 2**A, B). The proximal components are available in straight or tapered configurations and in diameters ranging from 28 to 42 mm and lengths from 120 to 216 mm. The distal component is available in the nontapered configuration only and the diameter ranges between 28 and 42 mm, the length from 127 to 207 mm.

The Zenith TX2 is delivered through the H&L-B One-Shot Introduction System, either 20F or 22F depending on device diameter (**Fig. 2**C). All component between 28 and 34 mm in diameter are deployed using a 20F system, and those between 36 and 42 mm in diameter are deployed using a 22F system. The delivery system features the Flexor braided sheath with hydrophilic coating designed to resist kinking and improve trackability from the iliac arteries to the thoracic aorta. The trigger-wire release mechanisms of the delivery system work in tandem to deliver sequential, controlled release of the graft during deployment. Once the sheath is withdrawn, the proximal end of all main body components remain attached to the delivery system with the use of 3 trigger wires, which keep the proximal end of the graft in a trifold configuration, thus preventing the "windsock effect" by allowing for blood flow around the graft (**Fig. 2**D).

Most US experience with the Zenith TX2 device has been provided by two clinical trials.[15,16] Greenberg and colleagues first reported their intermediate-term results of endovascular repair in their first 100 consecutive patients using the TX1 and TX2 thoracic grafts under the guidance of a sponsored ODE (n = 97) or on a compassionate-use basis (n = 3). The inclusion criteria for these patients considered high risk for conventional surgery was similar to other study criteria except that only a 10-mm proximal and distal neck was required. The indication for treatment was aneurysm in 96 patients, including 15 patients with underlying chronic dissection. Adjunctive debranching procedures were required to create adequate landing zones in 29% of patients, including 14 elephant trunk/arch reconstructions, 18 carotid to subclavian bypasses, and four visceral arterial bypasses. At 1 year, the overall mortality rate was 17% and the aneurysm-related mortality rate was 14%. Secondary interventions were required in 15 patients, six of whom underwent successful endovascular treatments of various endoleaks.

The pivotal STARZ-TX2 clinical trial is a nonrandomized, controlled, multicenter, international study designed to evaluate the safety and efficacy of the Zenith TX2 by comparing 30-day survival and 30-day rupture-free survival with contemporary and prospective open surgical controls. Important secondary end points included morbidity, clinical usefulness measures, and freedom from device events. One hundred sixty patients with descending thoracic aortic aneurysm or penetrating ulcer underwent endovascular repair (TEVAR) and were compared with 70 open surgical control patients; follow-up is ongoing. The 30-day survival rate for TEVAR patients was noninferior to that of open surgical patients, 98.1% versus 94.3%, respectively. At 1 year, freedom from aneurysm-related mortality was 94% in the TEVAR group versus 88% in the open surgical group. TEVAR patients also had significantly lower markers of morbidity than open-surgical patients, including severe composite morbidity index, cumulative major morbidity scores, and fewer cardiovascular, pulmonary, and vascular events. All measures of clinical usefulness were superior in the TEVAR group ($P < .01$) including duration of intubation and ICU stay, days to ambulation, days to oral intake, and days to hospital discharge. Freedom from any device event, defined as technical failure, secondary intervention, conversion, type I or III endoleak, or migration, was 90.1% at 1 year and there was no difference in need for reintervention between the two groups.

Talent Thoracic

The Talent Thoracic Stent Graft System is composed of a polyester woven graft fabric sewn to a series of individual self-expanding M-shaped nitinol springs (**Fig. 3**). Between the individual stents is an area of unsupported graft to allow for conformability. The device has a longitudinal support bar throughout the length of the endograft, which provides columnar strength while maintaining device flexibility by carefully orienting the bar along the greater curve of the aorta. This device is also designed in a two-component modular fashion with slightly different proximal and a distal components (see **Fig. 3**A, B). The proximal component possesses an uncovered nitinol spring and a mini-support spring proximally to allow for implantation across the origin of the left common carotid artery or the left subclavian artery while maintaining patency of the covered branch. These components are available in diameters ranging from 22 to 46 mm and lengths from 112 to 116 mm. The distal component has a "closed-web" design in which the most proximal spring is covered with fabric leaving a "tulip" appearance, which helps to ensure fixation within the region of overlap with the proximal component. The distal components are available in straight and tapered configurations with diameters ranging from 26 to 46 mm and 110 to 114 mm in length. All devices are deployed through the self-contained Xcelerant delivery system

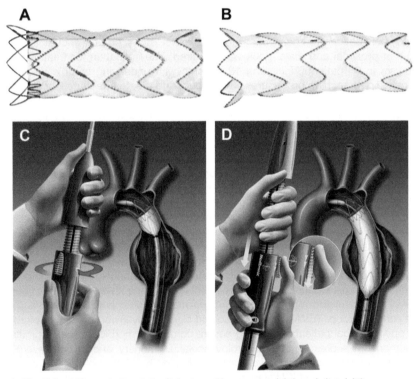

Fig. 3. The Talent Thoracic Stent Graft System. The proximal (*A*) and distal (*B*) components. (*C, D*) The deployment technique using the self-contained Xcelerant delivery system, which allows for controlled ratcheted deployment initially (*C*) and fast "zip" deployment (*D*). (*Courtesy of* Medtronic Vascular, Minneapolis, MN; with permission.)

(see **Fig. 3**C, D), which allows for controlled ratcheted precise deployment initially and fast "zip" deployment to prevent the "windsock effect" or proximal graft collapse while deploying. The delivery system for the Talent has profiles between 22F and 25F depending on device diameters.

Despite extensive experience with the Talent Thoracic stent graft internationally,[17,18] the device has only recently received FDA approval following submission of the pivotal results of the VALOR trial.[19] The study was a prospective, nonrandomized, multicenter trial conducted at 38 sites, which enrolled patients from December 2003 to June 2005 and compared TEVAR in low surgical risk patients to retrospective open surgical data from three centers of excellence. One hundred ninety-five patients underwent TEVAR and were compared with 189 open surgical patients. Vessel access and successful deployment of the device was accomplished in all but one patient (99.5%) who did not receive a device secondary to access failure. Iliac conduits were required in 21.1% and preemptive left subclavian revascularization was performed in 5.2% of patients. The TEVAR group demonstrated significantly better outcomes than the open-surgery group, including a 30-day mortality of 2% versus 8% ($P < .010$), 30-day MAE of 41% versus 84.4% ($P < .001$), and aneurysm-related mortality at 1 year of 3.1% versus 11.6% ($P < .002$). All measures of clinical usefulness were significantly better in the TEVAR group. Further, at 1 year, conversion to open surgery was 0.5%, device migration was 3.9%, endoleak was 12.2%, and a stable or decreasing aneurysm was noted in 91.5% of patients.

PREOPERATIVE EVALUATION

There are few surgical procedures for which the proverb "if you fail to plan, you plan to fail" rings truer than in the case of endovascular repair of the thoracic aorta, and the planning for such a repair begins with imaging. Most centers use contrast-enhanced, thin-cut helical computed tomography angiography (CTA) or magnetic resonance angiography (MRA) timed to the arterial phase extending from the base of the neck through the femoral heads. In patients who may require coverage of the left subclavian artery (LSCA), a CTA of the head and neck is obtained to establish the presence of a patent circle of Willis and a nondominant left vertebral artery. Imaging software that allows the creation of multiplanar and three-dimensional reconstructions, as well as centerline flow algorithms, is critical to establishing the presence of suitable anatomy for endovascular repair and for proper device selection and sizing. This imaging includes not only the thoracic aorta but also the size and characteristics of the femoral and iliac arteries, which serve as access vessels. From a planning standpoint, this imaging also helps determine the optimal projection to open up the aortic arch and profile the origins of the great vessels. Cross-sectional imaging also provides useful clinical information such as degree of atheromatous burden which may allow estimation of a patient's risk for embolic complications.

General Sizing and Anatomic Requirements

Although the exact anatomy required by the instructions for use of each individual device may vary slightly, the general principles are the same. Adequate proximal and distal landing zones of normal aorta must be present to allow for adequate seal and subsequent exclusion of the aneurysm. Equally as important are sufficient access vessels to allow for passage of the device into the thoracic aorta. This requirement also varies somewhat by device brand and size as dictated by the outer diameter of each individual device delivery system. Oversizing of the device to the aorta aids device fixation and seal. **Table 1** details the specific anatomic requirements and sizing recommendations of the three available thoracic devices.

Specific Considerations

TEVAR may still be a viable therapy in patients who do not meet some of the above anatomic requirements. For example, the supra-aortic vessels may be covered to gain additional proximal landing zone length. Zones of proximal aortic endograft attachment sites, as defined by Criado and colleagues,[20] are depicted in **Fig. 4**. Obviously, if deployment of the stent graft will extend into zones 0 or 1, debranching procedures must be performed before stent graft placement. The need for revascularization before planned coverage of the LSCA (zone 2), however, has been debated. Some investigators have advocated preprocedural revascularization for all of these patients.[21] At our institution, a policy of selective revascularization is used. Following thorough evaluation of the cerebrovascular blood supply using cross-sectional imaging, LSCA revascularization is performed before TEVAR in the presence of an incomplete posterior circulation, a left dominant vertebral artery, a stenosed or occluded right vertebral artery, a patent left internal mammary artery (LIMA) to left anterior descending artery coronary bypass graft, or an aberrant origin of the right subclavian artery. In addition, in recognizing that branches of the LSCA may contribute to spinal cord perfusion,[22,23] the authors have also begun revascularizing the LSCA if exclusion of a long length of descending thoracic aorta is planned, especially if the patient has undergone prior abdominal aortic repair. LSCA revascularization is most commonly accomplished by left carotid to LSCA bypass, although occasional LSCA transposition has been performed. Bypass techniques and staged embolization of the LSCA origin at time of TEVAR, as described by Woo and colleagues,[24] obviates the need for dissection and clamping of the LSCA proximal to the origins of the LIMA and left vertebral artery, thereby minimizing ischemic and bleeding risks. Postprocedural LSCA revascularization is performed for patients with ischemic symptoms such as left arm claudication or subclavian steal phenomenon, and doing so in a delayed fashion does not seem to have any untoward consequences.

Table 1
Indications and sizing guidelines for the three FDA approved thoracic aortic devices

Indication and Size Parameters	TAG	Zenith TX2	Talent Thoracic
FDA-approved indication	Descending thoracic aneurysm	Descending thoracic aneurysm and PAU	Descending thoracic aneurysm and PAU
Length of proximal and distal landing zones (mm)	≥20	≥25	≥20
Range of treatable aortic diameters (mm)	23–37	24–38	18–42
% of oversizing to aorta	6–19[a]	10–20	12–22
Required delivery sheath size (Fr)	20, 22, 24	20 or 22	22, 24, 25

[a] TAG device instructions for use recommend inner-wall to inner-wall measurement of diameter.

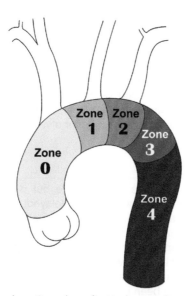

Fig. 4. The zones of proximal aortic endograft attachment sites.

Insertion of a lumbar catheter for cerebral spinal fluid (CSF) drainage is performed preoperatively by anesthesiologists at the discretion of the surgeon based on assessment of risk factors for spinal ischemia including region of planned aortic exclusion, length of planned aortic exclusion, and history of prior aortic procedure. Spinal drains are managed according to protocol in the ICU setting and are discontinued usually in 48 to 72 hours, before transfer to the acute care unit.

Vascular access to the thoracic aorta continues to be a significant issue with TEVAR. In most cases the bilateral iliofemoral vessels are accessed to allow for introduction of the delivery sheath from one groin and a pigtail catheter for diagnostic injection of contrast agent from the other groin. The caliber, degree of atherosclerotic disease, and the tortuosity are preoperatively assessed using CTA or MRA. Usually the larger diameter, less calcified and less tortuous iliofemoral arterial tree is selected as the main device delivery route. If femoral vessels are not heavily calcified and are of adequate diameter to accommodate the delivery sheath, totally percutaneous access utilizing the "preclose" technique, first described by Lee and colleagues[25] in 2007, can be used safely and effectively with the Perclose Proglide 6F suture-mediated closure system (Abbott Vascular, Redwood City, California). Briefly, this technique places two individual 3-0 polypropylene sutures with preformed slipknots through the anterior wall of the artery, which are cinched down at the conclusion of the case with the provided knot pusher. This method is a modification of the original technique described by Haas and colleagues[26] in 1999, employing the 10F Prostar XL suture-mediated closure system. In a follow-up review published 1 year later, Lee and colleagues[27] reported their mid-term outcomes of 292 patients who underwent percutaneous aortic endovascular repairs with successful closure of 408 of the attempted 432 (94.4%) common femoral arterial puncture sites. One hundred of those patients had an adequate CTA at 6 months or greater postprocedure to assess the 156 preclosed puncture sites and revealed a late complication rate of only 1.92% (3/156), including one asymptomatic femoral artery dissection and two femoral psuedoaneurysms requiring surgical repair.

Operative surgical control and exposure of the common femoral arteries should be performed in the setting of heavily calcified vessels or if the operating physician has not had adequate training in the "preclose" technique. If the common femoral arteries are not of a size that will accommodate the delivery system, a surgical conduit, most commonly a 10-mm diameter polyester tube graft, may be sewn to the iliac artery or less commonly the aorta. Decreasing vascular complications secondary to access issues are likely an appreciation of the critical value of using a graft conduit as a preemptive measure rather than a bailout after a vascular injury has occurred.

COMPLICATIONS
Neurologic Complications

Neurologic complications continue to be a rare but devastating complication of TEVAR. Spinal cord ischemia, immediate and delayed, resulting in paraplegia has been reported in multiple series, most commonly ranging between 3% and 5% and seems to be a multifactorial event.[28] Multiple risk factors have been implicated including an aortic exclusion greater than 20 cm in length, coverage of the LSCA, exclusion of the distal thoracic aorta with the T8 to L2 region most commonly quoted, and history of prior abdominal aortic repair.[29] Perioperative hypotension (mean arterial pressure [MAP] <70) has also been implicated as a risk factor for immediate and delayed spinal cord injury.[30] Like many investigators, the authors advocate the use of prophylactic CSF drainage in patients with these preoperative risk factors and closely manage blood pressure in the perioperative period to maintain an MAP greater than 90. What is more concerning within the literature is the significant numbers of patients who present weeks following the procedure and likely represent the further loss of collateral pathways. It is clear in this case, as it is with the spontaneous resolution of some endoleaks, that the dynamic state of the circulatory bed plays a significant role in the outcomes of certain patients.

Cerebrovascular accidents (CVA) have also been reported following thoracic stent graft procedures in the range of 3% to 5%,[6,15,19] especially in patients requiring extensive aortic arch manipulation or extension of endografting into zones 0 through 2.[31] Specifically, coverage of the LSCA (zone 2 deployment) seems to pose a higher stroke risk than TEVAR within all other zones, 8.6% as reported by Woo and colleagues[32] in their review of 70 patients undergoing zone 2 TEVAR. Risks of embolic cerebrovascular events are likely related to the severity and composition of the aortic atherosclerotic plaques and the extent of wire, catheter, and device manipulation within the arch, including balloon molding of the endograft.

TEVAR IN SPECIFIC AORTIC PATHOLOGIES

With commercial availability, several centers have expanded the indications beyond those of descending thoracic aneurysms and penetrating aortic ulcers. Recently, the authors reported their single institution experience with TEVAR using the TAG endoprosthesis in the post-FDA approval era,[33] comparing the outcomes of treating multiple aortic pathologies, such as atherosclerotic aneurysms, pseudoaneurysms, type B aortic dissections, traumatic aortic injuries, penetrating aortic ulcers, and lesions related to connective tissue disorders, with those of the pivotal study,[6] which was governed by strict anatomic constraints and permitted treatment of patients with descending thoracic aneurysm exclusively. With the exception of a higher endoleak rate at 30 days, 26% versus 4% ($P < .01$), our results compared favorably with those of the pivotal study, reporting no significant difference in length of stay (7.5 days versus 7.6 days), ICU days (3.7 days versus 2.6 days), 30-day mortality (2.0% versus

1.5%) spinal cord injury (2% versus 3%) and stroke (4% versus 4%). At 1 year, overall survival was 92% in our patients compared with 82% in the pivotal study. The authors concluded that the higher early endoleaks, most of which were small proximal type I visualized on postdeployment aortography or predischarge CTA, were a result of our willingness to challenge more hostile aortic arch anatomy than that permitted by the pivotal study protocols. The majority (67%, 6/9) of these endoleaks resolved spontaneously by 6 months, 1 patient was successfully treated endovascularly, and one patient underwent surgical conversion.

PENETRATING AORTIC ULCER

Penetrating atherosclerotic ulcer (PAU) refers to an ulcerating atherosclerotic lesion that penetrates the elastic lamina and is associated with hematoma formation within the media of the aortic wall and was first described as a distinct clinical and pathologic entity by Stanson and colleagues[34] in 1986 and has more recently been further characterized as one of the subgroups of acute aortic syndrome.[35] With reported rupture rates as high as 40% in symptomatic patients, urgent intervention is justified.[36] The focal nature of the PAUs, which are often present in older, high-risk surgical patients, makes them an ideal candidate for endovascular repair (**Fig. 5**). As previously stated, there are two devices currently approved by the FDA to treat symptomatic PAUs, the Zenith TX2 and the Talent Thoracic, and a comparable study in which patients with PAUs were treated under a single site IDE at the Arizona Heart Hospital with the TAG endoprosthesis to treat PAUs.[37] Subgroup analysis of the TX2 ulcer patients included 23 patients and reported 30-day and 365-day all-cause mortality survival of 100% with no severe morbid events within 30 days of treatment and a 365-day estimate of freedom from severe morbid events of 91.1%. Twenty-one patients with PAU were treated under the IDE at the Arizona Heart Hospital with 0% 30-day mortality and 4.8% overall mortality with a mean follow-up of 14 ± 18 months. With the exception of 1 vascular access complication, no perioperative morbidity was reported and the

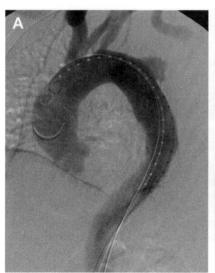
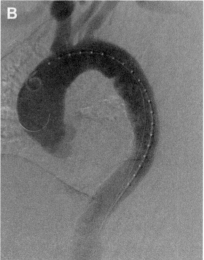

Fig. 5. Digital subtraction angiography of a focal penetrating aortic ulcer before (A) and after (B) successful endovascular repair.

incidence of endoleak or device migration during follow-up was 0%. Further, the use of just one device in 20 (95%) of 21 patients substantiates that the focal area of pathology in penetrating aortic ulcers is optimal for treatment by endovascular grafts.

TYPE B AORTIC DISSECTIONS

TEVAR has also been investigated as a treatment of acute Stanford type B aortic dissections. Due to mortality rates ranging from 35% to greater than 50% with surgical repair, medical therapy has been the preferred mode of treatment of most of these dissections. Surgery, and more recently TEVAR, has been reserved for patients with dissections complicated by extension of the dissection flap, refractory hypertension, localized pseudoaneurysm, impending rupture, persistent pain, and end-organ ischemia.[38] In 1999, Dake and colleagues[39] and Nienaber and colleagues[40] were the first to report their results with TEVAR in this patient population. Dake treated four patients with Stanford type A dissections and 15 patients with Stanford type B dissections with a 16% early mortality rate and no subsequent deaths or aortic rupture during the 13-month follow-up period. Nienaber compared the results of TEVAR in 12 consecutive patients to open surgical repair in 12 matched controls. Open surgery was associated with a 1-year mortality rate of 33% and serious adverse events in 42% of patients within 12 months, whereas TEVAR resulted in no significant morbidity or mortality during this same time. Both groups concluded that the key to success in this population was endograft coverage of the primary entry tear, which leads to at least partial thrombosis of the false lumen nearly all of the time. **Figs. 6** and **7** demonstrate a patient with acute dissection who underwent TEVAR for increased aneurysmal degeneration with remarkable results at 6-months follow-up. Xu and colleagues[41] looked to extending the indication for TEVAR to include asymptomatic type B aortic dissections because even medical management carried with it a mortality rate approaching 20% and significant likelihood of disease progression.[42] They treated 63 type B dissections with TEVAR resulting in 3.2% early mortality, complete

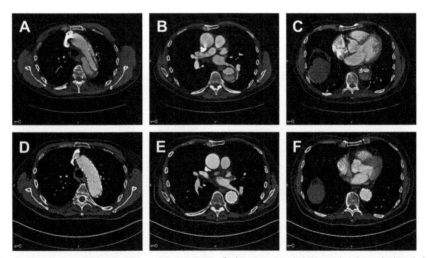

Fig. 6. Contrast-enhanced CTA axial images of the proximal (*A*), mid (*B*) and distal (*C*) thoracic aorta before treatment of a patient with acute type B thoracic dissection. Contrast-enhanced CTA axial images of the proximal (*D*), mid (*E*) and distal (*F*) thoracic aorta of the same patient at 6 months after successful endovascular repair.

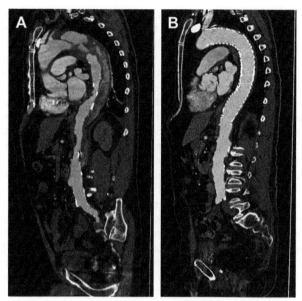

Fig. 7. (A) Multiplanar reconstruction of a patient with acute type B aortic dissection. (B) Multiplanar reconstruction of the same patient at 6 months after successful endovascular repair.

thrombosis of the false lumen in 98.4% of patients at 1 year, and 4-year survival rate of 89.4%.

Less is known about the efficacy of TEVAR in chronic Stanford type B dissections. Many investigators believe that this remains the least favorable indication for TEVAR secondary to fibrotic changes of the intimal flap and aortic wall, which can limit expansion of the true lumen following endograft placement. To combat this, some investigators have advocated use of covered endografts at the point of entry site with subsequent placement of uncovered Z-stents, which possess increased radial force, to further obliterate the false lumen.[43] However, this may carry with it a risk of creating intimal tears at the distal landing zone with potential for dissection extension. The predictability of intimal flap movement and subsequent true lumen expansion is difficult, however. Regardless, further studies are required to evaluate TEVAR as a treatment modality for chronic dissection.

TRAUMATIC AORTIC INJURY

In the last decade, endovascular treatment of blunt injury of the thoracic aorta has replaced open surgical repair to a great extent in most trauma centers. Demetriates and colleagues[44] recently reported on the observed changes in paradigm by comparing the American Association for the Surgery of Trauma study completed in 1997 to a similar study completed in 2007. The comparisons included the method of definitive diagnosis of the aortic injury, the method of aortic repair and outcomes, including overall mortality and procedure-related paraplegia. Aortic injury was diagnosed by CT scan in 34% of patients in 1997 versus 93.3% in 2007; all patients were managed with open surgical repair in 1997 versus only 35.2% in 2007 with the remaining 64.8% undergoing endovascular repair. The average time from injury to aortic repair increased from 16.5 hours in 1997 versus 54.6 hours in the 2007 study. Comparisons of outcomes between the two studies revealed that overall mortality decreased from 22% to 13% and the incidence of procedure-related paraplegia decreased from 8.7% to 1.6%. Although not all of these significant improvements in outcomes could be attributed to the shift toward endovascular repair alone, the investigators concluded that trauma surgeons should consider acquiring training in endovascular procedures. This specific patient population does have characteristics that make endovascular repair more difficult than in standard aneurysm patients. In general, proximal landing zones tended to be much smaller in young trauma patients than in other aortic pathologies, thereby requiring smaller devices to prevent endograft collapse, which has previously been linked to significant oversizing.[45] Currently the smallest thoracic endovascular device available is the Talent Thoracic stent graft, which is 22 mm in diameter and can treat aortas as small as 18 mm. It is also recognized that tighter arch angles are a significant obstacle to overcome in this population. Tighter arch angles can lead to lack of device apposition along the inner curve of the aortic wall as it enters the horizontal segment of the aortic arch, which subjects the device to extreme tangential forces and can also lead to collapse (**Fig. 8**). If the initial device is placed in zone 2, there may be no room to extend the endograft proximally without covering the left common carotid artery. In this case, the proximal aspect of the endograft can be reinforced with a balloon expandable stent (see **Fig. 8**E, F). This is one area in which future device development is needed to provide the next generation of endograft with the ability to accommodate an aorta with a smaller diameter and a tight radius of curvature. Ideas to combat these issues may include flared

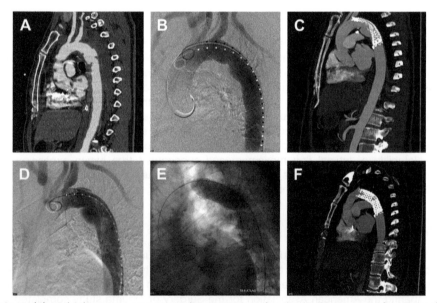

Fig. 8. (*A*) Multiplanar reconstruction demonstrating the classic appearance of contained thoracic aortic injury in the setting of blunt trauma. (*B*) Digital subtraction angiogram of the same patient following endovascular repair. Maximum intensity projection image (*C*) and digital subtraction angiogram (*D*) illustrating collapse of the endograft. (*E*) Endovascular placement of a balloon-mounted Palmaz stent to reinforce the previously placed endograft. (*F*) Maximum intensity projection image demonstrating the final result after placement of 2 Palmaz stents.

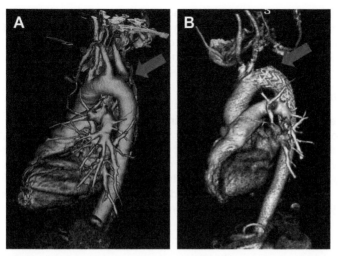

Fig. 9. Three-dimensional color reconstructions demonstrating aberrant origin of the right subclavian artery (*red arrows*) before endovascular exclusion (*A*) and following successful placement of the endograft (*B*).

endografts or smaller articulations, which would allow the endograft to conform better to the natural arch angle.

INTENTIONAL AORTIC BRANCH EXCLUSION

Less common indications for endograft placement in the thoracic aorta may include purposeful exclusion of vascular pathology within various aortic branches as adjunctive procedures to more peripheral surgical bypass, thereby precluding the need for sternotomy and medistinal dissection. For example, as demonstrated in **Fig. 9**, an endograft can be used to exclude a retroesophageal aberrant right subclavian artery

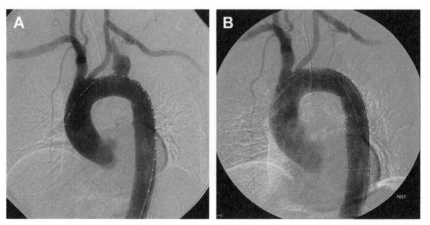

Fig. 10. (*A*) Digital subtraction angiogram demonstrating an aneurysm of the origin of the left subclavian artery. Also note the patent left carotid to left subclavian bypass graft with surgical ligation of the subclavian artery. (*B*) Digital subtraction angiography of the same patient following placement of endograft.

causing dysphagia, following right common carotid to distal right subclavian artery bypass. Another patient presented with an aneurysm of the proximal LSCA found incidentally on CT. She was treated with left carotid to LSCA bypass and ligation of the proximal LSCA and staged coverage of the LSCA origin with an endograft (**Fig. 10**).

FUTURE DEVICE DEVELOPMENT

In the 15 years since the first primitive hand-made endograft was used to repair the thoracic aorta, devices have undergone extensive and rapid evolvement to date. Anatomic characteristics continue to limit the suitability for endovascular repair with currently available devices. Future device designs will continue to increase the range of available device sizes, improve device trackability and conformability, and eventually include fenestrated and branched endografts, which will continue to expand the applicability of endovascular repair to more patients.

SUMMARY

The use of endovascular stent grafts for treatment of the descending thoracic aorta is reviewed. Currently, three devices have been approved by the US FDA for the treatment of descending thoracic aneurysms, and multiple studies are ongoing to investigate the efficacy of endovascular treatment in such pathologies as traumatic aortic injury and Stanford type B dissection. Outcomes are highly dependent on good case planning and patient selection and will likely continue to improve as newer-generation devices and delivery systems are designed and made available.

REFERENCES

1. DeBakey ME, Cooley DA. Successful resection of aneurysm of the thoracic aorta and replacement by graft. JAMA 1953;152:673–6.
2. Achneck HE, Rizzo JA, Tranquilli M, et al. Safety of thoracic aortic surgery in the present era. Ann Thorac Surg 2007;84:1180–5.
3. Parodi JC, Palmaz JC, Barone HD. Transfemoral intraluminal graft implantation for abdominal aortic aneurysms. Ann Vasc Surg 1991;5:491–9.
4. Dake MD, Miller DC, Semba CP, et al. Transluminal placement of endovascular stent-grafts for the treatment of descending thoracic aortic aneurysms. N Engl J Med 1994;331:1729–34.
5. Dake MD, Miller DC, Mitchell RS, et al. The "first generation" of endovascular stent-grafts for patients with aneurysms of the descending thoracic aorta. J Thorac Cardiovasc Surg 1998;116:689–703.
6. Makaroun MS, Dillavou ED, Kee ST, et al. Endovascular treatment of thoracic aortic aneurysms: results of the phase II multicenter trial of the GORE TAG thoracic endoprosthesis. J Vasc Surg 2005;41:1–9.
7. Greenberg R, Resch T, Nyman U, et al. Endovascular repair of descending thoracic aortic aneurysms: an early experience with intermediate-term follow-up. J Vasc Surg 2000;31:147–56.
8. Czerny M, Grimm M, Zimpfer D, et al. Results after endovascular stent graft placement in atherosclerotic aneurysms involving the descending aorta. Ann Thorac Surg 2007;83:450–5.
9. Dagenais F, Shetty R, Normand JP, et al. Extended applications of thoracic aortic stent grafts. Ann Thorac Surg 2006;82:567–72.

10. Verhoye JP, de Latour B, Heautot JF, et al. Mid-term results of endovascular treatment for descending thoracic aorta diseases in high-surgical risk patients. Ann Vasc Surg 2006;20:714–22.
11. Ince H, Rehders TC, Petzsch M, et al. Stent-grafts in patients with Marfan syndrome. J Endovasc Ther 2005;12:82–8.
12. Ehrlich M, Grabenwoeger M, Cartes-Zumelzu F, et al. Endovascular stent graft repair for aneurysms of the descending thoracic aorta. Ann Thorac Surg 1998;66:19–24.
13. Mitchell R, Dake M, Semba C, et al. Endovascular stent-graft repair of thoracic aortic aneurysms. J Thorac Cardiovasc Surg 1996;111:1054–62.
14. GORE TAG Thoracic endoprosthesis annual clinical update. April 2008.
15. Greenberg RK, O'Neill S, Walker E, et al. Endovascular repair of thoracic aortic lesions with the Zenith TX1 and TX2 thoracic grafts: intermediate-term results. J Vasc Surg 2005;41:589–96.
16. Matsumura JS, Cambria RP, Dake MD, et al. International controlled clinical trial of thoracic endovascular aneurysm repair with the Zenith TX2 endovascular graft: 1-year results. J Vasc Surg 2008;47:247–57.
17. Leurs LJ, Bell R, Degrieck Y, et al. Endovascular treatment of thoracic aortic diseases: combined experience from the EUROSTAR and United Kingdom Thoracic Endograft registries. J Vasc Surg 2004;40:670–9.
18. Fattori R, Nienaber CA, Rousseau H, et al. Results of endovascular repair of the thoracic aorta with the Talent thoracic stent graft: the Talent Thoracic Retrospective Registry. J Thorac Cardiovasc Surg 2006;132:332–9.
19. Fairman RM, Criado F, Farber M, et al. Pivotal results of the Medtronic Vascular Talent Thoracic Stent Graft System: the VALOR trial. J Vasc Surg 2008;48:546–54.
20. Criado F, Abul-Khoudoud O, Domer G, et al. Endovascular repair of the thoracic aorta: lessons learned. Ann Thorac Surg 2005;80:857–63.
21. Woo EY, Carpenter JP, Jackson BM, et-al. Left subclavian artery coverage during thoracic endovascular aortic repair: a single-center experience. J Vasc Surg 2008;48:555–60.
22. Buth J, Harris PL, Hovo R, et al. Neurologic complications associated with endovascular repair of thoracic aortic pathology: incidence and risk factors. A study from the European Collaborators on Stent/Graft Techniques for Aortic Aneurysm Repair (EUROSTAR) registry. J Vasc Surg 2007;46:1103–10, e2.
23. Noor N, Sadat U, Hayes PD, et al. Management of the left subclavian artery during endovascular repair of the thoracic aorta. J Endovasc Ther 2008;15:168–76.
24. Woo EY, Bavaria JE, Pochettino A, et al. Techniques for preserving vertebral artery perfusion during thoracic aortic stent grafting requiring aortic arch landing. Vasc Endovascular Surg 2006;40(5):367–73.
25. Lee WA, Brown MP, Nelson PR, et al. Total percutaneous access for endovascular aortic aneurysm repair ("Preclose" technique). J Vasc Surg 2007;45:1095–101.
26. Haas PC, Kracjer Z, Dietrich EB. Closure of large percutaneous access sites using the Prostar XL percutaneous vascular surgery device. J Endovasc Surg 1999;6:168–70.
27. Lee WA, Brown MP, Nelson PR, et al. Midterm outcomes of femoral arteries after percutaneous endovascular aortic repair using the Preclose technique. J Vasc Surg 2008;47(5):919–23.
28. Gravereaux EC, Faries PL, Burks JA, et al. Risk of spinal cord ischemia after endograft repair of thoracic aortic aneurysms. J Vasc Surg 2001;34:997–1003.
29. Baril DT, Carroccio A, Ellozy SH, et al. Endovascular thoracic aortic repair and previous or concomitant abdominal aortic repair: is the increased risk of spinal cord ischemia real? Ann Vasc Surg 2006;20:188–94.

30. Chiesa R, Melissano G, Marrocco-Trischitta MM, et al. Spinal cord ischemia after elective stent-graft repair of the thoracic aorta. J Vasc Surg 2005;42:11–7.
31. Feezor RJ, Martin TD, Hess PJ, et al. Risk factors for perioperative stroke during thoracic endovascular aortic repairs (TEVAR). J Endovasc Ther 2007;14:568–73.
32. Woo EY, Carpenter JP, Jackson BM, et al. Left subclavian artery coverage during thoracic endovascular aortic repair: a single-center experience. J Vasc Surg 2008;48:555–60.
33. Adams JD, Angle JF, Matsumoto AH, et al. Endovascular repair of the thoracic aorta in the post-FDA approval era. J Thorac Cardiovasc Surg 2009;137:117–23.
34. Stanson AW, Kazmier FJ, Hollier LH, et al. Penetrating atherosclerotic ulcers of the thoracic aorta: natural history and clinicopathologic correlations. Ann Vasc Surg 1986;1:15–23.
35. Vilacosta I, San Roman JA. Acute aortic syndrome. Heart 2001;85:365–8.
36. Coady MA, Rizzo JA, Hammond GL, et al. Penetrating ulcer of the thoracic aorta: what is it? How do we recognize it? How do we manage it? J Vasc Surg 1998;27:1006–15.
37. Brinster DR, Wheatley GH 3rd, Williams J, et al. Are penetrating aortic ulcers best treated using an endovascular approach? Ann Thorac Surg 2006;82:1688–91.
38. Fann JI, Miller DC. Aortic dissection. Ann Vasc Surg 1995;9:311–23.
39. Dake MD, Kato N, Mitchell RS, et al. Endovascular stent-graft placement for the treatment of acute aortic dissection. N Engl J Med 1999;340:1546–52.
40. Nienaber CA, Fattori R, Lund F, et al. Nonsurgical reconstruction of thoracic aortic dissection by stent-graft placement. N Engl J Med 1999;340:1539–45.
41. Xu SD, Huang FJ, Yang JF, et al. Endovascular repair of acute type B aortic dissection: early and mid-term results. J Vasc Surg 2006;43:1090–5.
42. Juvonen T, Ergin MA, Galla JD, et al. Risk factors for rupture of chronic type B dissections. J Thorac Cardiovasc Surg 1999;117:776–86.
43. Nienaber CA, Kische S, Zeller T, et al. Provisional extension to induce complete attachment after stent-graft placement in type B aortic dissection: the PETTICOAT concept. J Endovasc Ther 2006;13:738–46.
44. Demetriades D, Velmahos GC, Scalea TM, et al. Diagnosis and treatment of blunt thoracic aortic injuries: changing perspectives. J Trauma 2008;64:1415–8.
45. Muhs BE, Balm R, White GH, et al. Anatomic factors associated with acute endograft collapse after Gore TAG treatment of thoracic aortic dissection or traumatic rupture. J Vasc Surg 2007;45:655–61.

Off-Pump Versus On-Pump Coronary Artery Bypass Grafting

Michael E. Halkos, MD, John D. Puskas, MD*

KEYWORDS

- Off-pump • Coronary artery bypass grafting
- Cardiopulmonary bypass • Beating heart • Outcomes

Off-pump coronary artery bypass grafting (OPCAB) has been increasingly used over the past decade for surgical coronary revascularization. The interest in off-pump techniques has largely been driven by the increased awareness of the deleterious effects of cardiopulmonary bypass. Although many centers have adopted this technique, OPCAB use seems to have reached a plateau in recent years and currently accounts for approximately 20% of coronary artery bypass cases (Data Analyses of the Society of Thoracic Surgeons National Adult Cardiac Database, 2007). Technical considerations, surgeon comfort level, practice patterns, and the excellent reported outcomes with on-pump coronary artery bypass surgery (ONCAB) are common reasons cited by surgeons who continue to perform most of their operations on-pump. Although several centers perform the majority of their procedures off-pump, some surgeons prefer to implement this technique in low-risk patients or in patients requiring only 1- or 2-vessel grafting. This article summarizes the literature comparing outcomes of off-pump versus on-pump coronary artery bypass surgery.

OUTCOMES ANALYSIS

Clinical outcomes between OPCAB and ONCAB have been compared and reported for several years. These studies can generally be divided into smaller prospective randomized trials and larger observational or retrospective analyses. Prospective randomized trials provide the most accurate comparison between groups and avoid selection bias inherent in retrospective and observational analyses. However, these smaller studies are often statistically underpowered to detect incremental improvements in morbidity or mortality rates that are already low with ONCAB. This situation is especially true when predominantly low-risk patients are enrolled. Furthermore, the

Division of Cardiothoracic Surgery, Emory University Hospital-Midtown, Emory University School of Medicine, 550 Peachtree Street, 6th Floor, Medical Office Tower, Atlanta, GA 30308, USA
* Corresponding author.
E-mail address: john.puskas@emoryhealthcare.org (J.D. Puskas).

doi:10.1016/j.suc.2009.06.015
0039-6109/09/$ – see front matter © 2009 Elsevier Inc. All rights reserved.
surgical.theclinics.com

cost associated with randomized trials usually prevents patients from being followed for extended periods of time after surgery. Retrospective and observational analyses provide much larger sample sizes with longer duration of follow-up but are limited by their retrospective nature and inherent selection bias despite the use of propensity matching or other advanced statistical methodologies designed to control for this effect. Because of their larger size, small differences in outcomes can often be detected. Taken together, however, both types of studies can provide valuable information to guide clinical practice.

CARDIOPULMONARY BYPASS

Whereas a detailed discussion of the effects of cardiopulmonary bypass is beyond the scope of this review, a brief comment is warranted. Although cardiopulmonary bypass with cardioplegic arrest can be safely used in most patients, there are well-recognized complications and limitations to this approach. The use of cardiopulmonary bypass is associated with derangements in the coagulation pathways, inflammatory cell activation, generation and delivery of microemboli, variation in regional organ perfusion, hemodilution and hypothermia, and alterations in acid-base balance.[1] These effects are due in part to the exposure of blood to nonendothelialized surfaces (the pump and circuit) and to components within the surgical wound. An intense systemic inflammatory activation occurs that may ultimately result in neurologic impairment, renal dysfunction, or pulmonary insufficiency. Despite these potentially precarious consequences, the large majority of patients tolerate cardiopulmonary bypass without clinically apparent adverse outcomes.

TECHNICAL AND INTRAOPERATIVE CONSIDERATIONS

Improvements in exposure and retraction techniques and the development of specialized stabilizers and positioners allow surgeons to readily perform more complex coronary artery anastomoses that previously required cardiopulmonary bypass and an arrested heart.[2] Furthermore, the attention and diligence of experienced anesthesia personnel are required to minimize and address hemodynamic fluctuations that may occur with cardiac positioning, retraction, and regional ischemia. Careful attention must be paid to the sequence of grafting because regional myocardial perfusion is temporarily interrupted in the beating heart. For example, in a patient with an occluded right coronary artery with collateral flow supplied by the left anterior descending coronary artery, temporary occlusion of the left anterior descending would not only interrupt flow to the anterior wall but also to the inferior wall and right ventricle. Therefore grafting and restoring blood flow to the right coronary territory first would be more appropriate in this situation. Although concern for myocardial protection during OPCAB stems from the brief periods of coronary occlusion necessary to visualize distal target vessels, adequate perfusion can be achieved by maintaining adequate systemic perfusion pressure, selective use of coronary artery shunts, careful use of traction sutures and stabilizers, and proper sequencing of graft anastomoses.[3] Serum markers of myocardial injury have consistently been found to be lower in patients undergoing OPCAB compared with ONCAB,[4–6] which suggests a limited injury compared with the more global ischemic injury induced when cardioplegic arrest is used.

RANDOMIZED CLINICAL TRIALS

Over the past decade, several randomized trials have documented the safety and efficacy of OPCAB.[4,5,7–12] Although these relatively smaller trials did not show a mortality benefit for OPCAB compared with ONCAB, they did consistently demonstrate lower blood transfusion requirements, decreased ventilator times, and a shorter intensive care and hospital length of stay. However, at least one study has challenged these findings, reporting equivalent morbidity outcomes between OPCAB and ONCAB,[13] although this trial was small with only 150 patients in each group.

Paramount to these trials has been the importance of graft patency. It is clear that for off-pump techniques to be justified and beneficial, grafts sewn on the beating heart must have equivalent patency rates to those performed on-pump. Whereas one study found a lower graft patency in OPCAB patients at 3 months,[14] others have demonstrated equivalent early[8,15] angiographic patency in randomized patients undergoing OPCAB versus ONCAB. Short-term angiographic results have also been published by the groups of Widimsky,[11] Nathoe,[16] and Puskas,[17] which have shown equivalent angiographic graft patency at 1 year. Long-term graft patency has also been evaluated. Angelini and colleagues[12] recently presented 7-year results of a randomized trial comparing OPCAB to ONCAB, using computed tomographic angiography to assess graft patency. Overall long-term graft patency was excellent in both groups with no difference between ONCAB (89.4%) and OPCAB (89.0%) patients. Therefore, most evidence suggests that graft patency is not influenced by the technique of revascularization.

Several reports have raised concerns about the completeness of revascularization, suggesting that patients undergoing OPCAB were more likely to receive fewer grafts compared with those undergoing ONCAB.[11,18,19] However, using the number of grafts performed to determine completeness of revascularization may be erroneous, especially in nonrandomized retrospective series in which surgeons may selectively choose to perform OPCAB for patients requiring few grafts (1–3) and ONCAB for those requiring multiple (>3) grafts.[20] Instead, other studies have used an index score that compares the number of grafts performed to the number of diseased vessels on preoperative angiographic assessment. In these analyses, patients undergoing OPCAB had equivalent completeness of revascularization indices compared with ONCAB patients.[5,9,10,13–16]

RETROSPECTIVE AND OBSERVATIONAL TRIALS

Retrospective, observational, and registry trials, although limited by selection bias and lack of randomized comparisons, provide important insight into results that can only be appreciated with large sample sizes. Several registry studies have been published recently that are adequately powered to detect differences in adverse outcomes that occur relatively infrequently. Similar to the New York state registry data comparing survival outcomes of coronary artery bypass surgery to drug-eluting stents in multivessel disease,[21] these studies, powered by their large sample size, are able to detect significant differences in adverse outcomes among a broad population of patients. In a similar study by Hannan and colleagues,[22] 49,830 patients from the New York state registry underwent risk-adjusted analysis (Cox proportional hazard models and propensity analysis) comparing outcomes after OPCAB versus ONCAB. In this study, OPCAB patients had significantly lower 30-day mortality, as well as a lower incidence of postoperative stroke and respiratory failure. Three-year follow-up revealed that OPCAB patients had a higher rate of repeat revascularization, but 3-year survival was equivalent between the two groups.[22] An intention-to-treat retrospective analysis of 42,477 patients from the Society of Thoracic Surgeons National Database showed a reduction in risk-adjusted operative mortality as well as numerous morbidity outcomes favoring patients undergoing OPCAB.[23] In a large registry study of California coronary artery bypass grafting outcomes, Li and colleagues[24] also demonstrated a significant improvement in operative survival with OPCAB compared with ONCAB. These studies and others[25–28] have demonstrated that operative mortality may be reduced in patients undergoing OPCAB compared with ONCAB and that long-term survival is equivalent between the 2 groups.

Completeness of revascularization has been critical for the success of coronary artery bypass surgery.[29,30] At present the ability to provide complete revascularization with OPCAB techniques has been challenged in the aforementioned randomized trials as well as in larger retrospective databases, although most evidence from randomized studies suggests equivalent revascularization. Lattouf and colleagues[26] revealed that patients requiring more than three grafts were more likely to be revascularized on-pump. In this study, completeness of revascularization rather than number of grafts was associated with an improved long-term survival, and there was no difference in completeness of revascularization between groups. The detrimental effect of incomplete revascularization on long-term mortality was also reported in a study by Synnergren and colleagues.[30] In the Society of Thoracic Surgeons National Cardiac Database study by Puskas and colleagues,[23] OPCAB patients had a slightly lower index of completeness of revascularization than ONCAB patients, although operative morbidity and mortality were significantly reduced in patients undergoing OPCAB. Within the authors' own institution, 10-year survival of more than 12,000 patients was equivalent between OPCAB and ONCAB groups.[25] Thus, the issue of completeness of revascularization during OPCAB and its impact on long-term survival remains unsettled. Comparisons with older trials may not account for significant improvements in secondary medical prevention strategies or for advances in percutaneous coronary intervention. It is the policy of the authors that completeness of revascularization should not be compromised when deciding whether to use or avoid cardiopulmonary bypass unless the use of cardiopulmonary bypass poses significant risk for postoperative complications or mortality, which may be the case in patients with severe atherosclerotic disease of the ascending aorta. Because the authors perform the large majority of their coronary operations without cardiopulmonary bypass, complete revascularization, even in the more difficult lateral wall territory, is readily accomplished.

EMERGENT CORONARY REVASCULARIZATION

The safety and feasibility of OPCAB in select emergency situations has been confirmed in several series.[31–33] In a randomized trial, Fattouch and colleagues[31] reported that patients undergoing emergency off-pump revascularization for acute ST elevation myocardial infarction had a significantly lower in-hospital mortality and lower incidence of low cardiac output syndrome. However, this study included patients operated on within 48 hours of presentation, suggesting an urgent rather than emergent presentation in at least some patients. Locker and colleagues[33] also reported a survival advantage for emergent patients undergoing revascularization without cardiopulmonary bypass. In their study there was a similar incidence of preoperative cardiogenic shock in both groups. In hemodynamically stable patients taken to the operating room during an evolving infarct, off-pump revascularization seems to be feasible. However, this must be approached with caution for several reasons. Data on patients undergoing truly emergent revascularization off-pump is sparse. In addition, unloading the ventricle with cardiopulmonary bypass lowers the workload and decreases oxygen demand of an already ischemic heart. Finally, these studies are limited by selection bias; the most unstable patients are likely to be revascularized using cardiopulmonary bypass, whereas hemodynamically stable patients may be revascularized off-pump. As always, good surgical judgment based on individual patient risk factors and surgeon experience must guide decision making.

NEUROLOGIC OUTCOMES

Although the etiology of postoperative stroke after coronary artery bypass surgery is multifactorial, atheromatous aortic emboli is a major factor.[34] Emboli can arise from intraoperative manipulation of the aorta during (1) aortic cannulation, (2) institution and maintenance of cardiopulmonary bypass, or (3) application and removal of the aortic cross-clamp for cardioplegic arrest or partial clamping for proximal anastomoses. In the larger retrospective analyses, the incidence of adverse neurologic events has been lower in patients undergoing off-pump surgery. Mishra and colleagues[35] performed a propensity-matched comparison of OPCAB versus ONCAB in 6991 patients with atheromatous aortic disease and found a significant decrease in hospital mortality and stroke incidence, with OPCAB being the only independent predictor of a decreased stroke rate. Other large studies demonstrated a reduction in stroke in patients undergoing OPCAB versus ONCAB.[23,25,36] However, some trials have failed to demonstrate a reduction in neurologic events.[37–41] These analyses[37–41] included studies with a small sample size that individually were underpowered to detect a significant difference in a relatively infrequent although devastating complication. It is important to consider that in patients with a relatively low atherosclerotic burden of the ascending aorta, the risk of aortic emboli is low and thus it is unlikely that a difference in postoperative stroke will be appreciated between OPCAB and ONCAB without a very large sample size. It is possible that other variables, such as intraoperative hemodynamic instability resulting in hypoperfusion, or postoperative atrial fibrillation, may contribute to postoperative stroke. In addition, partial aortic clamping for construction of proximal anastomoses is still used selectively for patients undergoing OPCAB. Kim and colleagues[42] reported a lower incidence of postoperative stroke in patients undergoing OPCAB without any manipulation of the aorta (no partial clamping) compared with patients undergoing OPCAB with partial clamping and patients undergoing ONCAB. Hammon and colleagues[43] reported reduced neuropsychological deficits in patients undergoing ONCAB via single cross-clamp compared with patients undergoing ONCAB with multiple cross-clamping or patients undergoing OPCAB and partial clamping. Furthermore, Kapetanakis and colleagues[44] and Calafiore and colleagues[45] concluded that aortic manipulation is independently associated with an increased risk of postoperative stroke. Thus the potential benefits of OPCAB may not be fully realized if it is performed with partial aortic clamping. It therefore seems intuitive that this would be especially true in high-risk patients with severe atherosclerosis of the ascending aorta. Mere palpation of the ascending aorta is an inadequate means to assess the presence, absence, or extent of atherosclerosis. Intraoperative epiaortic ultrasound scanning is a quick, easy, and readily available technique that provides reliable measurement of the thickness and degree of atherosclerosis of the ascending aorta. This technique is used for every patient undergoing cardiac surgery at the authors' institution and guides the selective use or avoidance of partial aortic clamping.

Avoiding partial clamping during proximal anastomoses during OPCAB can be achieved by performing proximal anastomoses to in situ arterial grafts, or using proximal automated anastomotic connectors (PAS-Port Proximal Anastomosis System, Cardica Inc., Redwood City, California), or facilitating devices (hand-sewn anastomoses without partial clamping such as the Heartstring II proximal anastomosis system, Maquet Heartstring, Maquet Cardiovascular LLC, San Jose, California, or the Enclose II device, Novare Surgical Systems Inc., Cupertino, California), both of which can be performed without a partial aortic clamp. A recent study evaluating the production of solid microemboli using transcranial Doppler revealed a significant reduction in the proportion of solid microemboli with these devices (used without aortic clamping) compared with a strategy of partial aortic clamping.[46] The investigators concluded that the use of the Enclose and Heartstring devices may represent an important strategy for minimizing cerebral injury during proximal aortic anastomoses. In a recent randomized clinical trial evaluating the PAS-Port proximal anastomotic connector versus construction of hand-sewn proximal anastomoses with partial clamping, all of the reported strokes occurred in patients in whom an aortic clamp was used.[47] Other studies have also documented the efficacy of the PAS-Port proximal anastomotic connector.[48] The impact of these devices during OPCAB on postoperative neurologic outcomes needs to be addressed in clinical trials. In theory, however, avoiding manipulation of the aorta, especially in patients with advanced atherosclerotic aortic disease, would seem to favorably impact neurologic outcomes.

OPCAB IN HIGH-RISK PATIENTS

Several studies have documented improved outcomes in higher-risk patients undergoing off-pump bypass. In particular, well-known higher-risk groups such as women, patients with left ventricular dysfunction, prior stroke, renal insufficiency, and previous sternotomy have been investigated retrospectively. In a prospective randomized trial of patients with preoperative renal insufficiency, Sajja and colleagues[49] demonstrated that OPCAB was beneficial, with decreased postoperative serum creatinine values and increased glomerular filtration rate compared with ONCAB. Dewey and colleagues[50] showed improved operative mortality in favor of OPCAB among patients with dialysis-dependent renal failure. In patients with left ventricular dysfunction,[51] previous sternotomy,[52] advanced age,[53] previous stroke,[36] and in female patients,[27] more favorable outcomes have been reported with OPCAB compared with ONCAB.

MINIMALLY INVASIVE AND HYBRID APPROACHES

The use of off-pump techniques has facilitated the development and application of minimally invasive revascularization techniques. Endoscopic atraumatic coronary artery bypass has been well described and involves a thoracoscopic or robotic-assisted left internal mammary artery dissection and harvest, followed by a direct off-pump anastomosis to the left anterior descending coronary artery via a left anterior minithoracotomy.[54] Combining percutaneous intervention to non-left anterior descending targets, so-called hybrid revascularization, has also been described[55] and is gaining in popularity. Totally endoscopic coronary artery bypass, which is facilitated with off-pump and robotic techniques as well as anastomotic facilitating devices, has also been reported, but significant technical hurdles persist that have prevented broad adoption of this very demanding technique.[56] The feasibility of these alternative minimally invasive approaches has been demonstrated and the use of minimally invasive techniques has generated much enthusiasm in the surgical and interventional communities.

SUMMARY

Off-pump techniques can be safely used to perform coronary artery bypass operations on the beating heart without compromising short- or long-term graft patency. Although smaller prospective trials enrolling low-risk patients have been underpowered to show a mortality benefit, larger retrospective analyses demonstrate a significant reduction in mortality and morbidity after OPCAB compared with ONCAB. Patients with renal insufficiency, advanced age, chronic pulmonary disease, and ascending aortic disease are more likely to benefit from avoiding both the systemic effects of cardiopulmonary bypass and aortic manipulation with cross-clamping and cannulation. Therefore, the adoption of this technique in clinical practice provides surgeons with an effective option when cardiopulmonary bypass poses an excessive risk to the patient. On the contrary, it requires an astute clinician to understand the physiologic consequences of cardiac manipulation and regional ischemia necessary for off-pump anastomoses and to be able to predict and avoid hemodynamic instability. Finally, it is the policy of the authors to perform complete revascularization, regardless of whether the procedure is performed with or without cardiopulmonary bypass, because this remains the foundation of surgical revascularization.

REFERENCES

1. Hammon JW. Extracorporeal circulation. In: Cohn LH, editor. Cardiac surgery in the adult. 3rd edition. Columbus (OH): McGraw-Hill; 2008. p. 370–414.
2. Song HK, Puskas JD. Off-pump coronary artery bypass surgery. In: Kaiser R, Kron IL, Spray TL, editors. Mastery of cardiothoracic surgery. 2nd edition. Philadelphia: Lippincott Williams & Wilkins; 2007. p. 454–65.
3. Puskas JD, Vinten-Johansen J, Muraki S, et al. Myocardial protection for off-pump coronary artery bypass surgery. Semin Thorac Cardiovasc Surg 2001;13:82–8.
4. Gerola LR, Buffolo E, Jasbik W, et al. Off-pump versus on-pump myocardial revascularization in low-risk patients with one or two vessel disease: perioperative results in a multicenter randomized controlled trial. Ann Thorac Surg 2004;77(2): 569–73.
5. Puskas JD, Williams WH, Duke PG, et al. Off-pump coronary artery bypass grafting provides complete revascularization with reduced myocardial injury, transfusion requirements, and of length of stay: a prospective randomized comparison of two hundred unselected patients undergoing off-pump versus conventional coronary artery bypass grafting. J Thorac Cardiovasc Surg 2003;125:797–808.
6. Chowdhury UK, Malik V, Yadav R, et al. Myocardial injury in coronary artery bypass grafting: on-pump versus off-pump comparison by measuring high-sensitivity C-reactive protein, cardiac troponin I, heart-type fatty acid-binding protein, creatine kinase-MB, and myoglobin release. J Thorac Cardiovasc Surg 2008;135: 1110–9.
7. Angelini GD, Taylor FC, Reeves BC, et al. Early and midterm outcome after off-pump and on-pump surgery in Beating Heart Against Cardioplegic Arrest Studies (BHACAS 1 and 2): a pooled analysis of two randomised controlled trials. Lancet 2002;359(9313):1194–9.
8. Kobayashi J, Tashiro T, Ochi M, et al. Early outcome of a randomized comparison of off-pump and on-pump multiple arterial coronary revascularization. Circulation 2005;112(9 Suppl):I338–43.
9. Muneretto C, Bisleri G, Negri A, et al. Off-pump coronary artery bypass surgery technique for total arterial myocardial revascularization: a prospective randomized study. Ann Thorac Surg 2003;76:778–82.

10. van Dijk D, Nierich AP, Jansen EWL, et al. Early outcome after off-pump versus on-pump coronary bypass surgery—results from a randomized study. Circulation 2001;104:1761–6.
11. Widimsky P, Straka Z, Stros P, et al. One-year coronary bypass graft patency: a randomized comparison between off-pump and on-pump surgery angiographic results of the PRAGUE-4 trial. Circulation 2004;110:3418–23.
12. Angelini GD, Culliford L, Smith D, et al. Effects of on- and off-pump coronary artery surgery on graft patency, survival and quality of life: long term follow-up of two randomised controlled trials. American Association for Thoracic Surgery; San Diego, CA: 2008.
13. Legare JF, Buth KJ, King S, et al. Coronary bypass surgery performed off pump does not result in lower in-hospital morbidity than coronary artery bypass grafting performed on pump. Circulation 2004;109:887–92.
14. Khan NE, De Souza A, Mister R, et al. A randomized comparison of off-pump and on-pump multivessel coronary-artery bypass surgery. N Engl J Med 2004;350: 21–8.
15. Lingaas PS, Hol PK, Lundblad R, et al. Clinical and angiographic outcome of coronary surgery with and without cardiopulmonary bypass: a prospective randomized trial. Heart Surg Forum 2004;7:37–41.
16. Nathoe HM, van Dijk D, Jansen EW, et al. A comparison of on-pump and off-pump coronary bypass surgery in low-risk patients. N Engl J Med 2003; 348:394–402.
17. Puskas JD, Williams WH, Mahoney EM, et al. Off-pump vs conventional coronary artery bypass grafting: early and 1-year graft patency, cost, and quality-of-life outcomes. JAMA 2004;291:1841–9.
18. Carrier M, Perrault LP, Jeanmart H, et al. Randomized trial comparing off-pump to on-pump coronary artery bypass grafting in high-risk patients. Heart Surg Forum 2003;6:E89–92.
19. Czerny M, Baumer H, Kilo J, et al. Complete revascularization in coronary artery bypass grafting with and without cardiopulmonary bypass. Ann Thorac Surg 2001;71:165–9.
20. Alamanni F, Dainese L, Naliato M, et al. On- and off-pump coronary surgery and perioperative myocardial infarction: an issue between incomplete and extensive revascularization. Eur J Cardiothorac Surg 2008;34:118–26.
21. Hannan EL, Wu C, Walford G, et al. Drug-eluting stents vs. coronary artery bypass grafting in multivessel coronary disease. N Engl J Med 2008;358:331–41.
22. Hannan EL, Wu C, Smith CR, et al. Off-pump versus on-pump coronary artery bypass graft surgery: differences in short-term outcomes and in long-term mortality and need for subsequent revascularization. Circulation 2007;116: 1145–52.
23. Puskas JD, Edwards FH, Pappas PA, et al. Off-pump techniques benefit men and women and narrow the disparity in mortality after coronary bypass grafting. Ann Thorac Surg 2007;84:1447–54.
24. Li Z, Yeo KK, Parker JP, et al. Off-pump coronary artery bypass graft surgery in California, 2003 to 2005. Am Heart J 2008;156:1095–102.
25. Puskas JD, Kilgo PD, Lattouf OM, et al. Off-pump coronary bypass provides reduced mortality and morbidity and equivalent 10-year survival. Ann Thorac Surg 2008;86:1139–46.
26. Lattouf OM, Thourani VH, Kilgo PD, et al. Influence of on-pump versus off-pump techniques and completeness of revascularization on long-term survival after coronary artery bypass. Ann Thorac Surg 2008;86:797–805.

27. Puskas JD, Kilgo PD, Kutner M, et al. Off-pump techniques disproportionately benefit women and narrow the gender disparity in outcomes after coronary artery bypass surgery. Circulation 2007;116(Suppl 11):I192–9.

28. Puskas JD, Cheng D, Knight J, et al. Off-pump versus conventional coronary artery bypass grafting: a meta-analysis and consensus statement from the 2004 ISMICS consensus conference. Innovat Tech Tech Cardiothorac Vasc Surg 2005;1:3–27.

29. Jones EL, Weintraub WS. The importance of completeness of revascularization on long-term follow-up after coronary artery operations. J Thorac Cardiovasc Surg 1996;112:227–37.

30. Synnergren MJ, Ekroth R, Oden A, et al. Incomplete revascularization reduces survival benefit of coronary artery bypass grafting: role of off-pump surgery. J Thorac Cardiovasc Surg 2008;136:29–36.

31. Fattouch K, Bianco G, Sampognaro R, et al. Off-pump vs. on-pump CABG in patients with ST segment elevation myocardial infarction: a randomized, double blind study. American Association for Thoracic Surgery; San Diego, CA: 2008.

32. Kerendi F, Puskas JD, Craver JM, et al. Emergency coronary artery bypass grafting can be performed safely without cardiopulmonary bypass in selected patients. Ann Thorac Surg 2005;79:801–6.

33. Locker C, Mohr R, Paz Y, et al. Myocardial revascularization for acute myocardial infarction: benefits and drawbacks of avoiding cardiopulmonary bypass. Ann Thorac Surg 2003;76:771–6.

34. Likosky DS, Marrin CAS, Caplan LR, et al. Determination of etiologic mechanisms of strokes secondary to coronary artery bypass graft surgery. Stroke 2003;34:2830–4.

35. Mishra M, Malhotra R, Karlekar A, et al. Propensity case-matched analysis of off-pump versus on-pump coronary artery bypass grafting in patients with atheromatous aorta. Ann Thorac Surg 2006;82:608–14.

36. Halkos ME, Puskas JD, Lattouf OM, et al. Impact of preoperative neurologic events on outcomes after coronary artery bypass grafting. Ann Thorac Surg 2008;86:504–10.

37. Cheng DC, Bainbridge D, Martin JE, et al. Does off-pump coronary artery bypass reduce mortality, morbidity, and resource utilization when compared with conventional coronary artery bypass? a meta-analysis of randomized trials. Anesthesiology 2005;102:188–203.

38. Wijeysundera DN, Beattie S, Djaiani G, et al. Off-pump coronary artery surgery for reducing mortality and morbidity. J Am Coll Cardiol 2005;46:872–82.

39. Biancari F, Mosorin M, Rasinaho E, et al. Postoperative stroke after off-pump versus on-pump coronary artery bypass surgery. J Thorac Cardiovasc Surg 2007;133:169–73.

40. van Dijk D, Spoor M, Hijman R, et al. Cognitive and cardiac outcomes 5 years after off-pump vs on-pump coronary artery bypass graft surgery. JAMA 2007;297:701–8.

41. Jensen BO, Hughes P, Rasmussen LS, et al. Cognitive outcomes in elderly high-risk patients after off-pump versus conventional coronary artery bypass grafting: a randomized trial. Circulation 2006;113:2790–5.

42. Kim KB, Kang CH, Chang WI, et al. Off-pump coronary artery bypass with complete avoidance of aortic manipulation. Ann Thorac Surg 2002;74(Suppl):S1377–82.

43. Hammon JW, Stump DA, Butterworth JF, et al. Coronary artery bypass grafting with single cross-clamp results in fewer persistent neuropsychological deficits

than multiple clamp or off-pump coronary artery bypass grafting. Ann Thorac Surg 2007;84:1174–8.

44. Kapetanakis EI, Stamou SC, Dullum MKC, et al. The impact of aortic manipulation on neurologic outcomes after coronary artery bypass surgery: a risk-adjusted study. Ann Thorac Surg 2004;78:1564–71.

45. Calafiore AM, Di Mauro M, Teodori G, et al. Impact of aortic manipulation on incidence of cerebrovascular accidents after surgical myocardial revascularization. Ann Thorac Surg 2002;73:1387–93.

46. Guerrieri Wolf L, Abu-Omar Y, Choudhary BP, et al. Gaseous and solid cerebral microembolization during proximal aortic anastomoses in off-pump coronary surgery: the effect of an aortic side-biting clamp and two clampless devices. J Thorac Cardiovasc Surg 2007;133:485–93.

47. Puskas JD, Halkos ME, Connolly M, et al. Evaluation of the PAS-port proximal anastomosis system in coronary artery bypass surgery (the EPIC Trial). J Thorac Cardiovasc Surg 2009;138:125–32.

48. Kempfert J, Opfermann UT, Richter M, et al. Twelve-month patency with the PAS-port proximal connector device: a single center prospective randomized trial. Ann Thorac Surg 2008;85:1579–84.

49. Sajja LR, Mannam G, Chakravarthi RM, et al. Coronary artery bypass grafting with or without cardiopulmonary bypass in patients with preoperative non-dialysis dependent renal insufficiency: a randomized study. J Thorac Cardiovasc Surg 2007;133:378–88.

50. Dewey TM, Herbert MA, Prince SL, et al. Does coronary artery bypass graft surgery improve survival among patients with end-stage renal disease? Ann Thorac Surg 2006;81:591–8.

51. Youn YN, Chang BC, Hong YS, et al. Early and mid-term impacts of cardiopulmonary bypass on coronary artery bypass grafting in patients with poor left ventricular dysfunction: a propensity score analysis. Circ J 2007;71:1387–94.

52. Mishra YK, Collison SP, Malhotra R, et al. Ten-year experience with single-vessel and multivessel reoperative off-pump coronary artery bypass grafting. J Thorac Cardiovasc Surg 2008;135:527–32.

53. Panesar SS, Athanasiou T, Nair S, et al. Early outcomes in the elderly: a meta-analysis of 4921 patients undergoing coronary artery bypass grafting—comparison between off-pump and on-pump techniques. Heart 2006;92:1808–16.

54. Vassiliades TA Jr, Reddy VS, Puskas JD, et al. Long-term results of the endoscopic atraumatic coronary artery bypass. Ann Thorac Surg 2007;83:979–84.

55. Vassiliades TA Jr, Douglas JS, Morris DC, et al. Integrated coronary revascularization with drug-eluting stents: immediate and seven-month outcome. J Thorac Cardiovasc Surg 2006;131:956–62.

56. Argenziano M, Katz M, Bonatti J, et al. Results of the prospective multicenter trial of robotically assisted totally endoscopic coronary artery bypass grafting. Ann Thorac Surg 2006;81:1666–74.

Minimally Invasive Valve Surgery

Y. Joseph Woo, MD

KEYWORDS

- Valve surgery • Minimally-invasive • Mitral • Aortic
- Valvuloplasty

Cardiac valve surgery is in the midst of undergoing rapid evolution. For several decades, valve surgery consisted of replacement of a diseased valve with a mechanical or biologic prosthesis by way of a full sternotomy using cardiopulmonary bypass (CPB), performed on a cardioplegia arrested heart. During the past decade, this fundamental paradigm has shifted to now encompass preferential valve repair instead of replacement, alternate minimal access incisions, on-pump beating heart techniques, off-pump valve repair devices,[1–6] robotics, and transcatheter valve devices[7,8] Multiple combinations and permutations of these approaches abound.[9] This has been fueled on one front by technological advances in peripheral vessel-based CPB perfusion systems, imaging modalities, and intracardiac devices, and on the other by surgical creativity and innovation. Rapid dissemination of knowledge and information in the electronic era has further fueled this evolution, and referring cardiologists and patients often have specific pre-existing concepts of what minimally invasive heart valve repair operation they are seeking.

Recently there have been further improvements in the conduct of valve operations, with more anatomically and physiologically correct repair techniques, extremely small micro-access incisions, and a range of new intracardiac devices.[10] This article reviews the benefits of minimally invasive approaches to valve surgery and concentrates on detailing the technical aspects of this surgery, the advanced repair techniques that have evolved around minimal access approaches, and the adjunctive devices. The focus is on the mitral and aortic valves, with some discussion of the tricuspid and pulmonary valves.

MITRAL VALVE

Decades ago some of the earliest mitral valve surgeries, involving closed mitral commissurotomy for rheumatic mitral stenosis, were often performed by nonsternotomy repair, albeit using larger thoracotomy approaches, often by left thoracotomy and through the left atrial appendage.[11,12] With the application of CPB as a routine component of mitral valve surgery, excellent access to the heart and the great vessels for

Division of Cardiovascular Surgery, Department of Surgery, University of Pennsylvania, Silverstein 6, 3400 Spruce Street, Philadelphia, PA 19104, USA
E-mail address: wooy@uphs.upenn.edu

Surg Clin N Am 89 (2009) 923–949
doi:10.1016/j.suc.2009.05.005
0039-6109/09/$ – see front matter © 2009 Elsevier Inc. All rights reserved.

cannulation provided by median sternotomy made this approach the obvious preferred cardiac surgery incision.

Because the mitral valve lies in an annular plane that nearly approximates the sagittal plane of the body, it is particularly well suited to a right lateral approach. In the mid-to-late 1990s, with the development of an advanced circulatory system with peripheral arterial and venous perfusion, cardioplegia, and venting cannulas, the use of minimally invasive mitral valve procedures became widespread.[13–19] Since then multiple large retrospective studies, a small prospective, randomized study,[20] and a meta-analysis have been published. These studies have shown the advantages of minimally invasive mitral valve surgery to be:[21–42]

1. Equivalent mitral valve repair capability and quality
2. Long-term durability of mitral valve repair and freedom from reoperation
3. Certain concomitant procedures are possible
4. Reduced blood loss and transfusion requirements
5. Reduced postoperative pain
6. Shorter duration of mechanical ventilation
7. Shorter duration of intensive care unit time
8. Shorter length of hospitalization
9. Quicker recovery
10. Greater satisfaction
11. Improved cosmesis, especially in women in whom the incision can be hidden within the right inframammary crease

DETRIMENTS INCLUDE:

1. Significant surgeon and operating room team learning curves
2. Increased infrastructural requirements
3. Increased cross-clamp and CPB times
4. Potential aortovascular injury with femoral cannulation, particularly with the use of the endoballoon aortic occlusion device

Patient Selection

Typically, patients present with a preconceived notion of, a specific interest in, or instructions from their cardiologist regarding a minimally invasive approach to their mitral valve surgery. With the wide access to digital information, patients often have extensive knowledge about minimally invasive valve operations before consultation with a cardiac surgeon. Nevertheless, there are multiple issues to consider when deciding on a patient's candidacy for a minimally invasive approach. These include disease process, cardiac operation needed, comorbidities, body habitus, patient/cardiologist expectations, and overall risk/benefit ratio.[43–45]

Beyond the standard preoperative evaluation including echocardiography, coronary angiography, carotid duplex ultrasonography, laboratory evaluation, and detailed history and physical examination, generally no additional specific diagnostic studies are necessary to prepare a patient for a minimally invasive operation. Under rare circumstances, if there is need for information regarding the size and position of the heart within and in relation to the other intrathoracic structures and the chest wall, a contrast CT scan can be particularly useful. If there is a history of peripheral vascular disease or diminished femoral pulses on examination, further analysis of peripheral circulation using pulse volume recordings or CT angiography may be useful in determining the suitability of the femoral arterial vessels for cannulation. Patients with relative contraindications to femoral vessel cannulation are still candidates for minimally invasive surgery. Alternative cannulation strategies are detailed later.

Anesthetic Preparation

In addition to the standard monitoring lines, the anesthesiologist can place a double-lumen endotracheal tube to facilitate isolated single left lung ventilation and right lung deflation during certain periods of the operation. External defibrillator cardioversion pads are placed on the patient, usually under the right scapula and over the left antero-lateral chest. A right internal jugular superior vena caval cannula (usually a 16FR wire reinforced cannula) is placed using the Seldinger wire technique and cervical surface ultrasonographic guidance. The catheter is flush-locked with heparin saline and the patient is administered a small dose of intravenous heparin to aid in preventing thrombus formation in this large catheter (**Fig. 1**).

If preferred, a percutaneous retrograde pulmonary sinus cannula and a pulmonary arterial venting cannula can also be placed by the anesthesiologist through the right internal jugular vein.[46,47] If an endoaortic balloon occlusion catheter is planned, bilateral radial arterial line placement provides additional assurance by offering immediate recognition of distal migration of the inflated balloon and subsequent obstruction of the innominate artery. Inadvertent endoballoon migration occurs in up to 40% of operations and has been associated with higher complication rates than transthoracic clamping. Most notably, intravascular injuries including aortic dissection have contributed to a decrease in use of this approach. It is our institutional preference to employ the transthoracic Chitwood aortic cross-clamp and standard antegrade cardioplegia, retrograde cardioplegia, and right superior pulmonary vein venting cannulas placed across the thoracic wall or directly through the access incision. This approach not only generates a cannulation strategy that much more closely resembles a standard sternotomy operation but also greatly simplifies and expedites the anesthetic preparation.

Whereas thoracic epidural placement may assist in the management of postoperative pain, these are generally not used because pain has been reported to be mild after minimally invasive incisions. The patient is placed in a supine position and a small inflatable pillow is placed under the right scapula to slightly elevate the right hemithorax. The right arm is padded and placed along the right side of the body. The patient is prepped down beyond the right mid-axillary line and into the axilla. The anterior chest is prepped for potential sternotomy and both groins are prepped. The operating table is placed in reverse Trendelenburg position and rotated slightly to the left. This position maximizes the direct visualization of the mitral valve through the incision.

Incision

Although multiple options exist, the right anterolateral mini-thoracic incision has become the approach of choice for most surgeons performing minimally invasive mitral valve surgery.[48] This incision offers a tremendous advantage over the lower partial sternotomy in that it presents a more en face view of the mitral valve and avoids any surgery in the xiphosternal region, the area most prone to wound breakdown and infection after sternotomy.[49,50] The right chest approach is extremely resistant to infection as there is always overlying pectoralis muscle and other soft tissue to aid in sealing and healing the wound. In men, the skin incision is usually made medial and inferior to the right nipple. A 4-cm skin incision usually suffices. The pectoralis muscle is divided with electrocautery and the third intercostal space is entered, staying lateral of the right internal thoracic artery and veins. In women, the skin incision

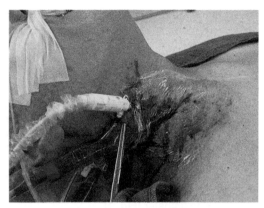

Fig. 1. Superior vena caval venous drainage cannula inserted percutaneously via the right internal jugular vein, along with pulmonary artery catheter.

is placed in the right inframammary crease and the soft tissue dissection is angled cephalad to reach the third interspace. To facilitate this exposure in women, the right breast is retracted superiorly during placement of the adhesive clear plastic drapes. The medial aspect of the fourth rib is then sharply divided with an orthopedic microsaw while preserving the fourth intercostal neurovascular bundle. Later, during closure, this rib is restabilized by internally fixating the medial cut edges with a #2 Dexon suture driven directly through the rib edges, then also more laterally with another #2 Dexon suture wrapped around the third and fourth ribs.

After intercostal entry and rib division, a minimally invasive mitral retractor is placed into the interspace and gentle spreading reveals an excellent view of the right-sided pericardium. An excessively large right pericardial fat pad should be removed, and the right hemidiaphragm can be retracted inferiorly with a single suture placed into the dome of the right hemidiaphragm and externalized through the right chest wall around the sixth or seventh intercostal space by using a thin suture hook. A longitudinal pericardiotomy is performed at least 3 cm anterior to the right phrenic nerve and extended from the diaphragmatic surface cephalad to the pericardial reflection on the aorta. The inferior pericardial edge of the pericardium is then retracted laterally with two sutures externalized along the mid-axillary line and the anterior pericardial edge is sutured tightly to the medial aspect of the skin incision. These maneuvers

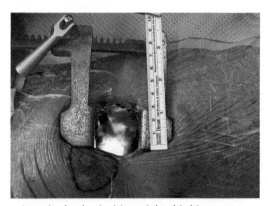

Fig. 2. Minimally invasive mitral valve incision, right third interspace.

retract the mediastinum toward and rotate the heart toward the right chest incision, providing an outstanding exposure of the right atrium, interatrial groove, right pulmonary venous confluence, superior vena cava (SVC), inferior vena cava (IVC), and the aortic root and ascending aorta (**Fig. 2**). A small Satinsky clamp placed onto the lateral aspect of the skin incision to hook the skin edge and then attached tightly to the operating room table further shifts the incision onto a sagittal plane and thus presents a more en face view of the mitral valve through the incision.

With the incision completed, adjunctive sites are created to introduce additional equipment. A small port is placed through the chest wall inferior and lateral to the skin incision, through which carbon dioxide is insufflated into the right hemithorax. This significantly simplifies deairing procedures later. A small suction catheter can be placed through this port to help maintain field visualization during the operation. A 30-degree standard thoracic videoscope can be placed into the chest superior and lateral to the skin incision to aid in illuminating the operative field and provide additional visualization, particularly for everyone in the operating room other than the surgeon. The scope is also especially useful in aiding visualization of the anterolateral aspect of the mitral valve annulus as well as the papillary muscles and intraventricular structures when performing Gore-Tex neochordal procedures. The transthoracic Chitwood aortic cross-clamp is introduced into the chest by way of the right third interspace at the mid-axillary line and positioned near the ascending aorta. The vertical post of the left atrial retractor can be introduced through the chest wall just medial to the incision and secured to the operating table attachment arm in a location slightly anterior to the heart. Performing as many of these equipment positioning and preparatory actions in advance decreases CPB and aortic cross-clamp times. The patient is now ready for system anticoagulation and cannulation.

Cannulation

Femoral arterial and venous structures are cannulated using Seldinger wire techniques and purse-string sutures placed on the anterior surface of the vessels. The vessels themselves are not dissected out, nor are they encircled with snares. Using the appropriately sized cannulas, intravascular flow around and beyond the cannula is preserved, albeit somewhat reduced. Nevertheless, this is a more favorable situation than the use of an overly large arterial or venous cannula or vessel snares. Cannulation is performed with transesophageal echocardiography (TEE) guidance. During arterial cannulation, the distal descending thoracic aorta is imaged to confirm the intraluminal position of the wire and, thus, markedly reduce the risk of intramural wire malpositioning and aortic dissection. Depending on the size of the patient and the artery, an 18, 16, or 14FR wire wrapped cannula provides adequate flow rate for CPB. By using a transthoracic aortic cross-clamp and avoiding the endoballoon system, the much larger obligatory 23 and 21FR arterial cannulas are thus avoided.

During venous cannulation, TEE is used to confirm wire position inside the right atrium and aid in exact positioning of the venous cannula. A 22FR long venous cannula always provides sufficient venous drainage. When positioned with the tip in the SVC and additional drainage holes in the body of the right atrium and the IVC, this cannula may provide adequate venous drainage for mitral valve surgery using a left atrial approach. The addition of a superior vena caval venous drainage cannula introduced through the right internal jugular vein adds significant additional drainage capacity, particularly when retracting anteriorly on the interatrial septum, to provide additional exposure to the mitral valve and thus effectively separate the superior and inferior vena caval circulation. Adding this SVC drainage cannula also permits one to position more of the holes of the long IVC cannula into the IVC itself, thus improving IVC drainage. This approach also facilitates potential transseptal approaches to the mitral valve as well as concomitant tricuspid valve surgery.

When a contraindication to direct femoral arterial cannulation exists, such as small vessel size or significant peripheral vascular disease, alternatives include graft attachment in the case of small size, and axillary or ascending aortic cannulation in the case of small vessel size or peripheral vascular disease. Ascending aortic cannulation can be facilitated by use of a wire wrapped cannula introduced using the Seldinger wire and sequential dilator technique, either across the chest wall or through a slightly larger access incision. In the setting of a femoral venous cannulation contraindication, such as a patient with an inferior vena caval filter placed for deep venous thrombosis/pulmonary embolism, the inferior vena caval/right atrial junction can be cannulated directly through the access incision. Seldinger wire techniques and TEE guidance are again used.

Retrograde coronary sinus cannulation can be performed by the surgeon through the access incision and with TEE guidance. Occasionally, an additional backward bend to the metal stilette is necessary to compensate for the lateral incision. Just before the initiation of CPB, the aortic line is retrograde primed and the venous line is antegrade primed with the patient's blood. Depending on the size of the patient and the hemoglobin level, a liter of whole autologous blood can be sequestered now for use after discontinuation of CPB, thus providing a source of fresh whole blood with coagulation factors and intact platelets that have not been exposed to the membrane oxygenator. CPB is first initiated by way of the SVC cannula to generate flow rates of at least 1 L per minute, confirming proper positioning of this cannula. Vacuum- or kinetic-assisted venous return is used.[51,52] After initiating full bicaval bypass, a left ventricular venting cannula can also be introduced through the right superior pulmonary vein, if desired. On completely decompressing the heart, the aortic root is easily visualized and an ascending aortic cardioplegia and venting cannula can be placed. Application of the transthoracic aortic clamp is aided by significantly lowering the systemic blood pressure with volume removal and reduction of pump flow. Adequate visualization around the ascending aorta prevents inadvertent clamp malposition, pulmonary artery injury, or left atrial appendage injury. The conduct of CPB and cardioplegic arrest can now be managed as in a standard operation (**Fig. 3**).

Mitral Valve Surgery

The mitral valve can now be exposed using a standard interatrial groove left atriotomy. The anterior left atrium and interatrial septum are retracted anteriorly with a table-mounted arm. To collect any blood returning into the operative field and thereby improve visualization, the right superior pulmonary vein vent can be placed across the posterior left atrium and into the left inferior pulmonary vein. This position is usually the deepest portion of the left atrium. Additional left atrial drainage can be facilitated by placing the tip of the pericardial suction catheter, introduced through the carbon dioxide insufflator port, into the right inferior pulmonary vein. These maneuvers, combined with venting of the aortic root cannula, usually provide a completely bloodless operative field. The surgeon's view through the incision is outstanding (**Fig. 4**). The inferior margin of the left atriotomy may obscure some of the mitral valve annulus. This problem can easily be addressed by first placing the mitral valve annular ring sutures underneath the P3 scallop or from 3 to 6 o'clock and attaching these tightly to the drape. Because the focus nowadays is to preserve as much mitral valve leaflet tissue

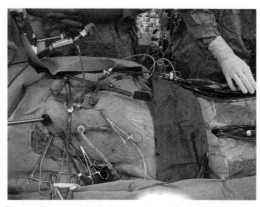

Fig. 3. Exposure and cannulation technique in minimally invasive mitral valve surgery.

as possible and remodel, as opposed to resect, leaflet tissue, there is rarely a need for annular plication or sliding annuloplasty, thus all of the mitral ring annuloplasty sutures can be placed at the beginning of the operation and do not need to be removed or adjusted. These are placed under tension and further present the mitral valve for inspection.

At this point, aortic root venting is temporarily discontinued and the left ventricle is rapidly filled with saline to reveal the mitral valve pathology. In the setting of functional ischemic mitral regurgitation, this usually reveals centrally directed regurgitation due to inadequate leaflet coaptation from a combination of annular enlargement and chordal tethering from left ventricular dilatation. In the setting of myxomatous mitral valve disease, the specific leaflet pathology can now be demonstrated and further examined.

For functional ischemic mitral regurgitation cases, grasping 1 or 2 mitral ring annuloplasty sutures underneath the P2 scallop around 6 o'clock and pulling anteriorly toward the anterior annulus simulates the effect of a ring annuloplasty. Refilling the ventricle with saline usually now demonstrates competence of the mitral valve, providing a high level of confidence that a standard ring annuloplasty will achieve a successful mitral valve repair. Ring sizing in this setting is done to approximate

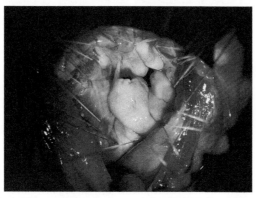

Fig. 4. Operative view of the mitral valve in a minimally invasive approach exceeds that of a standard sternotomy.

the size of the anterior leaflet to ensure proper reduction of the size of and anterior traction on the posterior mitral annulus as well as providing adequate length of leaflet coaptation across the entire coaptation plane. One must be careful not to excessively undersize the mitral ring, as there have been increasing reports of functional dynamic mitral stenosis after aggressive ring annuloplasty mitral valve repair.[53]

For myxomatous degenerative mitral valves, repair is focused on the leaflets. In the setting of a routine posterior leaflet P2 chordal rupture and flail segment, the standard Carpentier repair has entailed a quadrangular resection of the involved region followed by annular plication or sliding annuloplasty of P1 and P3, followed by reapproximation of the residual P2 components, and then augmented by a ring annuloplasty. This technique usually results in a highly reproducible, reliable, and durable mitral valve repair, albeit with essentially minimal posterior leaflet function.

More recently, out of concern for potentially producing functional mitral stenosis, there has been a surge in interest in preserving posterior leaflet tissue with the goal of preserving bileaflet function and avoiding small annuloplasty rings.[54,55] Various techniques have been developed. Perhaps the most common technique is that of chordal reconstruction. Chordal reconstruction can be done by fashioning a Gore-Tex neochord at the time of surgery and adjusting the length intraoperatively or, by using TEE, predetermining the appropriate length of the chord, prefashioning these before surgery, sterilizing, and implanting.[56–58] Another technique that has been described is Brigham foldoplasty.[59] In this technique, a U-stitch suture is placed in the leading edge of the flail segment and then brought out through the body of P2

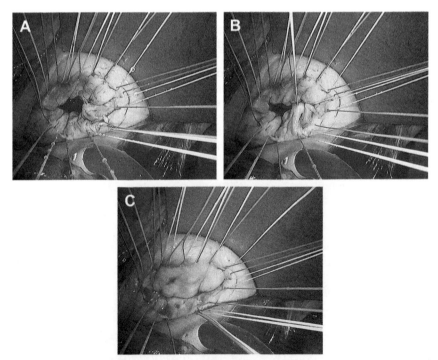

Fig. 5. (A) Ruptured P2 chord and flail segment. (B) Flail segment inverted into ventricular side of mitral valve and repair initiated with CV-5 Gore-Tex suture. (C) Left ventricle pressurized and competency of mitral valve repair examined.

close to or at the level of the annulus so as to fold the flail segment underneath. This technique is particularly useful in addressing the potential risk for systolic anterior motion (SAM) of the mitral valve when the height of the posterior leaflet is large.

Two techniques have been specifically designed to help preserve as much posterior leaflet tissue as possible. These techniques have evolved within the context of conducting minimally invasive mitral repairs and are particularly efficient methods for this environment. The first applies to situations whereby the leaflet disease involves primarily the P2 scallop (**Fig. 5A**). The inversionplasty entails grasping the leading edge of the ruptured chordal segment with forceps and inverting into the left ventricle. This procedure moves a small triangular piece of posterior leaflet tissue below the plane of the mitral valve annulus and presents 2 opposing short lines of tissue along the residual P2 segment (**Fig. 5B**). These 2 lines are then reapproximated with the double running CV-5 Gore-Tex suture. Static pressure testing of the ventricle at this point almost uniformly demonstrates a competent mitral valve with preservation of nearly the entire posterior leaflet (**Fig. 5C**). Furthermore, the appearance of the mitral valve in this setting almost mimics that of a normal mitral valve seen in a nonpathologic state.

If the disease is in the P1 or P3 scallop or the lateral or medial aspect of P2, it can be addressed by linking the diseased portion of the scallop to the nondiseased adjoining scallop using a CV-5 Gore-Tex suture (**Fig. 6A and B**). With this technique, the flail or prolapsed unsupported leaflet tissue is now supported by the structurally intact adjoining posterior leaflet tissue. This technique also preserves all of the posterior leaflet tissue and again yields, when pressurized, a mitral valve that appears completely normal or typically as shown in an anatomy textbook (**Fig. 6C**).

These two types of repairs are then reinforced with ring annuloplasty, paying careful attention to size the annuloplasty ring appropriately to the entire mitral valve orifice, including the pressurized anterior and posterior leaflet areas (**Fig. 7**). This procedure usually yields a large annuloplasty ring and a large functional mitral valve area with zero risk of inducing potential mitral stenosis. Furthermore, by reestablishing the proper normal relationship of the posterior leaflet to the anterior leaflet, specifically with respect to leaflet height, the risk of SAM also becomes negligible. These two techniques yield a repair of natural appearance and have been highly effective in practice; thus far they have been extremely durable with no reoperations for recurrent mitral regurgitation.

Anterior leaflet pathology has typically presented a greater repair challenge. The anterior leaflet serves a greater overall role in mitral valvular function, especially after standard repairs. It's proximity to the left ventricular outflow tract is of great importance. Often there is markedly less excess anterior leaflet tissue compared with the posterior leaflet and thus it is much less tolerant of resection and reapproximation. Neochords or transposed posterior chords must be shortened or lengthened precisely to avoid positioning the leaflet even slightly above or below the plane of coaptation. When properly executed, a highly competent repair of the mitral valve can be established (**Fig. 8A–C**). Occasionally, billowing leaflets in Barlow pathology present significant risk of movement into the left ventricular outflow tract and induction of SAM after overcorrection. This entity can often be repaired with variations of inversionplasty and foldoplasty, as demonstrated with this curling leaflet repair (**Fig. 9A and B**). Alternatively, aggressively reducing the size and height of the posterior leaflet can unfurl the billowing anterior leaflet and transfer the plane of coaptation posteriorly, thereby fully employing the anterior leaflet and avoiding the risk of SAM (**Fig. 10A–C**).

To further test the competency of the mitral valve repair, one can also add a form of dynamic testing whereby antegrade cardioplegia is used to highly pressurize the left

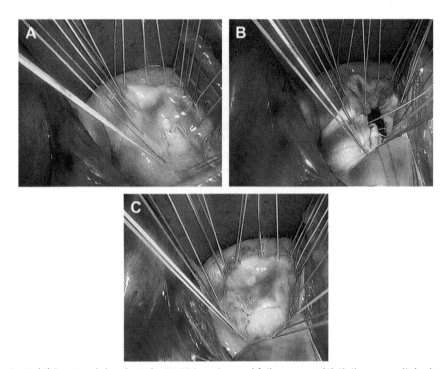

Fig. 6. (*A*) Ruptured chords at the P1-P2 junction and fail segment. (*B*) Flail segment linked to structurally intact P1 component. (*C*) Repaired mitral valve resembling normal anatomy.

ventricle. With the heart retracted anteriorly, the aortic valve is made mildly incompetent regardless of its pre-existing competency. The antegrade cardioplegia fully pressurizes and distends the left ventricle beyond what would normally be achievable with injection of saline through the mitral valve. This technique can even generate suprasystemic ventricular pressures and provide extreme confidence that the mitral valve repair will be highly competent.

Deairing and Closure

On completion of the mitral valve procedure, the right superior pulmonary vein vent is placed across the mitral valve annulus to a depth within the ventricle whereby venting

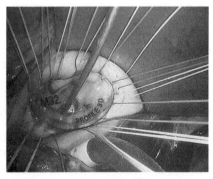

Fig. 7. Mitral ring sizing focusing on entire mitral orifice, anterior and posterior leaflet area.

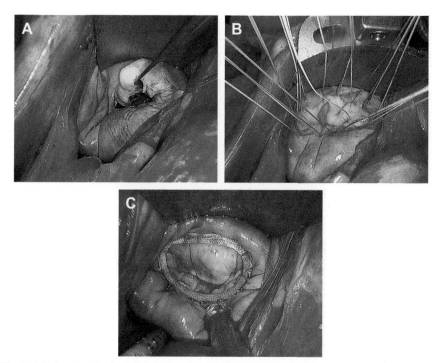

Fig. 8. (*A*) Ruptured A2 chord and flail segment. (*B*) Neochord construction for anterior repair. (*C*) Repaired mitral valve with ring annuloplasty for an anterior flail segment.

holes in the cannula are present in the ventricle and the left atrium. The operating table is tilted further to the left and in this simulated semi-thoracotomy position, the left ventricle is in a dependent position. Blood enters the left atrium, arising from the pulmonary veins, and because the mitral valve is made incompetent by the venting cannula, the blood pools into the deep end of the left ventricle, and air rises out into the left atrium and toward the atrial closure. Just before tying the left atriotomy suture, a bilateral lung Valsalva maneuver is performed to extrude any remaining pulmonary venous air into the left atrium. The heart is then deaired in standard fashion by

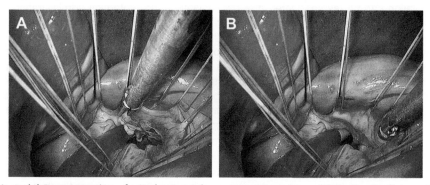

Fig. 9. (*A*) Demonstration of a Barlow's syndrome anterior prolapse. (*B*) Curling leaflet repair of the prolapsed A3 segment.

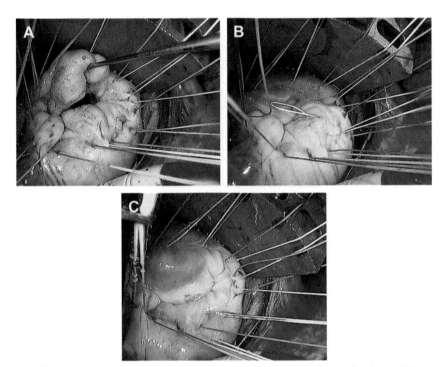

Fig. 10. (*A*) Demonstration of a Barlow's syndrome anterior prolapse with a large billowing anterior leaflet. (*B*) Addressing anterior leaflet prolapse by posterior leaflet height reduction repair. (*C*) Fully pressurized, competent mitral repair.

ventilating both lungs, filling the heart, and turning on the aortic root vent. The aortic cross-clamp is removed and the heart is reperfused. At this time, atrial and ventricular pacing wires should be placed because exposure to the right ventricle becomes progressively more difficult as the heart fills and beats. Because the hemithorax has been flushed with CO_2 throughout the entire operation, any residual bubbles or pockets of air consist of CO_2 and are rapidly metabolized by carbonic anhydrase. One usually finds during subsequent TEE-guided deairing maneuvers that there is minimal intracardiac air.

Separation from CPB is usually facilitated by dual lung ventilation. Single left lung ventilation can be resumed later after decannulation and protamine administration, if necessary, to examine the operative field for hemostasis. The divided edges of the pericardium are sutured at one location over the right atrium to eliminate the potentially devastating complication of cardiac herniation. Thoracostomy tubes are placed through any of the various small stab incisions. A long-acting local anesthetic, bupivicaine 0.25%, is then infused into the thoracic incision as an intercostal nerve block to markedly reduce initial postoperative pain. Postoperative management is essentially identical to that of a standard sternotomy procedure with specific advantages such as less bleeding, earlier extubation, and others listed previously, typically becoming apparent.

Beating Heart

There are certain complex clinical situations whereby a right chest minimally invasive incision and avoidance of aortic cross-clamping provide an optimal surgical approach.[60-63] The most common scenario is that of a patient with multivessel coronary artery disease who has undergone coronary artery bypass grafting (CABG) and has developed progressive ischemic cardiomyopathy with resultant mitral regurgitation. The patient is now presenting for mitral valve repair in the setting of prior CABG and patent grafts. Patients generally prefer to avoid a reoperative sternotomy and mediastinal reentry.[64-67] Also, there is the potential for bypass graft injury particularly if there is a midline patent left internal mammary artery graft. Furthermore, manipulation of old venous bypass grafts during dissection of adhesions risks distal embolization. Another setting is that of a patient with severe left ventricular dysfunction in which a period of aortic cross-clamping would typically be accompanied by prolonged weaning from CPB, significant inotropic support requirements, and occasional intra-aortic balloon pump placement after mitral valve repair. Finally, patients with significant atheromatous disease of the ascending aorta may be better approached by this method. Anterior retraction of the left atrium to expose the mitral valve during minimally invasive right chest approaches tends to displace the heart less and result in less induction of aortic valve incompetence; thus, beating heart non-cross-clamp techniques are generally better tolerated. In contrast to cold fibrillating noncross-clamp techniques, this warm beating heart technique is highly myoprotective, and on completion of the procedure the patient can be immediately weaned from CPB.[68]

CPB is established with peripheral cannulation as previously described. A small deairing needle cannula is placed into the aortic root and maintained at a continuous rate of 500 mL per minute to ensure that any small amount of air ejected out of the ventricle is captured. Even a small amount of air that escapes the root vent is unlikely to be propagated antegrade into the cerebral or systemic circulation because the aortic perfusion occurs in retrograde fashion from the femoral artery and therefore any blood arriving in the aortic root travels retrograde down into the coronary arteries. Immediately after performing a left atriotomy, a venting cannula is placed across the mitral valve to eliminate the ability of the ventricle to fill with blood and eject blood and air. With appropriately positioned intra-atrial suction catheters, even in a fully perfused heart, the mitral valve can be perfectly and bloodlessly exposed (Fig. 11).

The mitral valve repair is then conducted as described earlier. The only difference is that whenever the competence of the mitral valve is undergoing testing, this should be done carefully by filling the ventricle slowly with saline and ensuring that no air is accidentally injected into the ventricle. A venting cannula with multiple holes is placed just slightly across the mitral valve into the left ventricle but not actively placed on suction. The ventricle is then filled with saline. The ventricle begins to eject any residual air through the vent into the left atrium. The slightly incompetent aortic valve and resultant aortic regurgitation then continues to fill and pressurize the ventricle, and test the competency of the mitral valve repair at systemic pressure. During this period, the aortic root venting rate is increased to 1.5 L per minute to capture any residual ejected air. During closure of the left atriotomy, the right superior pulmonary vein venting cannula is placed across the competent mitral valve such that venting holes are in the ventricle and the atrium. Thus, any ventricular ejection occurs into the left atrium. These maneuvers coupled with CO_2 insufflation markedly minimize risks of air embolism and greatly simplify deairing. As the heart has been actively beating throughout the entire operation and has not received any cardioplegia or been exposed to ischemia, there is essentially minimal time needed to wean from CPB.

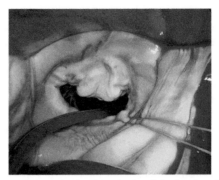

Fig. 11. Excellent exposure of the mitral valve obtained during beating heart valve surgery. Note the essentially bloodless field in this fully perfused heart. Also note the 2 tiny Thebesian veins draining on the anterior surface of the left atrium just above the mitral valve.

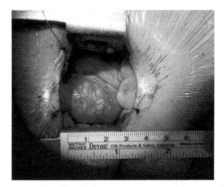

Fig. 12. Minimally invasive aortic valve incision, upper partial sternal division into the right fourth interspace.

AORTIC VALVE

Surgery of the aortic valve has been performed through a variety of incisions other than the standard full sternotomy. Whereas some surgeons still advocate a right parasternotomy or right mini-thoracotomy, most minimally invasive surgeons are now using a partial upper sternal division with entry into the right third or fourth intercostal space and preservation of the right internal thoracic artery. Multiple studies have been

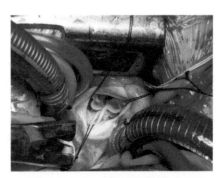

Fig. 13. Exposure and cannulation technique for minimally invasive aortic valve surgery.

published describing minimally invasive approaches to aortic valve surgery. Several comparative studies have likewise been published, usually describing a standard sternotomy versus a partial right upper sternotomy. There have been small prospective randomized trials as well as large retrospective studies. In general, these studies have shown the advantages of minimally invasive aortic valve surgery to be:[69–87]

1. Equivalent aortic valve replacement capability
2. Possibility of certain concomitant procedures
3. Reduced blood loss and transfusion requirements
4. Reduced postoperative pain
5. Preservation of chest wall integrity and improved pulmonary function
6. Reduced wound infections
7. Shorter length of hospitalization
8. Quicker recovery

Patient Selection

Whereas most patients who are candidates for standard aortic valve replacement by sternotomy would likely be eligible for a minimally invasive approach, there are some groups in which this approach presents greater difficulties.[88] Obese patients may have abundant adipose and soft tissue overlying the sternum. Here, a short incision creates a challenging, deep tunnel through which to visualize the aortic root and to conduct the operation. Patients with unclear but potential need for concomitant procedures such as coronary bypass grafting or mitral valve repair during aortic valve replacement, based on intraoperative indications, may be better served with an initial standard sternotomy. Finally, patients with severe left ventricular dysfunction who would likely benefit from an expeditious operation and hence brief myocardial ischemic time, may be better served with the increased exposure of a standard sternotomy.

Anesthetic Preparation

The anesthetic preparation for minimally invasive valve surgery is essentially identical to that of a standard sternotomy procedure with the only addition being the placement of transcutaneous defibrillator pads because of the decreased access to the ventricles through the minimally invasive incision. The patient is placed in a standard supine position. Because of the anterior anatomic localization of the ascending aorta and aortic root as well as the right atrial appendage, all cannulation can be easily achieved through the minimally invasive incision without the need for adjunctive femoral or jugular cannulas.

Incision

A skin incision beginning at the sternomanubrial junction and extending inferiorly for 4 to 5 cm is usually sufficient.[50] A standard sternal saw is used to divide the manubrium and the upper portion of the sternum and curve into the right third or fourth intercostal space. After pericardiotomy, the cut edges of the pericardium are sutured to the skin edge and a pediatric sternal retractor is placed. This procedure allows significant anterior retraction of the upper mediastinal structures of interest (**Fig. 12**). The patient is now ready for systemic anticoagulation and cannulation.

Cannulation and CPB

Multiple cannulation options exist. On one end of the spectrum is the use of only peripheral vasculature to maximize space and visualization within the incision. On the other end is complete cannulation through the incision, just as in a standard sternotomy operation, for simplicity and to minimize peripheral vascular manipulation. Over time, I have found that the use of central cannulation has been expeditious and with proper positioning, does not interfere with space or visualization constraints. The ascending aorta, right atrial appendage, coronary sinus, and right superior pulmonary vein can all be cannulated directly as in a standard operation. The critical adjunctive maneuver is to position the venous cannula, coronary sinus cannula, and ventricular venting cannula in the right lower portion of the incision, sew a heavy suture around all 3 cannulas, and then through the pericardium underlying the divided right hemisternal junction. Tying this suture tightly while pushing the cannulas toward the right lung greatly increases the space between the right atrium and the aortic root, and provides excellent visualization to the aortic valve (**Fig. 13**). Retrograde aortic priming and antegrade venous priming, and blood sequestration are routinely employed. The aorta can be occluded with a standard cross-clamp. After the delivery of antegrade cardioplegia it is often useful to temporarily remove the ascending aortic cardioplegia cannula while leaving the purse-string suture in place. This procedure aids in visualization of the aortic root.

Aortic Valve Surgery

To optimize aortic valve exposure, a curvilinear aortotomy is made transversely and toward the left side of the aorta and more vertically into the noncoronary sinus of Valsalva toward the right of the aorta. Three silk sutures are placed through the top of each leaflet commissure and retracted under significant tension in a triangular fashion to retract the edges of the aortotomy and evert the aortic valve and annulus into the operative field. When operating on calcific aortic stenosis, the aortic valve leaflets should be excised with a single cut to each leaflet along the narrow plane between the calcification and the aortic annulus. If performed carefully and correctly, the entire valve leaflet and all annular calcification can be excised en bloc, obviating the need for any further annular debridement. This approach minimizes any potential spillage of calcific material into the ventricle and likely reduces the risk of stroke. The aortic annular sizing, replacement suture placement, and valve implantation are all performed as in a standard operation. With aggressive sizing and supra-annular positioning techniques, a large prosthetic aortic valve that clearly eclipses the entire aortic root can be successfully implanted even in this minimally invasive setting, particularly when using a flexible bioprosthetic valve (**Fig. 14**A and B).

Aortic Valve Repair

Recently there has been resurgent interest in aortic valve repair. What has been learned over years of failed aortic valve repair is that the pathologic process greatly impacts the likelihood of success. Whereas debridement and decalcification of heavily calcified valve leaflets portends a poor prognosis, other specific pathologies are much more readily repairable. Isolated sinotubular junction dilatation from ascending aortic aneurysmal disease and resultant leaflet malcoaptation are often readily addressable with ascending aortic graft replacement and reduction of sinotubular junction diameter, and reestablishment of leaflet coaptation. Concomitant aortic root aneurysmal disease with annular dilatation, sinotubular dilatation, and leaflet malcoaptation can be repaired with valve-sparing root replacement. Cusp prolapse from loss of architectural support at the commissure due to aortic dissection can be easily repaired with commissural resuspension and aortic dissection false lumen repair. Finally, isolated cusp prolapse in a trileaflet valve without aortic pathology can be addressed with primary suspension of the leaflet leading edge (**Fig. 15**A–C).

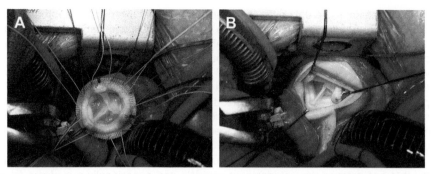

Fig. 14. (A) Oversizing bioprosthetic aortic valve replacement. (B) Implanted aortic valve bioprosthesis.

Partial resection and reapproximation of a prolapsed leaflet together with bilateral commissuroplasty for a prolapsed leaflet in a bicuspid aortic valve has been moderately successful, albeit at some expense of the induction of mild to moderate aortic stenosis postoperatively. These complex aortic valve leaflet repair and root reconstruction procedures have also been performed through minimally invasive approaches.[89–91]

Deairing and Closure

During aortotomy closure, left ventricular venting is discontinued early to aid in filling the atrium and ventricle with blood. Retrograde cardioplegia administration also

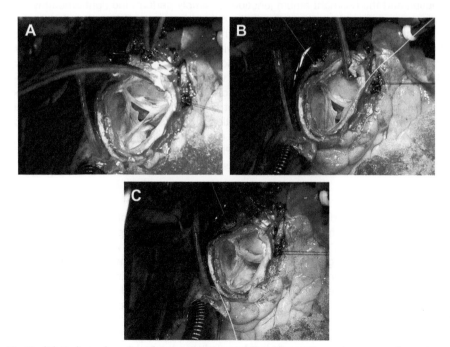

Fig. 15. (A) Prolapsed aortic valve noncoronary leaflet. (B) Leading edge suspension suture repair of prolapsed leaflet. (C) Successful repositioning of prolapsed leaflet into proper coaptation plane.

facilitates deairing. The only difference between a minimally invasive approach and a standard sternotomy is lack of access to the left ventricle and inability to physically manipulate the left ventricle to aid in deairing. Carbon dioxide insufflation into the operative field may be of some help, although a minimally invasive aortic procedure overall is a much more open operative field compared with a minimally invasive mitral procedure wherein there is essentially a closed hemithorax to entrap the CO_2. Epicardial pacing wires should be placed immediately after removal of the aortic cross-clamp as access to the right ventricle progressively decreases. Also at this time a thoracostomy tube should be placed. The patient is further deaired with TEE guidance and weaned from CPB.

Because of the partially undivided sternum, there is a region of the partial sternotomy that compresses the anterior right ventricle and occasionally provides a false image of an underfilled right ventricle on TEE. Yet the central venous pressure appears elevated and the right atrium dilated. This condition is easily addressed by releasing the pericardial traction sutures placed at the beginning of the operation to anteriorly elevate the heart, thereby lowering the heart back into the thorax. The partial sternotomy is then closed with stainless steel wire.

TRICUSPID VALVE

Tricuspid valve repair and replacement surgery can be conducted through a right chest minimally invasive incision. The same chest incision used for mitral valve surgery is used. The superior and inferior vena caval cannulas need to be placed precisely. To minimize obstruction of field visualization by caval snares, one can either introduce additional transthoracic clamps through the chest wall to clamp the SVC/right atrium junction and the IVC/right atrium junction, or simply perform the right atriotomy and then place purse-string sutures inside the right atrium at the SVC orifice and the IVC orifice, then remove these later. Because the tricuspid valve annulus is more anterior than the mitral valve annulus, the angle of view of the tricuspid valve is somewhat less optimal than the mitral valve using this incision. This problem can be mitigated by placing additional anterior traction sutures within the body of the right atrium to bring the tricuspid valve annulus into the field of vision (**Fig. 16**). Generally, when using a partial ring, placement of the sutures at the 7 o'clock position and then moving clockwise sequentially improves visualization. In this setting, the use of the videoscope to facilitate placement of sutures is extremely helpful. Tricuspid valve surgery is amenable to beating heart techniques. Placing a venting cannula into the coronary sinus and another into the right ventricle usually keeps the field free of blood.

PULMONIC VALVE

Pulmonic valve procedures are becoming somewhat more common in the adult population. The previous thought process that having only one competent valve within the right-sided circulation is sufficient is generally being replaced with the concept that having two functioning valves is superior and yields better long-term outcome for the right ventricle. Furthermore, the increasing use of screening echocardiography tends to detect incidental tumors such as fibroelastomas of the pulmonic valve. Finally, as patients who have undergone tetralogy of Fallot and other pulmonic procedures as infants are now growing into adulthood, there is an increasing population of adult patients in need of reoperative pulmonic valve surgery, which can be easily addressed by minimally invasive approaches similar to the aortic incision. However, the right sided J-incision is made into a left-sided L-incision, usually into the left third or fourth intercostal space. This procedure provides excellent exposure of the pulmonic

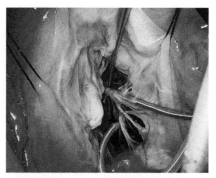

Fig. 16. Minimally invasive exposure and view of tricuspid valve. Note the pacing lead piercing the tricuspid leaflet tissue.

root as well as enough exposure of the ascending aorta and right atrium for central cannulation (**Fig. 17**). Venting of the left heart is accomplished through the open distal pulmonary artery.

ROBOTICS

Advanced operative three-dimensional visualization and telemanipulation systems have now come into routine use in urologic, gynecologic, general surgical, ear, nose, and throat, thoracic, and cardiac surgery.[92] Cardiac surgical applications include valve reconstruction, CABG, atrial septal defect closure, atrial fibrillation ablation, and left ventricular lead implantation, and others are in development.[93–128] The initial, and to date still the most common application for robotics in cardiac surgery, is minimally invasive mitral valve surgery.[129–131] Robotics provides a logical, stepwise progression from advanced minimally invasive mitral surgery by adding true three-dimensional optical visualization, multidirectional intracardiac instrument articulation, motion scaling, tremor filtration, potential force feedback, and a totally endoscopic approach.[132]

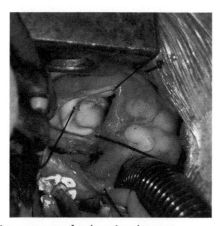

Fig. 17. Minimally invasive exposure of pulmonic valve root.

SUMMARY

Traditional cardiac valve replacement surgery is being rapidly supplanted by innovative, minimally invasive approaches toward the repair of these valves. Patients are experiencing benefits ranging from less bleeding and pain to faster recovery and greater satisfaction. These operations are proving to be safe, highly effective, and durable, and their use will likely continue to increase and become even more widely applicable.

REFERENCES

1. Fukamachi K, Inoue M, Popovic ZB, et al. Off-pump mitral valve repair using the Coapsys device: a pilot study in a pacing-induced mitral regurgitation model. Ann Thorac Surg 2004;77:688–92 [discussion: 692–3].
2. Grossi EA, Saunders PC, Woo YJ, et al. Intraoperative effects of the coapsys annuloplasty system in a randomized evaluation (RESTOR-MV) of functional ischemic mitral regurgitation. Ann Thorac Surg 2005;80:1706–11.
3. Grossi EA, Woo YJ, Schwartz CF, et al. Comparison of Coapsys annuloplasty and internal reduction mitral annuloplasty in the randomized treatment of functional ischemic mitral regurgitation: impact on the left ventricle. J Thorac Cardiovasc Surg 2006;131:1095–8.
4. Kollar A, Kekesi V, Soos P, et al. Left ventricular external subannular plication: an indirect off-pump mitral annuloplasty method in a canine model. J Thorac Cardiovasc Surg 2003;126:977–82.
5. Mishra YK, Mittal S, Jaguri P, et al. Coapsys mitral annuloplasty for chronic functional ischemic mitral regurgitation: 1-year results. Ann Thorac Surg 2006;81: 42–6.
6. Ramadan R, Al-Attar N, Mohammadi S, et al. Left ventricular infarct plication restores mitral function in chronic ischemic mitral regurgitation. J Thorac Cardiovasc Surg 2005;129:440–2.
7. Ma L, Tozzi P, Huber CH, et al. Double-crowned valved stents for off-pump mitral valve replacement. Eur J Cardiothorac Surg 2005;28:194–8 [discussion: 198–9].
8. Webb JG, Harnek J, Munt BI, et al. Percutaneous transvenous mitral annuloplasty: initial human experience with device implantation in the coronary sinus. Circulation 2006;113:851–5.
9. Rosengart TK, Feldman T, Borger MA, et al. Percutaneous and minimally invasive valve procedures: a scientific statement from the American Heart Association Council on Cardiovascular Surgery and Anesthesia, Council on Clinical Cardiology, Functional Genomics and Translational Biology Interdisciplinary Working Group, and Quality of Care and Outcomes Research Interdisciplinary Working Group. Circulation 2008;117:1750–67.
10. Shrestha M, Khaladj N, Bara C, et al. A staged approach towards interventional aortic valve implantation with a sutureless valve: initial human implants. Thorac Cardiovasc Surg 2008;56:398–400.
11. Cutler EC, Levine SA. Cardiotomy and valvotomy for mitral stenosis: experimental observations and clinical notes concerning an operated case with recovery. Boston Med Surg J 1923;5.
12. Harken DE, Ellis LB, Norman LR. The surgical treatment of mitral stenosis; progress in developing a controlled valvuloplastic technique. J Thorac Surg 1950;19: 1–15, illust [Discussion: 45–9].
13. Arom KV, Emery RW. Minimally invasive mitral operations. Ann Thorac Surg 1997;63:1219–20.

14. Chitwood WR Jr, Elbeery JR, Moran JF. Minimally invasive mitral valve repair using transthoracic aortic occlusion. Ann Thorac Surg 1997;63:1477–9.

15. Chitwood WR Jr, Wixon CL, Elbeery JR, et al. Video-assisted minimally invasive mitral valve surgery. J Thorac Cardiovasc Surg 1997;114:773–80 [discussion: 780–2].

16. Mohr FW, Falk V, Diegeler A, et al. Minimally invasive port-access mitral valve surgery. J Thorac Cardiovasc Surg 1998;115:567–74 [discussion: 574–6].

17. Mohr FW, Onnasch JF, Falk V, et al. The evolution of minimally invasive valve surgery–2 year experience. Eur J Cardiothorac Surg 1999;15:233–8 [discussion 238–9].

18. Navia JL, Cosgrove DM 3rd. Minimally invasive mitral valve operations. Ann Thorac Surg 1996;62:1542–4.

19. Schwartz DS, Ribakove GH, Grossi EA, et al. Minimally invasive cardiopulmonary bypass with cardioplegic arrest: a closed chest technique with equivalent myocardial protection. J Thorac Cardiovasc Surg 1996;111:556–66.

20. Dogan S, Aybek T, Risteski PS, et al. Minimally invasive port access versus conventional mitral valve surgery: prospective randomized study. Ann Thorac Surg 2005;79:492–8.

21. Asher CR, DiMengo JM, Arheart KL, et al. Atrial fibrillation early postoperatively following minimally invasive cardiac valvular surgery. Am J Cardiol 1999;84:744–7, A749.

22. Aybek T, Dogan S, Risteski PS, et al. Two hundred forty minimally invasive mitral operations through right minithoracotomy. Ann Thorac Surg 2006;81:1618–24.

23. Casselman FP, Van Slycke S, Dom H, et al. Endoscopic mitral valve repair: feasible, reproducible, and durable. J Thorac Cardiovasc Surg 2003;125:273–82.

24. de Vaumas C, Philip I, Daccache G, et al. Comparison of minithoracotomy and conventional sternotomy approaches for valve surgery. J Cardiothorac Vasc Anesth 2003;17:325–8.

25. Greco E, Zaballos JM, Alvarez L, et al. Video-assisted mitral surgery through a micro-access: a safe and reliable reality in the current era. J Heart Valve Dis 2008;17:48–53.

26. Greelish JP, Cohn LH, Leacche M, et al. Minimally invasive mitral valve repair suggests earlier operations for mitral valve disease. J Thorac Cardiovasc Surg 2003;126:365–71 [discussion: 371–3].

27. Grossi EA, Galloway AC, LaPietra A, et al. Minimally invasive mitral valve surgery: a 6-year experience with 714 patients. Ann Thorac Surg 2002;74:660–3 [discussion: 663–4].

28. Grossi EA, Zakow PK, Ribakove G, et al. Comparison of post-operative pain, stress response, and quality of life in port access vs. standard sternotomy coronary bypass patients. Eur J Cardiothorac Surg 1999;16(Suppl 2):S39–42.

29. Jeanmart H, Casselman F, Beelen R, et al. Modified maze during endoscopic mitral valve surgery: the OLV Clinic experience. Ann Thorac Surg 2006;82:1765–9.

30. Jeanmart H, Casselman FP, De Grieck Y, et al. Avoiding vascular complications during minimally invasive, totally endoscopic intracardiac surgery. J Thorac Cardiovasc Surg 2007;133:1066–70.

31. Maselli D, Pizio R, Borelli G, et al. Endovascular balloon versus transthoracic aortic clamping for minimally invasive mitral valve surgery: impact on cerebral microemboli. Interact Cardiovasc Thorac Surg 2006;5:183–6.

32. McClure RS, Cohn LH, Wiegerinck E, et al. Early and late outcomes in minimally invasive mitral valve repair: an eleven-year experience in 707 patients. J Thorac Cardiovasc Surg 2009;137:70–5.

33. Modi P, Hassan A, Chitwood WR Jr. Minimally invasive mitral valve surgery: a systematic review and meta-analysis. Eur J Cardiothorac Surg 2008;34:943–52.

34. Onnasch JF, Schneider F, Falk V, et al. Five years of less invasive mitral valve surgery: from experimental to routine approach. Heart Surg Forum 2002;5:132–5.

35. Reichenspurner H, Detter C, Deuse T, et al. Video and robotic-assisted minimally invasive mitral valve surgery: a comparison of the Port-Access and transthoracic clamp techniques. Ann Thorac Surg 2005;79:485–90 [discussion: 490–1].

36. Richardson L, Richardson M, Hunter S. Is a port-access mitral valve repair superior to the sternotomy approach in accelerating postoperative recovery? Interact Cardiovasc Thorac Surg 2008;7:678–83.

37. Schneider F, Onnasch JF, Falk V, et al. Cerebral microemboli during minimally invasive and conventional mitral valve operations. Ann Thorac Surg 2000;70:1094–7.

38. Seeburger J, Borger MA, Falk V, et al. Minimal invasive mitral valve repair for mitral regurgitation: results of 1339 consecutive patients. Eur J Cardiothorac Surg 2008;34:760–5.

39. Walther T, Falk V, Metz S, et al. Pain and quality of life after minimally invasive versus conventional cardiac surgery. Ann Thorac Surg 1999;67:1643–7.

40. Woo YJ, Rodriguez E, Atluri P, et al. Minimally invasive, robotic, and off-pump mitral valve surgery. Semin Thorac Cardiovasc Surg 2006;18:139–47.

41. Woo YJ, Seeburger J, Mohr FW. Minimally invasive valve surgery. Semin Thorac Cardiovasc Surg 2007;19:289–98.

42. Yamada T, Ochiai R, Takeda J, et al. Comparison of early postoperative quality of life in minimally invasive versus conventional valve surgery. J Anesth 2003;17:171–6.

43. Enriquez-Sarano M, Avierinos JF, Messika-Zeitoun D, et al. Quantitative determinants of the outcome of asymptomatic mitral regurgitation. N Engl J Med 2005;352:875–83.

44. Ling LH, Enriquez-Sarano M, Seward JB, et al. Early surgery in patients with mitral regurgitation due to flail leaflets: a long-term outcome study. Circulation 1997;96:1819–25.

45. Tribouilloy CM, Enriquez-Sarano M, Schaff HV, et al. Impact of preoperative symptoms on survival after surgical correction of organic mitral regurgitation: rationale for optimizing surgical indications. Circulation 1999;99:400–5.

46. Schachner T, Bonaros N, Feuchtner G, et al. How to handle remote access perfusion for endoscopic cardiac surgery. Heart Surg Forum 2005;8:E232–5.

47. Panagiotou M, Voutetakis K, Zarbis N, et al. Saving space for less invasive direct-vision, mitral valve surgery with altered cannulation protocol. J Cardiovasc Surg (Torino) 2007;48:523–5.

48. Saunders PC, Grossi EA, Sharony R, et al. Minimally invasive technology for mitral valve surgery via left thoracotomy: experience with forty cases. J Thorac Cardiovasc Surg 2004;127:1026–31 [discussion: 1031–2].

49. Gillinov AM, Cosgrove DM. Minimally invasive mitral valve surgery: mini-sternotomy with extended transseptal approach. Semin Thorac Cardiovasc Surg 1999;11:206–11.

50. Gillinov AM, Banbury MK, Cosgrove DM. Hemisternotomy approach for aortic and mitral valve surgery. J Card Surg 2000;15:15–20.

51. Colangelo N, Torracca L, Lapenna E, et al. Vacuum-assisted venous drainage in extrathoracic cardiopulmonary bypass management during minimally invasive cardiac surgery. Perfusion 2006;21:361–5.

52. Murai N, Cho M, Okada S, et al. Venous drainage method for cardiopulmonary bypass in single-access minimally invasive cardiac surgery: siphon and vacuum-assisted drainage. J Artif Organs 2005;8:91–4.
53. Magne J, Senechal M, Mathieu P, et al. Restrictive annuloplasty for ischemic mitral regurgitation may induce functional mitral stenosis. J Am Coll Cardiol 2008;51:1692–701.
54. Alfieri O, Maisano F, De Bonis M, et al. The double-orifice technique in mitral valve repair: a simple solution for complex problems. J Thorac Cardiovasc Surg 2001;122:674–81.
55. Chu MW, Gersch KA, Rodriguez E, et al. Robotic "haircut" mitral valve repair: posterior leaflet-plasty. Ann Thorac Surg 2008;85:1460–2.
56. Falk V, Seeburger J, Czesla M, et al. How does the use of polytetrafluoroethylene neochordae for posterior mitral valve prolapse (loop technique) compare with leaflet resection? A prospective randomized trial. J Thorac Cardiovasc Surg 2008;136:1200–5 [discussion: 1205–6].
57. Kudo M, Yozu R, Kokaji K, et al. Feasibility of mitral valve repair using the loop technique. Ann Thorac Cardiovasc Surg 2007;13:21–6.
58. Risteski PS, Aybek T, Dzemali O, et al. Artificial chordae for mitral valve repair: mid-term clinical and echocardiographic results. Thorac Cardiovasc Surg 2007;55:239–44.
59. Tabata M, Ghanta RK, Shekar PS, et al. Early and midterm outcomes of folding valvuloplasty without leaflet resection for myxomatous mitral valve disease. Ann Thorac Surg 2008;86:1388–90.
60. Sharony R, Grossi EA, Saunders PC, et al. Propensity score analysis of a six-year experience with minimally invasive isolated aortic valve replacement. J Heart Valve Dis 2004;13:887–93.
61. Sharony R, Grossi EA, Saunders PC, et al. Minimally invasive reoperative isolated valve surgery: early and mid-term results. J Card Surg 2006;21:240–4.
62. Umakanthan R, Leacche M, Petracek MR, et al. Safety of minimally invasive mitral valve surgery without aortic cross-clamp. Ann Thorac Surg 2008;85:1544–9 [discussion 1549–50].
63. Seeburger J, Borger MA, Falk V, et al. Minimally invasive mitral valve surgery after previous sternotomy: experience in 181 patients. Ann Thorac Surg 2009;87:709–14.
64. Bolotin G, Kypson AP, Reade CC, et al. Should a video-assisted mini-thoracotomy be the approach of choice for reoperative mitral valve surgery? J Heart Valve Dis 2004;13:155–8 [discussion: 158].
65. Burfeind WR, Glower DD, Davis RD, et al. Mitral surgery after prior cardiac operation: port-access versus sternotomy or thoracotomy. Ann Thorac Surg 2002;74:S1323–5.
66. Casselman FP, La Meir M, Jeanmart H, et al. Endoscopic mitral and tricuspid valve surgery after previous cardiac surgery. Circulation 2007;116:I270–5.
67. Onnasch JF, Schneider F, Falk V, et al. Minimally invasive approach for redo mitral valve surgery: a true benefit for the patient. J Card Surg 2002;17:14–9.
68. Loulmet DF, Patel NC, Jennings JM, et al. Less invasive intracardiac surgery performed without aortic clamping. Ann Thorac Surg 2008;85:1551–5.
69. Bakir I, Casselman FP, Wellens F, et al. Minimally invasive versus standard approach aortic valve replacement: a study in 506 patients. Ann Thorac Surg 2006;81:1599–604.

70. Bonacchi M, Prifti E, Giunti G, et al. Does ministernotomy improve postoperative outcome in aortic valve operation? A prospective randomized study. Ann Thorac Surg 2002;73:460–5 [discussion: 465–6].
71. Candaele S, Herijgers P, Demeyere R, et al. Chest pain after partial upper versus complete sternotomy for aortic valve surgery. Acta Cardiol 2003;58:17–21.
72. Cohn LH. Minimally invasive valve surgery. J Card Surg 2001;16:260–5.
73. Cohn LH, Adams DH, Couper GS, et al. Minimally invasive aortic valve replacement. Semin Thorac Cardiovasc Surg 1997;9:331–6.
74. Cosgrove DM 3rd, Sabik JF. Minimally invasive approach for aortic valve operations. Ann Thorac Surg 1996;62:596–7.
75. Detter C, Deuse T, Boehm DH, et al. Midterm results and quality of life after minimally invasive vs. conventional aortic valve replacement. Thorac Cardiovasc Surg 2002;50:337–41.
76. Doll N, Borger MA, Hain J, et al. Minimal access aortic valve replacement: effects on morbidity and resource utilization. Ann Thorac Surg 2002;74: S1318–22.
77. Ehrlich W, Skwara W, Klovekorn W, et al. Do patients want minimally invasive aortic valve replacement? Eur J Cardiothorac Surg 2000;17:714–7.
78. Hsu VM, Atluri P, Keane MG, et al. Minimally invasive aortic valve papillary fibroelastoma resection. Interact Cardiovasc Thorac Surg 2006;5:779–81.
79. Kim BS, Soltesz EG, Cohn LH. Minimally invasive approaches to aortic valve surgery: Brigham experience. Semin Thorac Cardiovasc Surg 2006;18:148–53.
80. Kolakowski S Jr, Woo YJ. Minimally invasive aortic valve replacement combined with radiofrequency-modified maze procedure. J Card Surg 2005;20:164–6.
81. Masiello P, Coscioni E, Panza A, et al. Surgical results of aortic valve replacement via partial upper sternotomy: comparison with median sternotomy. Cardiovasc Surg 2002;10:333–8.
82. Mihaljevic T, Cohn LH, Unic D, et al. One thousand minimally invasive valve operations: early and late results. Ann Surg 2004;240:529–34 [discussion: 534].
83. Murtuza B, Pepper JR, Stanbridge RD, et al. Minimal access aortic valve replacement: is it worth it? Ann Thorac Surg 2008;85:1121–31.
84. Tabata M, Khalpey Z, Shekar PS, et al. Reoperative minimal access aortic valve surgery: minimal mediastinal dissection and minimal injury risk. J Thorac Cardiovasc Surg 2008;136:1564–8.
85. Tabata M, Umakanthan R, Cohn LH, et al. Early and late outcomes of 1000 minimally invasive aortic valve operations. Eur J Cardiothorac Surg 2008;33: 537–41.
86. Tabata M, Umakanthan R, Khalpey Z, et al. Conversion to full sternotomy during minimal-access cardiac surgery: reasons and results during a 9.5-year experience. J Thorac Cardiovasc Surg 2007;134:165–9.
87. Dogan S, Dzemali O, Wimmer-Greinecker G, et al. Minimally invasive versus conventional aortic valve replacement: a prospective randomized trial. J Heart Valve Dis 2003;12:76–80.
88. De Smet JM, Rondelet B, Jansens JL, et al. Assessment based on EuroSCORE of ministernotomy for aortic valve replacement. Asian Cardiovasc Thorac Ann 2004;12:53–7.
89. Bakir I, Casselman F, De Geest R, et al. Minimally invasive aortic root replacement: a bridge too far? J Cardiovasc Surg (Torino) 2007;48:85–91.
90. Svensson LG. Minimally invasive surgery with a partial sternotomy "J" approach. Semin Thorac Cardiovasc Surg 2007;19:299–303.

91. Tabata M, Khalpey Z, Aranki SF, et al. Minimal access surgery of ascending and proximal arch of the aorta: a 9-year experience. Ann Thorac Surg 2007;84: 67–72.

92. Marescaux J, Leroy J, Gagner M, et al. Transatlantic robot-assisted telesurgery. Nature 2001;413:379–80.

93. Amin Z, Woo R, Danford DA, et al. Robotically assisted perventricular closure of perimembranous ventricular septal defects: preliminary results in Yucatan pigs. J Thorac Cardiovasc Surg 2006;131:427–32.

94. Argenziano M, Oz MC, Kohmoto T, et al. Totally endoscopic atrial septal defect repair with robotic assistance. Circulation 2003;108(Suppl 1):II191–4.

95. Argenziano M, Katz M, Bonatti J, et al. Results of the prospective multicenter trial of robotically assisted totally endoscopic coronary artery bypass grafting. Ann Thorac Surg 2006;81:1666–74 [discussion: 1674–5].

96. Bolotin G, Scott WW Jr, Austin TC, et al. Robotic skeletonizing of the internal thoracic artery: is it safe? Ann Thorac Surg 2004;77:1262–5.

97. Bonatti J, Schachner T, Bonaros N, et al. Technical challenges in totally endoscopic robotic coronary artery bypass grafting. J Thorac Cardiovasc Surg 2006;131:146–53.

98. Bonatti J, Schachner T, Bernecker O, et al. Robotic totally endoscopic coronary artery bypass: program development and learning curve issues. J Thorac Cardiovasc Surg 2004;127:504–10.

99. Casselman FP, Meco M, Dom H, et al. Multivessel distal sutureless off-pump coronary artery bypass grafting procedure using magnetic connectors. Ann Thorac Surg 2004;78:e38–40.

100. Cichon R, Kappert U, Schneider J, et al. Robotically enhanced "Dresden technique" with bilateral internal mammary artery grafting. Thorac Cardiovasc Surg 2000;48:189–92.

101. Derose JJ Jr, Belsley S, Swistel DG, et al. Robotically assisted left ventricular epicardial lead implantation for biventricular pacing: the posterior approach. Ann Thorac Surg 2004;77:1472–4.

102. Dogan S, Aybek T, Risteski P, et al. Totally endoscopic coronary artery bypass graft: initial experience with an additional instrument arm and an advanced camera system. Surg Endosc 2004;18:1587–91.

103. Falk V, Diegeler A, Walther T, et al. Total endoscopic off-pump coronary artery bypass grafting. Heart Surg Forum 2000;3:29–31.

104. Falk V, Diegeler A, Walther T, et al. Total endoscopic computer enhanced coronary artery bypass grafting. Eur J Cardiothorac Surg 2000;17:38–45.

105. Folliguet TA, Vanhuyse F, Konstantinos Z, et al. Early experience with robotic aortic valve replacement. Eur J Cardiothorac Surg 2005;28:172–3.

106. Folliguet T, Vanhuyse F, Constantino X, et al. Mitral valve repair robotic versus sternotomy. Eur J Cardiothorac Surg 2006;29:362–6.

107. Gerosa G, Bianco R, Buja G, et al. Totally endoscopic robotic-guided pulmonary veins ablation: an alternative method for the treatment of atrial fibrillation. Eur J Cardiothorac Surg 2004;26:450–2.

108. Kiaii B, McClure RS, Kostuk WJ, et al. Concurrent robotic hybrid revascularization using an enhanced operative suite. Chest 2005;128:4046–8.

109. Kypson AP, Nifong LW, Chitwood WR Jr. Robot-assisted surgery: training and re-training surgeons. Int J Med Robot 2004;1:70–6.

110. Mohr FW, Falk V, Diegeler A, et al. Computer-enhanced "robotic" cardiac surgery: experience in 148 patients. J Thorac Cardiovasc Surg 2001;121:842–53.

111. Morgan JA, Thornton BA, Peacock JC, et al. Does robotic technology make minimally invasive cardiac surgery too expensive? A hospital cost analysis of robotic and conventional techniques. J Card Surg 2005;20:246–51.

112. Morgan JA, Peacock JC, Kohmoto T, et al. Robotic techniques improve quality of life in patients undergoing atrial septal defect repair. Ann Thorac Surg 2004; 77:1328–33.

113. Murphy DA, Byrne JJ, Malave HA. Robotic endoscopic excision of accessory mitral leaflet. J Thorac Cardiovasc Surg 2006;131:468–9.

114. Nifong LW, Law YB, Reade CC, et al. 200 consecutive robotic mitral valve repairs. Circulation Supplement 2005;112:1.

115. Reade CC, Bower CE, Bailey BM, et al. Robotic mitral valve annuloplasty with double-arm nitinol U-clips. Ann Thorac Surg 2005;79:1372–6 [discussion: 1376–7].

116. Reade CC, Johnson JO, Bolotin G, et al. Combining robotic mitral valve repair and microwave atrial fibrillation ablation: techniques and initial results. Ann Thorac Surg 2005;79:480–4.

117. Reichenspurner H, Boehm DH, Welz A, et al. 3D-video- and robot-assisted minimally invasive ASD closure using the Port-Access techniques. Heart Surg Forum 1998;1:104–6.

118. Rodriguez E, Kypson AP, Moten SC, et al. Robotic mitral surgery at East Carolina University: a 6 year experience. Int J Med Robot 2006;2:211–5.

119. Srivastava S, Gadasalli S, Agusala M, et al. Use of bilateral internal thoracic arteries in CABG through lateral thoracotomy with robotic assistance in 150 patients. Ann Thorac Surg 2006;81:800–6 [discussion: 806].

120. Subramanian VA, Patel NU, Patel NC, et al. Robotic assisted multivessel minimally invasive direct coronary artery bypass with port-access stabilization and cardiac positioning: paving the way for outpatient coronary surgery? Ann Thorac Surg 2005;79:1590–6 [discussion: 1590–6].

121. Suematsu Y, del Nido PJ. Robotic pediatric cardiac surgery: present and future perspectives. Am J Surg 2004;188:98S–103S.

122. Tatooles AJ, Pappas PS, Gordon PJ, et al. Minimally invasive mitral valve repair using the da Vinci robotic system. Ann Thorac Surg 2004;77:1978–82 [discussion 1982–4].

123. Vassiliades TA Jr. Technical aids to performing thoracoscopic robotically-assisted internal mammary artery harvesting. Heart Surg Forum 2002;5:119–24.

124. Woo YJ, Nacke EA. Robotic minimally invasive mitral valve reconstruction yields less blood product transfusion and shorter length of stay. Surgery 2006;140: 263–7.

125. Woo YJ, Grand TJ, Weiss SJ. Robotic resection of an aortic valve papillary fibroelastoma. Ann Thorac Surg 2005;80:1100–2.

126. Woo YJ. Robotic cardiac surgery. Int J Med Robot 2006;2:225–32.

127. Wimmer-Greinecker G, Dogan S, Aybek T, et al. Totally endoscopic atrial septal repair in adults with computer-enhanced telemanipulation. J Thorac Cardiovasc Surg 2003;126:465–8.

128. Yuh DD, Simon BA, Fernandez-Bustamante A, et al. Totally endoscopic robot-assisted transmyocardial revascularization. J Thorac Cardiovasc Surg 2005; 130:120–4.

129. Falk V, Walther T, Autschbach R, et al. Robot-assisted minimally invasive solo mitral valve operation. J Thorac Cardiovasc Surg 1998;115:470–1.

130. Nifong LW, Chitwood WR, Pappas PS, et al. Robotic mitral valve surgery: a United States multicenter trial. J Thorac Cardiovasc Surg 2005;129: 1395–404.
131. Nifong LW, Chu VF, Bailey BM, et al. Robotic mitral valve repair: experience with the da Vinci system. Ann Thorac Surg 2003;75:438–42 [discussion: 443].
132. Bethea BT, Okamura AM, Kitagawa M, et al. Application of haptic feedback to robotic surgery. J Laparoendosc Adv Surg Tech A 2004;14:191–5.

Transcatheter Cardiac Valve Interventions

William T. Brinkman, MD[b], Michael J. Mack, MD[a,b],*

KEYWORDS

- Aortic valve replacement • Aortic stenosis • Mitral insufficiency
- Mitral valve repair • Transcatheter valve implantation

TRANSCATHETER AORTIC VALVE INTERVENTIONS
Background

Currently aortic valve replacement (AVR) is performed for patients with severe aortic stenosis and symptoms or objective pathophysiologic consequences such as left ventricular (LV) dysfunction.[1,2] Even in an elderly population, AVR can be performed with minimal morbidity and mortality with careful patient selection.[3,4] However, there is a significant population of patients meeting criteria for AVR who are not referred for surgery due to perceived high operative risks. In analysis of the Euro Heart Survey on valvular hear disease, surgery was denied in 33% of elderly patients with severe, symptomatic aortic stenosis. Old age and LV dysfunction were the most common characteristics of the patients denied surgery.[5]

Because of this unmet clinical need catheter-based interventions for aortic stenosis have become an area of intense study. Balloon aortic valvuloplasty (BAV) was initially met with enthusiasm,[6] but proved unsatisfactory due to limited long-term efficacy.[7,8] BAV currently has been relegated to a salvage procedure to bridge a patient to a definitive aortic valve (AV) intervention.[9] Since the "first in man" transcatheter aortic valve implantation (TAVI) in 2002 by Cribier and colleagues,[10] multiple devices and techniques for TAVI are undergoing development. Two devices, the Edwards Sapien valve (ESv, Edwards Lifesciences Inc, California) (**Fig. 1**) and the Medtronic CoreValve® System[11] (Medtronic, Inc., Minneapolis, Minnesota) (**Fig. 2**) have received commercial approval in Europe. In the United States, the ESv, is currently enrolling in the United States pivotal randomized trial against medical management and traditional AVR, PARTNER US. Commercial approval is expected in the United States possibly in 2011. Another device, the Medtronic CoreValve® System is preparing to initiate its own randomized clinical trial in the United States.

a Cardiovascular Surgery Baylor Health Care System, Dallas, TX, USA
b The Heart Hospital Baylor Plano, 1100 Allied Boulevard, Plano, TX 75093, USA
* Corresponding author. The Heart Hospital Baylor Plano, 1100 Allied Boulevard, Plano, TX 75093.
E-mail address: mmack@csant.com (M. J. Mack).

Surg Clin N Am 89 (2009) 951–966
doi:10.1016/j.suc.2009.06.004
0039-6109/09/$ – see front matter © 2009 Elsevier Inc. All rights reserved.

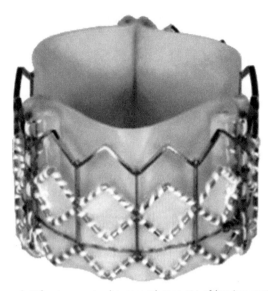

Fig. 1. Sapien (Edwards Lifesciences, Inc.) transcatheter AV of bovine pericardium mounted in a stainless steel, balloon deployable stent. (*Courtesy of* Edwards Lifesciences, Inc, Irvine, CA; with permission.)

Current Devices

ESv

The ESv is a trileaflet pericardial valve mounted on a balloon expandable stainless steel stent with a fabric sealing cuff. Initially equine pericardium was used, but this was later changed to bovine pericardium consistent with materials used for Edwards stented AVs used for surgical implantation. In vitro durability has repeatedly been demonstrated to be greater than 400 million cycles, corresponding to greater than 10 years of life. The valves are supplied uncrimped in sterile glutaraldehyde. The stent is tubular in shape, slotted, and comes in 2 sizes, 23 and 26 mm. For the retrograde

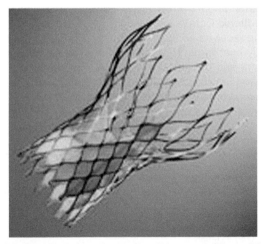

Fig. 2. CoreValve® (Medtronic, Inc) percutaneous AV mounted in a nitinol, self-expanding frame. (*Courtesy of* Medtronic, Inc, Minneapolis, MN; with permission.)

transfemoral (TF) approach, the 23-mm valve requires a 22F introducer sheath (8 mm optical density [OD]) and the 26 mm valve requires a 24F introducer sheath (9 mm OD). Transapical (TA) valves are inserted through a single 26F sheath.

CRS

The CoreValve uses 3 pericardial leaflets (porcine) mounted in a self-expanding, nitinol frame.[11–13] The CoreValve length is 55 mm for the 26 mm valve size and 53 mm for the 29 mm valve size, and it is specifically designed with a waist in its mid portion. The radial forces along the stent vary. The lower inflow portion of the frame has a high radial force. The mid portion, which contains the valve, is constrained to maintain coronary perfusion. The upper portion of the stent with modest radial forces then enables orientation to the annulus. Even though the frame spans the entire aortic root into the ascending aorta, coronary intervention post CoreValve has been reported.[14] The system is available in 2 sizes, 26 and 29 mm, that can be delivered through an 18F sheath for TF delivery. Because of the length of the frame and the small ventricular sizes frequently encountered in the setting of aortic stenosis, TA delivery of the CoreValve has been abandoned. This system with its 18F sheath is largely a percutaneous TF approach performed without general anesthesia.[12]

Other Devices

Many other devices intended for TAVI are in various stages of development. The Lotus Valve System (Sadra Medical Inc, Campbell, California), the percutaneous AV from Direct Flow Inc. (Santa Rosa, California), AorTx Inc (Palo Alto, California), and Heart Leaflet Inc (Maple Grove, Minnesota) have all entered early human trials. These second generation devices have been designed to improve ease of deliverability, valve positioning, and give the possibility of valve repositioning.[15] Recently, the Ventor® Transcatheter Aortic Valve (Medtronic, Inc, Minneapolis, Minnesota) has been found to be feasible by a TA approach in a limited number of patients (**Fig. 3**).

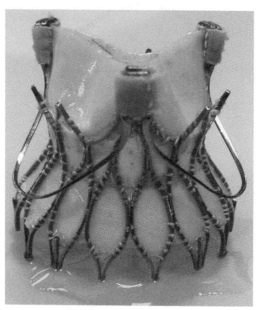

Fig. 3. Ventor® (Medtronic, Inc) transapical transcatheter aortic valve mounted in a nitinol, self expanding frame. (*Courtesy of* Medtronic, Inc., Minneapolis, MN; with permission.)

Techniques of Implantation

After feasibility studies in animals,[16] initial attempts at TAVI in humans were performed using an antegrade approach by the femoral vein.[17] This approach required access across the atrial septum and the mitral valve to reach the aortic root. Although TAVI was achieved, this approach proved complex and the ability to reproduce similar results in other centers was an issue. Therefore, 2 additional approaches for TAVI were developed, the retrograde transfemoral (TF-AVI) (**Fig. 4**) and the antegrade trans-apical (TA-AVI) (**Fig. 5**).[18–24] The TF approach was facilitated by the development of a flexible delivery catheter capable of negotiating the aortic arch and a stenotic AV in a retrograde fashion. Webb and colleagues[24] in Vancouver were instrumental in the development of this approach. The TA procedure was primarily developed by Walther and colleagues[19,21] in Leipzig and Lichtenstein[20] in Vancouver. These are 2 approaches being used for all current TAVI interventions.

These 2 approaches (TA-AVI and TF-AVI) share critical elements in strategy and technique:[25]

- The procedures are usually performed under general anesthesia. Optimally, these procedures should be performed in a hybrid environment with the imaging capabilities of a cardiac catheterization suite and the sterility of an operating room. The ability to accurately visualize and deploy the valve can be hampered by patient movement. Moreover, transient hemodynamic instability and the need for temporary mechanical hemodynamic support are not uncommon. However, the TF approach (specifically using the CoreValve System) has been performed with local anesthesia and moderate sedation.

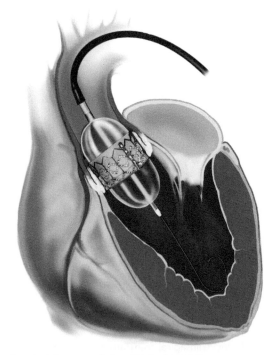

Fig. 4. TF retrograde arterial approach for AV deployment.

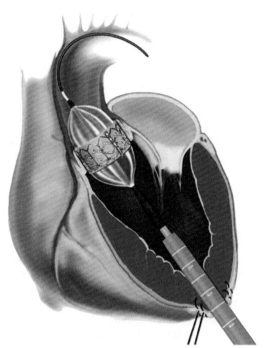

Fig. 5. TA antegrade approach for transcatheter AV deployment.

- Imaging is critical. Preoperative CT angiography with three-dimensional reconstructions of the aortic root can also be useful in screening patients for TAVI.
  Measurements from the aortic annulus to the sinotubular junction, the annulus
  to the coronary orifices, and the aortic annular diameter should be routinely
  measured.[26] The precision of these measurements, however, can be difficult in
  the presence of heavy calcification. Periprocedural transesophageal echocardiography (TEE) is mandatory for aortic sizing, valve positioning, and monitoring of
  valve/cardiac function post-TAVI. TEE is the most reliable tool to measure the
  diameter of the aortic root (long axis view) and the pattern of calcification on
  the valve cusps (short axis view). In general the aortic annulus is measured at
  mid systole from the insertion of the right coronary cusp at the junction between
  the interventricular septum, aortic annulus, and aortic root and the insertion of the
  noncoronary cusp just opposite the junction between the anterior mitral leaflet,
  aortic annulus, and aortic root.[27] Multiple measurements should be performed.
  If a coronary orifice measures less than 10 mm from the aortic annulus, placing
  a guide wire in the coronary should be considered before deploying the AV. TEE
  confirmation is also helpful for stent location before valve deployment. Real time
  three-dimensional TEE and intracardiac echocardiography are currently being
  studied, but they have not been commonly used.
- High-resolution fluoroscopy is also required for wire and sheath manipulation,
  valve positioning/deployment, emergent coronary intervention, and for diag-
  nosis/treatment of access vessel injury. Valve positioning can be performed
  using fluoroscopy to identify aortic leaflet/annular calcification, and when
  combined with aortography can be used to align the valve in the proper coaxial
  plane.

- TAVI requires a team effort. Periprocedural input from cardiology, cardiovascular surgery, and anesthesia is critical for successful outcomes. Moreover, careful disaster planning for various scenarios (access vessel injury, hemodynamic collapse, cardiac injury, and so forth) should be performed before TAVI. All necessary bailout equipment (cardiopulmonary bypass machine with appropriately sized arterial and venous cannulas, cardiovascular surgical instruments, intraaortic balloon pump, covered vascular stents, coronary stents, and so forth) should be readily available.
- Postprocedure monitoring should be done in an intensive care unit setting. Close monitoring of hemodynamics, evidence of hemorrhage, cardiac rhythm, and renal function is required.

Retrograde transfemoral aortic valve implantation

The major limitation for the application of retrograde TF-AVI is vascular access issues, which is important with the ESv. A 23-mm Sapien valve requires a 22F sheath (8 mm OD) and the 26-mm valve requires a 24F sheath (9 mm OD), which limits the application of this technology to patients with femoral and iliac arteries with a luminal diameter of at least 7 to 7.5 cm. In addition, heavily calcified arteries cause even greater limits to the TF route. Currently, the use of aortic or iliac conduits is not allowed in the PARTNER US pivotal trial of the ESv. In the future this restriction will be lifted allowing broader application of TF-AVI. The CoreValve, however, can now be deployed through an 18F system greatly expanding the patient population in whom this technology can be applied. Successful TAVI has been reported using right subclavian artery access using the 18F CoreValve.[28]

Another important factor specific to TF-AVI is the safe passage of large devices across the aortic arch, which has important implications for stroke risk. To address this Edwards has developed the retroflex delivery catheter, which allows the operator to bend the distal aspect of the catheter, allowing passage of the valve across the arch and decreasing the probability of scraping the greater curve of the arch.

The crossing of a calcified stenotic AV can be challenging from a retrograde approach. The catheter and valve tend to fall away from the center of the valve and toward the commisures. The retroflex catheter can help with wire orientation in the aortic root. The addition of a nose cone in front of the Sapien valve in the retroflex 2 system has aided greatly in decreasing valve crossing difficulties.

Antegrade transapical aortic valve implantation

TA-AVI is primarily a surgical procedure and should be performed in a hybrid operating room, which includes fluoroscopic equipment to cardiac catheterization laboratory quality. If high quality fluoroscopic equipment is not available in the operating room, then there should be consideration for conversion of a cardiac catheterization room into an operative setting. High quality imaging is the most important factor for TAVI.

A left anterolateral minithoracotomy is performed in the fifth or sixth intercostal space. A soft tissue retractor can be used along with minimal rib spreading. Palpation of the LV apex or point of maximal pulsation can be useful in planning your incision. Pacing wires can be placed directly on the ventricular surface. Two apical purse strings are then placed in the apex. The apex is then punctured with a soft guide wire followed by a 14F sheath, which is positioned across the AV. A stiff guide wire is then placed into the descending aorta using a right Judkins catheter to guide the stiff wire across the aortic arch. A BAV is then performed during rapid ventricular pacing (RVP). Following this the delivery sheath is positioned with the stent in the aortic annulus and deployed under RVP. Positioning of the valve in the annulus is more straightforward in the TA technique compared with the TF technique. The TA-AVI is a valve on stick; in TF-AVI the valve is at the end of a long stiff curved wire with variable amounts of stored energy. For an excellent step-by-step review of TA-AVI, see the recent review by Walther and colleagues.[27]

Results

Edwards Sapien

Early results of TF-AVI[24] and TA-AVI[21] have been reported. Webb and colleagues have reported on their initial 50 patients using the ESv deployed from the femoral artery. The patients enrolled were a high-risk population with a mean logistic EuroSCORE of 28%. Valve implantation was successful in 86% of patients with an intraprocedural mortality of 2%. Results improved greatly with operator experience from 76% procedural success and 16% 30-day mortality in the first 25 patients to 96% procedural success and 8% 30-day mortality in the second 25 patients. Mild paravalvular regurgitation was common, but was well tolerated. They also demonstrated significant improvement in the LV ejection fraction ($P<.0001$), mitral regurgitation ($P = .01$), and functional class ($P<.0001$). This improvement was maintained at 1 year and no structural valve deterioration was demonstrated (medial follow-up of 359 days).

Walther and colleagues[21] in Leipzig have reported on their first 50 TA-AVI patients. The average EuroSCORE predicted risk for mortality in this high-risk population was 27.6%. Overall procedural success was 94%. Echocardiography demonstrated good hemodynamic function in all patients and minor valvular incompetence (primarily paravalvular without signs of hemolysis) was demonstrated in 23 patients. Mortality was due to overall health condition and nonvalve related in all patients. Actuarial survival at 1 month, 6 months, and 1 year was 92%, 74%, and 71%, respectively.

CoreValve

Procedural and 30-day outcomes following implantation of the 18F CoreValve® System have recently been reported. This study enrolled a population at high risk for conventional AVR with a mean logistic EuroSCORE of 23%.[12] Following implantation mean transvalvular gradients decreased from 49.4 mm Hg to 3 mm Hg. The procedural and 30-day mortality rates were 1.5% and 8%, respectively. The 30-day combined rate of death, stroke, and myocardial infarction was 9.3%.

TRANSCATHETER MITRAL VALVE INTERVENTIONS

Percutaneous catheter-based treatment of valvular heart disease began in the early 1980s with the introduction of percutaneous mitral commissurotomy for mitral stenosis.[29,30] This catheter-based approach has achieved comparable results with closed surgical commissurotomy in the short- and long-term.[31] Percutaneous treatments for mitral regurgitation, however, have not progressed rapidly. The complex pathophysiology of mitral regurgitation with varying causes along with challenging imaging and delivery issues has led to slower than anticipated clinical introduction, limited early device success, required iterative changes in device design, and caused some devices with early promise to be shelved.[32]

Pathophysiology of Mitral Regurgitation

Mitral regurgitation can be classified as a primary leaflet problem (primary MR) or as secondary to another process such as ventricular dysfunction (functional MR [FMR]). In primary MR there is a derangement of the components of the mitral valve itself, which permits regurgitation causing a pure volume overload on the LV. If the regurgitant volume is significant over time, LV remodeling, dysfunction, pulmonary hypertension, and eventual heart failure can result. There is a definite causal relation between primary MR and LV dysfunction. Timely correction of significant primary MR is well accepted. In general, regurgitant fractions (RF) less than 0.4 are well tolerated indefinitely in animal and human studies, but RF greater than 0.5 usually lead to heart failure.[33] Patients with moderate MR who are asymptomatic generally are managed medically. However, with the onset of even mild symptoms or LV dysfunction surgery, preferably mitral repair is indicated.[1]

The pathophysiology of secondary MR (or FMR) is more complex than primary. The advantage of correcting secondary MR is less clear. Myocardial damage from ischemic insults or other causes of dilated cardiomyopathies cause an anatomically normal valve to become incompetent. So, even if the valve leakage can be improved the primary pathophysiology had not been altered. If secondary MR is a cause for worsened prognosis, then attempts to correct it are reasonable. However, if secondary MR is only a byproduct of altered LV function and morphology, the treatment of secondary MR may be inconsequential.

The surgical correction of secondary MR has indeed shown some beneficial effects. Bolling and Bach reported on the use of a restrictive annuloplasty to reduce secondary MR. With an operative mortality of less than 5%, they demonstrated LV volume reductions and modest increases in LV ejection fraction.[34] The use of LV external restraint devices has also demonstrated substantial reverse remodeling effects for the diseased LV in the setting of secondary MR.[35] However, there is no proof yet that these surgical interventions improve survival or quality of life.[36,37]

Percutaneous Treatment of Mitral Regurgitation

Because of this debate, the use of nonsurgical mechanical interventions for the treatment of secondary MR and primary MR is an area of intense investigation. Percutaneous therapies for mitral repair include coronary sinus (CS) annuloplasty, direct annuloplasty, leaflet repair, LV chamber remodeling, and some involve combinations of these tactics.

Percutaneous Edge-to-Edge Repair

Two devices are based on the surgical edge-to-edge repair technique of Alfieri. This technique has been applied for the treatment of primary and secondary MR. The MitraClip (Evalve, Menlo Park, California) and Mobius II leaflet repair system (Edwards Life Sciences, Irving, California) simulate the surgical edge-to-edge repair technique of Alfieri,[38] the former by placement of a clip between the free edges of the mitral leaflets and the latter with a suture-based system. The Edwards Mobius device underwent an early clinical feasibility trial in 15 patients, and because of the disappointing results and arduous delivery and placement, further clinical development of this device was abandoned.

The MitraClip is a polyester-covered device with 2 arms that engage the anterior and posterior leaflets of the mitral valve, creating a double orifice mitral valve in a bow-tie configuration. The MitraClip is delivered by a transseptal puncture using a 24F guide catheter. For effective deployment the clip must be aligned in the center of the mitral valve orifice with the clip arms perpendicular to the mitral annular plane (**Fig. 6**). This procedure is accomplished with the use of steering knobs on the guide catheter and the clip delivery catheter. Using fluoroscopy and TEE the clip is passed into the ventricle and then pulled back to grasp the leaflet margins (**Fig. 7**). The device can be repositioned and an additional clip may be delivered if control of MR is not adequate. The phase I clinical trial, Everest I, enrolled 55 patients and demonstrated safety and efficacy of the device.[39] Two-year freedom from death, mitral valve surgery,

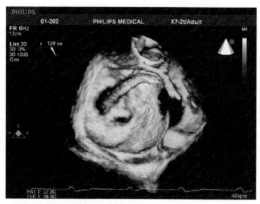

Fig. 6. Three-dimensional echocardiogram demonstrating the Evalve Mitraclip in position across the mitral valve ready for deployment.

or recurrent MR greater than 2+ has been 80% among patients with successfully deployed clips.[40] If the results were poor, standard surgical mitral repair techniques were possible as late as 18 months post procedure.[41] The pivotal trial, Everest II, enrolled 60 patients in a roll-in phase and 279 patients in a 2:1 randomization between the clip and surgery. This trial has been completely enrolled with 184 patients receiving the device and 95 patients randomized to surgery. In addition, another 78 patients have been enrolled in a high-risk registry giving a total of 472 patients now enrolled in the Everest I and Everest II trials (Feldman T, presented at TCT 2008; October 2008) The EVEREST II trial will be important not only for assessing percutaneous mitral therapy but will also be the first prospective, echocardiography, core laboratory evaluated trial of mitral valve repair in the surgical literature. The results of this are eagerly awaited by cardiologist and cardiac surgeons.

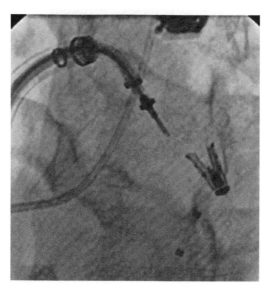

Fig. 7. Fluoroscopic image with the recently deployed Mitraclip in place on the mitral valve leaflets.

Functional Mitral Regurgitation

As mentioned previously secondary MR or FMR has been most frequently treated by a surgical annuloplasty with an undersized, complete, rigid ring. Although the whole annulus dilates in patients with FMR, the greatest degree of dilation is in the posterior annulus and the greatest increase in dimension is the septal-lateral (or anterior-posterior) diameter. Key to this strategy is the anchoring of the ring to the central fibrous skeleton of the heart at the fibrous trigones. Anchoring the ring away from the mitral annulus (MA) in the atrial wall or in the leaflet tissue itself yields suboptimal results.[42] Correction of the septal-lateral dimension by as little as 5 to 8 mm has been demonstrated to reconstitute leaflet coaptation and decrease mitral regurgitation in FMR patients. Percutaneous approaches to FMR are based on this concept of altering mitral annular morphology in an effort to decrease the septal-lateral diameter.[43] There has been a plethora of strategies applied to this problem FMR. Some systems use the anatomic relationship between the posterior MA and the CS to deliver devices. Others take a more direct approach by actually plicating the posterior annulus. Still others rely on distraction of the LV or left atrium to secondarily decrease the septal-lateral diameter of the annulus.

Coronary Sinus Devices

Due to its anatomic vicinity to the MA, the CS has been targeted for use in transcatheter mitral interventions. The relationship of the CS to the MA has substantial variability from person to person (**Fig. 8**). Most commonly the CS is located along the wall of the left atrium superior to the MA. The smallest separation between the CS and the MA is typically at the anterolateral commisure. CS separation from the MA is maximal at the posteromedial commisure. Masselli and colleagues reported on CS anatomy in 61 normal cadaveric human hearts. Distances between the inferior border of the CS and the MA at the P2 and P3 segments were reported. Average CS to MA distance at P3 was 9.7 mm (±3.2) (range 5–19 mm) and at P2 5.7 mm (±3.3) (range 1–15 mm).[44] Patients

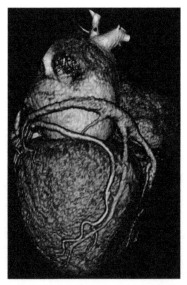

Fig. 8. Three-dimensional reconstruction of a CT demonstrating the relationship between the posterior MA and the CS.

with severe MR have been shown to have significantly increased CS to MA distances when compared with patients without severe MR.[45] Another potential concern with the use of the CS is its relationship to the left circumflex coronary artery. Left circumflex artery interposition between the CS and MA has been reported in up to 80% of patients.[44,45] Despite these anatomic limitations, the use of the CS for the performance of percutaneous mitral repair is an area of active clinical investigation.

There is now clinical experience with at least 3 devices that use the CS to perform an annuloplasty.[46] The Monarc device (Edwards Life Sciences) has been placed in more than 80 patients in studies outside the United States. With this device, the CS is cannulated from the right internal jugular vein and distal and proximal self-expanding stent anchors separated by a connecting bridge element are deployed. The connecting member is a spring held open by a bioabsorbable suture. Tension on the CS and performance of the annuloplasty occurs as the spring shortens over a 3- to 6-week period of time after implantation. Initial feasibility trials were stopped because of early bridge fracture.[47] After redesign, a second prospective, multicenter feasibility study was initiated. Enrollment criteria included at least 2+ FMR with a dilated cardiomyopathy or myocardial ischemia. Patients with significant mitral calcification, an LV ejection fraction less than 25%, mitral valve prolapse, a history of intracardiac defibrillator or pacing leads in the CS, or patients 3 months pre- or postcoronary revascularization were excluded. Of the 55 patients enrolled, 49 (89%) had the device implanted. Of these 49 patients, 42 (70%) had the device implanted in the intended location without major adverse cardiac events. Three events were judged to be device or procedure related: 1 myocardial infarction due to coronary compression and 2 instances of cardiac tamponade. Efficacy (MR reduction >1 grade) improved significantly from 30 days post implantation to 180 days post implantation (48.5% and 92.3% of patients, respectively). The improvement in efficacy is understandable due to the device's delayed bridge mechanism and possible LV remodeling.[46,48]

Another device, the Carillon Mitral Contour System (Cardiac Dimensions, Kirkland, Washington) is a nitinol wire between distal and proximal anchors in the CS. During deployment, it is progressively shortened until an appropriate reduction in mitral regurgitation is achieved.[49] In the first-generation cases with this device there were issues with the distal anchoring device requiring redesign. Subsequently, implantation has resumed and early results in 34 patients in 6 European centers in the AMADEUS trial have been reported.[50] The device was successfully implanted in 21 (62%) patients and demonstrated improvement in mitral regurgitation by at least 1 grade in 14 (67%) of the patients with successful implants. Two patients required recapture of the device after the coronary arteriography demonstrated coronary compression. So, because the device can be recaptured, the documentation of the crossed coronary arteries does not necessarily preclude device implantation.

A third device, the percutaneous transvenous mitral annuloplasty (PTMA) system (Viacor Inc, Wilmington, Massachusetts) is another CS delivered device, which is a polytetrafluoroethylene (PTFE) catheter with a distal atraumatic silicone tip. Up to 3 nitinol rods of variable stiffness can be inserted to affect the conformation of the CS. The rods compress the mid portion of the CS to diminish the septal-lateral dimension, and reduce the severity of mitral regurgitation. These rods can be interchanged at the time of implantation as well as subsequently after implantation by varying the shape and stiffness to achieve the appropriate reduction in mitral regurgitation. A small series of temporary implants have been inserted in the operating room to demonstrate proof of concept.[51] The Viacor device in short-term studies has demonstrated safety. The potential for retrieval and later adjustment make it an attractive concept. Permanent implantation studies are underway.

Other Devices with Clinical Experience

Although no other devices have clinical experience at the present time, other unique concepts have shown proof of concept in animal studies. One device, the Mitralign (Mitralign, Inc, Tewkesbury, Massachusetts) bypasses the CS and its limitations to perform a direct annuloplasty by the LV side of the MA. This concept was based on early suture plication annuloplasty performed in the 1970s. The device uses anchoring pledgets placed directly into the MA with a drawstring between the anchors cinching the annulus. This device has been demonstrated in preclinical models, but clinical studies have not yet been reported. According to the company's Web site, the first 2 implants in its European pilot study were successful resulting in significant reductions in mitral regurgitation.[52]

The Quantam Cor (Quantam Cor, Inc San Clemente, California) proposes to shrink the posterior annulus of the mitral valve by direct application of radiofrequency energy. The ability to shrink the posterior annulus has been demonstrated in animal studies.[53] Another intriguing concept is percutaneous mitral valve replacement (Endovalve, Princeton, New Jersey). To obviate the recurrence of mitral regurgitation, and the complexity of delivery of some of the repair techniques, this system is designed to totally replace the mitral valve by a percutaneous approach. By a transseptal delivery and anchoring on the atrial side, this device is designed to simplify delivery, placement, and obviate the recurrence of mitral regurgitation. The device has undergone some early iterative changes, and has achieved proof of concept in animals.

All of the devices mentioned earlier effect FMR by manipulation of the posterior MA or leaflet coaptation. The Coapsys System (Myocor, Maple Grove, Minnesota) and the Ample PS3 system (Ample Medical, Foster City, California) aim to affect FMR by directly causing a decrease in the septal-lateral dimension. The Coapsys system consists of an epicardial posterior pad, an epicardial anterior pad, and a PTFE-coated braided subvalvular chord. The 2 pads are placed on the epicardial surface with the load bearing subvalvular chord passing through the ventricle. Currently the device is implanted with an open chest approach on a beating heart and adjusted using echocardiography. The iCoapsys device (based on the same technology) was subsequently developed for implantation by a percutaneous subxiphoid approach. Early clinical results with the Coapsys device have been encouraging with significant improvements in MR grade and New York Heart Association (NYHA) functional status.[54–56] The Ample PS3 system is a truly a percutaneous endovascular system. Anchors are situated in the CS and the fossa ovalis with a tether in between. The tether is cinched to manipulate the septal-lateral distance. Although the use of septal-lateral cinching techniques (such Coapsys and PS3) is an attractive concept with good early results, there are concerns that extreme shortening of the septal-lateral distance with tethering adversely effects systolic wall thickening adjacent to the MA. These alterations in LV strain could have a deleterious effect on remodeling.[57]

TRANSCATHETER PULMONARY VALVE INTERVENTIONS

Percutaneous pulmonary valve implantation was introduced in 2000 for the treatment of right ventricular outflow tract dysfunction. This technology was primarily designed to treat the difficult problem of right ventricular to pulmonary artery conduit stenosis in the congenital population. Initial attempts at nonsurgical pulmonary valve implantation in animals and then humans were pioneered by Bonhoeffer and colleagues[58,59] Since these initial experiences, Bonhoeffer and colleagues have percutaneously placed stented pulmonary valves in over 155 patients. Significant reductions in right ventricular pressures and outflow gradients were demonstrated. Freedom from reoperation at 10 and 50 months were 95% and 84%, respectively.[60] This technology was then acquired by Medtronic and became known as the Melody valve.

The Melody transcatheter pulmonary valve (Medtronic, Minneapolis, MN) is an 18-mm modified Contegra bovine jugular vein valve mounted in a platinum iridium stent. The stent is 28 mm in length and is crimped down to 6 mm. The balloon expandable stent can then be re-expanded on 18- to 22-mm balloons. Results after the first 300 implantations were good with a 97% technical success rate. In December 2006 the Melody valve received approval for Canadian use becoming the first available transcatheter valve in North America. As of August 2008, 636 Melody pulmonary valves have been implanted in 58 centers worldwide. A feasibility study is ongoing in the United States.

REFERENCES

1. Bonow RO, Carabello BA, Chatterjee K, et al. 2008 Focused update incorporated into the ACC/AHA 2006 guidelines for the management of patients with valvular heart disease: a report of the American College of Cardiology/American Heart Association Task Force on Practice Guidelines (writing committee to revise the 1998 guidelines for the management of patients with valvular heart disease): endorsed by the Society of Cardiovascular Anesthesiologists, Society for Cardiovascular Angiography and Interventions, and Society of Thoracic Surgeons. Circulation 2008;118(15):e523–661.
2. Bonow RO, Carabello BA, Kanu C, et al. ACC/AHA 2006 guidelines for the management of patients with valvular heart disease: a report of the American College of Cardiology/American Heart Association Task Force on Practice Guidelines (writing committee to revise the 1998 guidelines for the management of patients with valvular heart disease): developed in collaboration with the Society of Cardiovascular Anesthesiologists: endorsed by the Society for Cardiovascular Angiography and Interventions and the Society of Thoracic Surgeons. Circulation 2006;114(5):e84–231.
3. Kolh P, Kerzmann A, Honore C, et al. Aortic valve surgery in octogenarians: predictive factors for operative and long-term results. Eur J Cardiothorac Surg 2007;31(4):600–6.
4. Melby SJ, Zierer A, Kaiser SP, et al. Aortic valve replacement in octogenarians: risk factors for early and late mortality. Ann Thorac Surg 2007;83(5):1651–6 [discussion: 1656–7].
5. Iung B, Cachier A, Baron G, et al. Decision-making in elderly patients with severe aortic stenosis: why are so many denied surgery? Eur Heart J 2005;26(24):2714–20.
6. Cribier A, Savin T, Saoudi N, et al. Percutaneous transluminal valvuloplasty of acquired aortic stenosis in elderly patients: an alternative to valve replacement? Lancet 1986;1(8472):63–7.
7. Iung B, Baron G, Butchart EG, et al. A prospective survey of patients with valvular heart disease in Europe: the Euro Heart Survey on Valvular Heart Disease. Eur Heart J 2003;24(13):1231–43.
8. Jabbour RJ, Dick R, Walton AS. Aortic balloon valvuloplasty—review and case series. Heart Lung Circ 2008;17(Suppl 4):S73–81.
9. To AC, Zeng I, Coverdale HA. Balloon aortic valvuloplasty in adults—a 10-year review of Auckland's experience. Heart Lung Circ 2008;17(6):468–74.
10. Cribier A, Eltchaninoff H, Bash A, et al. Percutaneous transcatheter implantation of an aortic valve prosthesis for calcific aortic stenosis: first human case description. Circulation 2002;106(24):3006–8.

11. Grube E, Schuler G, Buellesfeld L, et al. Percutaneous aortic valve replacement for severe aortic stenosis in high-risk patients using the second- and current third-generation self-expanding CoreValve prosthesis: device success and 30-day clinical outcome. J Am Coll Cardiol 2007;50(1):69–76.

12. Piazza N, Grube E, Gerckens U, et al. Procedural and 30-day outcomes following transcatheter aortic valve implantation using the third generation (18 Fr) core-valve revalving system: results from the multicentre, expanded evaluation registry 1-year following CE mark approval. EuroIntervention 2008;4(2):242–9.

13. Grube E, Laborde JC, Gerckens U, et al. Percutaneous implantation of the CoreValve self-expanding valve prosthesis in high-risk patients with aortic valve disease: the Siegburg first-in-man study. Circulation 2006;114(15):1616–24.

14. Geist V, Sherif MA, Khattab AA. Successful percutaneous coronary intervention after implantation of a CoreValve percutaneous aortic valve. Catheter Cardiovasc Interv 2009;73(1):61–7.

15. Del Valle-Fernandez R, Ruiz CE. Transcatheter heart valves for the treatment of aortic stenosis: state-of-the-art. Minerva Cardioangiol 2008;56(5):543–56.

16. Andersen HR, Knudsen LL, Hasenkam JM. Transluminal implantation of artificial heart valves. Description of a new expandable aortic valve and initial results with implantation by catheter technique in closed chest pigs. Eur Heart J 1992;13(5):704–8.

17. Cribier A, Eltchaninoff H, Tron C, et al. Early experience with percutaneous transcatheter implantation of heart valve prosthesis for the treatment of end-stage inoperable patients with calcific aortic stenosis. J Am Coll Cardiol 2004;43(4):698–703.

18. Walther T, Simon P, Dewey T, et al. Transapical minimally invasive aortic valve implantation: multicenter experience. Circulation 2007;116(11 Suppl):I240–5.

19. Walther T, Falk V, Borger MA, et al. Minimally invasive transapical beating heart aortic valve implantation—proof of concept. Eur J Cardiothorac Surg 2007; 31(1):9–15.

20. Lichtenstein SV, Cheung A, Ye J, et al. Transapical transcatheter aortic valve implantation in humans: initial clinical experience. Circulation 2006;114(6):591–6.

21. Walther T, Falk V, Kempfert J, et al. Transapical minimally invasive aortic valve implantation: the initial 50 patients. Eur J Cardiothorac Surg 2008;33(6):983–8.

22. Leon MB, Kodali S, Williams M, et al. Transcatheter aortic valve replacement in patients with critical aortic stenosis: rationale, device descriptions, early clinical experiences, and perspectives. Semin Thorac Cardiovasc Surg 2006;18(2): 165–74.

23. Svensson LG, Dewey T, Kapadia S, et al. United States feasibility study of transcatheter insertion of a stented aortic valve by the left ventricular apex. Ann Thorac Surg 2008;86(1):46–54 [discussion: 54–5].

24. Webb JG, Pasupati S, Humphries K, et al. Percutaneous transarterial aortic valve replacement in selected high-risk patients with aortic stenosis. Circulation 2007; 116(7):755–63.

25. Vahanian A, Alfieri OR, Al-Attar N, et al. Transcatheter valve implantation for patients with aortic stenosis: a position statement from the European Association of Cardio-Thoracic Surgery (EACTS) and the European Society of Cardiology (ESC), in collaboration with the European Association of Percutaneous Cardiovascular Interventions (EAPCI). Eur J Cardiothorac Surg 2008;34(1):1–8.

26. Lu TL, Huber CH, Rizzo E, et al. Ascending aorta measurements as assessed by ECG-gated multi-detector computed tomography: a pilot study to establish normative values for transcatheter therapies. Eur Radiol 2009;19(3):664–9.

27. Walther T, Dewey T, Borger MA, et al. Transapical aortic valve implantation: step by step. Ann Thorac Surg 2009;87(1):276–83.

28. Ruge H, Lange R, Bleiziffer S, et al. First successful aortic valve implantation with the CoreValve Revalving System via right subclavian artery access: a case report. Heart Surg Forum 2008;11(5):E323–4.

29. Inoue K. [Percutaneous transvenous mitral commissurotomy (PTMC) by using Inoue-balloon]. Kyobu Geka 1989;42(8 Suppl):596–602 [Japanese].

30. Lock JE, Khalilullah M, Shrivastava S, et al. Percutaneous catheter commissurotomy in rheumatic mitral stenosis. N Engl J Med 1985;313(24):1515–8.

31. Rifaie O, Abdel-Dayem MK, Ramzy A, et al. Percutaneous mitral valvotomy versus closed surgical commissurotomy. Up to 15 years of follow-up of a prospective randomized study. J Cardiol 2009;53(1):28–34.

32. Mack MJ. Percutaneous treatment of mitral regurgitation: so near, yet so far! J Thorac Cardiovasc Surg 2008;135(2):237–9.

33. Carabello BA. The current therapy for mitral regurgitation. J Am Coll Cardiol 2008; 52(5):319–26.

34. Bach DS, Bolling SF. Improvement following correction of secondary mitral regurgitation in end-stage cardiomyopathy with mitral annuloplasty. Am J Cardiol 1996; 78(8):966–9.

35. Acker MA, Bolling S, Shemin R, et al. Mitral valve surgery in heart failure: insights from the Acorn Clinical Trial. J Thorac Cardiovasc Surg 2006;132(3):568–77, 577.e1–4.

36. Mihaljevic T, Lam BK, Rajeswaran J, et al. Impact of mitral valve annuloplasty combined with revascularization in patients with functional ischemic mitral regurgitation. J Am Coll Cardiol 2007;49(22):2191–201.

37. Wu AH, Aaronson KD, Bolling SF, et al. Impact of mitral valve annuloplasty on mortality risk in patients with mitral regurgitation and left ventricular systolic dysfunction. J Am Coll Cardiol 2005;45(3):381–7.

38. Alfieri O, Elefteriades JA, Chapolini RJ, et al. Novel suture device for beating-heart mitral leaflet approximation. Ann Thorac Surg 2002;74(5):1488–93.

39. Feldman T, Wasserman HS, Herrmann HC, et al. Percutaneous mitral valve repair using the edge-to-edge technique: six-month results of the EVEREST Phase I Clinical Trial. J Am Coll Cardiol 2005;46(11):2134–40.

40. Feldman T. Percutaneous mitral valve repair. J Interv Cardiol 2007;20(6):488–94.

41. Dang NC, Aboodi MS, Sakaguchi T, et al. Surgical revision after percutaneous mitral valve repair with a clip: initial multicenter experience. Ann Thorac Surg 2005;80(6):2338–42.

42. Carpentier A. Cardiac valve surgery—the "French correction". J Thorac Cardiovasc Surg 1983;86(3):323–37.

43. Fukamachi K. Percutaneous and off-pump treatments for functional mitral regurgitation. J Artif Organs 2008;11(1):12–8.

44. Maselli D, Guarracino F, Chiaramonti F, et al. Percutaneous mitral annuloplasty: an anatomic study of human coronary sinus and its relation with mitral valve annulus and coronary arteries. Circulation 2006;114(5):377–80.

45. Tops LF, Van de Veire NR, Schuijf JD, et al. Noninvasive evaluation of coronary sinus anatomy and its relation to the mitral valve annulus: implications for percutaneous mitral annuloplasty. Circulation 2007;115(11):1426–32.

46. Piazza N, Bonan R. Transcatheter mitral valve repair for functional mitral regurgitation: coronary sinus approach. J Interv Cardiol 2007;20(6):495–508.

47. Webb JG, Harnek J, Munt BI, et al. Percutaneous transvenous mitral annuloplasty: initial human experience with device implantation in the coronary sinus. Circulation 2006;113(6):851–5.

48. Harnek J. The Monarc Experience. Barcelona; Presented at the EuroPCR 2007.

49. Siminiak T, Firek L, Jerzykowska O, et al. Percutaneous valve repair for mitral regurgitation using the Carillon Mitral Contour System. Description of the method and case report. Kardiol Pol 2007;65(3):272–8 [discussion: 279].

50. Schofer J. The Carillon Experience. Barcelona, Presented at the EuroPCR 2007.

51. Dubreuil O, Basmadjian A, Ducharme A, et al. Percutaneous mitral valve annuloplasty for ischemic mitral regurgitation: first in man experience with a temporary implant. Catheter Cardiovasc Interv 2007;69(7):1053–61.

52. Available at: http://www.mitralign.com/eurostudy.shtml. Tewksbury (MA), 2008. Accessed July 12, 2009.

53. Williams JL, Toyoda Y, Ota T, et al. Feasibility of myxomatous mitral valve repair using direct leaflet and chordal radiofrequency ablation. J Interv Cardiol 2008; 21(6):547–54.

54. Fukamachi K, Inoue M, Popovic ZB, et al. Off-pump mitral valve repair using the Coapsys device: a pilot study in a pacing-induced mitral regurgitation model. Ann Thorac Surg 2004;77(2):688–92 [discussion: 692–3].

55. Fukamachi K, Popovic ZB, Inoue M, et al. Changes in mitral annular and left ventricular dimensions and left ventricular pressure-volume relations after offpump treatment of mitral regurgitation with the Coapsys device. Eur J Cardiothorac Surg 2004;25(3):352–7.

56. Inoue M, McCarthy PM, Popovic ZB, et al. The Coapsys device to treat functional mitral regurgitation: in vivo long-term canine study. J Thorac Cardiovasc Surg 2004;127(4):1068–76 [discussion: 1076–7].

57. Nguyen TC, Cheng A, Tibayan FA, et al. Septal-lateral annnular cinching perturbs basal left ventricular transmural strains. Eur J Cardiothorac Surg 2007;31(3): 423–9.

58. Bonhoeffer P, Boudjemline Y, Saliba Z, et al. Transcatheter implantation of a bovine valve in pulmonary position: a lamb study. Circulation 2000;102(7): 813–6.

59. Bonhoeffer P, Boudjemline Y, Saliba Z, et al. Percutaneous replacement of pulmonary valve in a right-ventricle to pulmonary-artery prosthetic conduit with valve dysfunction. Lancet 2000;356(9239):1403–5.

60. Lurz P, Coats L, Khambadkone S, et al. Percutaneous pulmonary valve implantation: impact of evolving technology and learning curve on clinical outcome. Circulation 2008;117(15):1964–72.

Surgical Treatments for Advanced Heart Failure

Mani A. Daneshmand, MD, Carmelo A. Milano, MD*

KEYWORDS

- Heart failure • Ventricular assist device • Transplantation
- Surgical ventricular restoration • Immunosuppression

In the United States one in eight deaths are due to heart failure or its sequelae, and the prevalence of this disease exceeds 5 million people.[1] Patients with heart failure represent a significantly ill cohort, approximately 80% of men and 70% of women under the age of 65 with heart failure will die within 8 years; one in five will die within 1 year.[1,2] During the last 20 years, hospital admissions for this disease have increased almost threefold (**Fig. 1**). Moreover, in 2008, the management of heart failure exceeded $34 billion in direct and indirect costs.[1] Although medical management with diuretics, β-blockers, angiotensin-converting enzyme inhibitors, and other afterload reduction agents has provided symptomatic relief and survival benefit, the survival of the most advanced heart failure patients is dismal with medical management alone.[3–7] This cohort of advanced heart failure patients benefits from several surgical treatments. Historically, the first successful surgical therapy for end-stage cardiomyopathy was cardiac allograft transplantation.[8–11] Soon thereafter, the first reports of mechanical cardiac support and replacement were issued.[12–14] Although several techniques for surgical ventricular restoration (SVR) in the setting of left ventricular (LV) aneurysms have been described over the years, the broader application of these techniques to patients with ischemic cardiomyopathy has occurred during the last decade.

This review focuses on LV aneurysm (LVA) repair and SVR, ventricular assist devices (VADs), and cardiac allograft transplantation for the treatment of advanced heart failure. Indications for these procedures are addressed, as well as intraoperative technical features and postoperative management strategies.

SVR

In 1996, working in South America, Dr Randas J. V. Batista first described partial left ventriculectomy with linear reapproximation to restore ventricular function in patients with dilated cardiomyopathy secondary to Chagas Disease.[15] Efforts in this country extended his procedure to individuals with idiopathic dilated cardiomyopathy.[16–20]

Department of General and Thoracic Surgery, Duke University Medical Center, DUMC 3043, Durham, NC 27710, USA
* Corresponding author.
E-mail address: milan002@mc.duke.edu (C.A. Milano).

Surg Clin N Am 89 (2009) 967–999
doi:10.1016/j.suc.2009.06.007
0039-6109/09/$ – see front matter © 2009 Published by Elsevier Inc.

surgical.theclinics.com

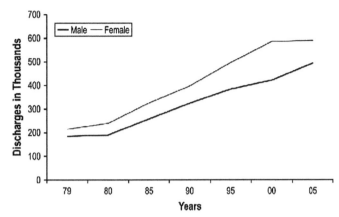

Fig. 1. Hospital discharges for heart failure (by sex) from 1979 through 2005, including patients characterized as "alive", "dead", or "status unknown" at time of discharge. (*Data from* The Centers for Disease Control National Center for Health Statistics; and the National Heart Lung and Blood Institute. Circulation 2008;117:e25; with permission.)

Unfortunately, approximately 45% of his patients were deceased within the first 2 years.[21] Before Dr Batista's report on partial left ventriculectomy, in the early 1980s, Dr Vincent Dor developed the endoventricular circular patch plasty for repair of LVAs.[22] A decade later, after observation of the effects of this procedure on LV remodeling, he advocated its usefulness in the treatment of advanced ischemic cardiomyopathy.[23,24] Although the Batista operation is no longer implemented in the treatment of dilated cardiomyopathy, the Dor procedure has gained popularity due to the promising results of the RESTORE trial and is an integral component of the recently reported Surgical Treatment for Ischemic Heart Failure (STICH) trial.[25–27]

Ventricular restoration with surgery is built on the observation that the left ventricle undergoes negative remodeling after infarction. This remodeling occurs in the setting of no revascularization and (to a lesser extent) in the setting of appropriate and timely revascularization.[28] After transmural infarction, the diseased area may undergo 3 transformations: (1) necrosis; (2) fibrosis; (3) calcification and often mural thrombosis.[29] Although the infarcted area of the ventricle undergoes these changes, the surrounding "normal tissue" also remodels. Immediately post infarct, the surrounding myocardium is normal. During subsequent months, the remaining myocardium first hypertrophies in compensation for the akinetic/dyskinetic infarcted zone, and then dilates because of increased volumes and wall tension (based on Starling's and Laplace's laws respectively).[30] Increased wall tension may trigger myocyte apoptosis in the remote myocardium, resulting grossly in wall thinning and dilation.[31,32]

Because the viable myocardium is in essence normal and is "remodeled" in response to the changes that occur within the infarcted zone, it logically follows that "restoration" of normal ventricular anatomy should halt further deleterious "remodeling" of normal myocardium. This concept is the fundamental basis for LV reconstruction by endoventricular circular patch plasty.[33] The main goals of this therapy are: (1) removal of the abnormal ventricular wall (the scar); (2) normalization of myocardial fiber alignment; (3) decrease in ventricular wall tension; and (4) restoration of a normal ventricular anatomy (reduce LV volume and restore a more ellipsoid shape).[34]

Patient Selection

SVR is most commonly applied in patients with the following features: (1) anteroseptal myocardial infarction secondary to left anterior descending (LAD) occlusion, resulting in a dilated left ventricle (end-diastolic volume index > 100 mL/m^2); (2) decreased LV function; (3) focal antero-apical and septal wall motion abnormalities (dyskinesis or akinesis); (4) symptomatic heart failure.[34] Patients who have focal LV antero-apical and septal dysfunction with preservation of function in basal segments may benefit the most from SVR. Furthermore, preserved right ventricular (RV) function is favorable; severe RV dysfunction and pulmonary hypertension have been defined as factors associated with increased procedural risk.[35,36] Patients in whom SVR is being considered should undergo echocardiography, right- and left-heart catheterization, and cardiac magnetic resonance with late gadolinium enhancement. The goal of these examinations is to assess the viability profile of the LV myocardium, define the extent of scar, as well as to determine areas suitable for revascularization.[29]

Procedure

Surgical revascularization of any remaining ischemic areas is typically combined with SVR. Furthermore most surgeons advocate revascularization of the LAD with the internal mammary artery (IMA). Although many of these patients have apical regions of transmural scar, viable regions of septal myocardium invariably remain and benefit from LAD revascularization. Although mild mitral insufficiency may resolve with SVR, moderate and severe mitral insufficiency is also typically addressed surgically.[37–39] Usually, mitral valve replacement is not necessary and ischemic mitral regurgitation can be addressed with complete ring annuloplasty.[29,40]

Therefore, the SVR procedure is typically performed with concomitant coronary artery bypass graft (CABG) revascularization in patients with ischemic cardiomyopathy. The first step of the procedure consists of conduit harvesting (IMA, SVG, and so forth). Next, cardiopulmonary bypass (CPB) is established, typically using ascending aortic and right atrial canulae. Bicaval venous canulation is employed for those cases that require concomitant mitral valve procedures. Most surgeons also use an LV vent introduced by way of the right superior pulmonary vein. The vent enables better visualization of the inside of the LV and facilitates the deairing process. Aortic cross-clamping and cardioplegic arrest with antegrade and retrograde cardioplegia are typically used to perform the distal coronary anastamoses. After the distal anastamoses are completed, the SVR procedure is undertaken. Some surgeons advocate continued cardioplegic arrest, whereas others have described benefits to performing the SVR after release of the aortic cross-clamp with the heart reperfused.[41] Important steps of the SVR include:

1) The LV is opened through the center of the apical scar, intraventricular thrombus is carefully removed.
2) Endocardium is carefully inspected and palpated to define the border between normal myocardium and scar.
3) At the border of the endocardial scar and normal myocardium, an endoventricular purse string suture is placed (known as the Fontan stitch). Typically a 2-0 polypropylene suture is used; some surgeons prefer to place a double purse string (**Figs. 2 and 3B**). Usually, the purse string is at least 1 cm distal to the papillary muscle insertions. Placing the purse string too close to the base may result in an LV with inadequate volume. The authors advocate placing this stitch just within the scar tissue, giving the purse string greater strength and avoiding undersizing the ventricular volume.

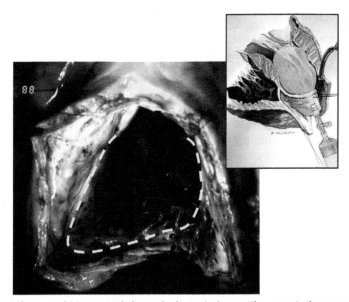

Fig. 2. The left ventricle is opened through the apical scar. The margin between scar and healthy myocardium (the "contractility trail") is identified (*yellow dotted line*) and a purse-string suture is inserted within this margin. A balloon ventricular sizer (*inset*) may be used to control ventricular reshaping as the purse string is tied down. (*From* Dor V, Civaia F, Alexandrescu C, et al. The post-myocardial infarction scarred ventricle and congestive heart failure: the preeminence of magnetic resonance imaging for preoperative, intraoperative, and postoperative assessment. J Thorac Cardiovasc Surg 2008;136(6):1405–12; with permission.)

4) A rubber balloon can be inserted through the purse string and inflated to the theoretical "normal" end-diastolic volume of the patient's left ventricle (50–60 mL/m^2 body surface area [BSA]). The Fontan stitch(es) is (are) tied, restoring "normal" ventricular size. The balloon is then deflated and removed (see **Fig. 2** inset and see **Fig. 3**C). Alternatively, some investigators forego "balloon sizing" and base the new ventricle size on preoperative imaging and intraoperative judgment.[41]

5) Based on the remaining orifice, an endoventricular patch (of either synthetic or autologous material) is fashioned and secured over the orifice (see **Fig. 3**D). The authors use a Hemashield patch (Boston Scientific, Natick, Massachusetts, USA) secured with a running 2-0 polypropylene suture.

6) The excluded areas of the ventricle can be partially resected and sutured over the patch for further hemostasis.

The procedure continues with placement of the proximal anastamoses of the coronary grafts, usually accomplished with a partial aortic occlusion clamp. The heart is deaired, atrial and ventricular temporary pacing wires are placed, and the patient is carefully weaned from CPB.

Postoperative Management

The initial postoperative management for SVR is similar to other cardiac procedures, with a focus on hemostasis and resolution of coagulopathy and bleeding. Patients who undergo SVR generally have significantly reduced LV function, and postoperative hemodynamic stabilization is another critical goal. Almost all patients are supported

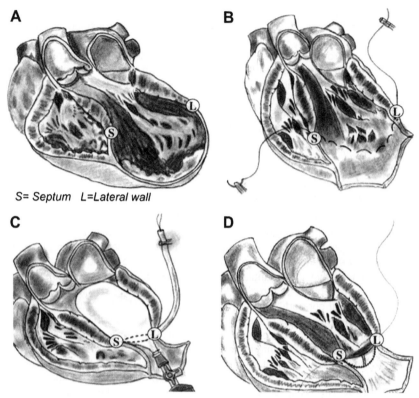

S= Septum   L=Lateral wall

Fig. 3. (A) Postmyocardial infarction ventricular remodeling. (B) Through a ventriculotomy made within the myocardial scar region, a purse-string suture is placed along the border of normal myocardium and scar. (C) A ventriculoplasty balloon may be used to ensure proper sizing of the ventricular reconstruction. (D) An endoventricular patch is used to close the remaining defect in the apex of the left ventricle, the scar tissue can be closed over this patch to improve hemostasis. (*From* Dor V, Civaia F, Alexandrescu C, et al. The post-myocardial infarction scarred ventricle and congestive heart failure: the preeminence of magnetic resonance imaging for preoperative, intraoperative, and postoperative assessment. J Thorac Cardiovasc Surg 2008;136(6):1405–12; with permission.)

with intravenous inotropes, usually low-dose epinephrine or intraaortic balloon counterpulstation therapy. Fortunately, this support is typically weaned off within the first 24 to 48 hours.

Another important perioperative problem is the management of ventricular arrhythmias. Ventricular resection may result in greater postoperative myocardial irritability. Avoidance of hypokalemia, hypomagnesemia, early discontinuation of β-adrenergic agonists, and use of β-blockers seems to help reduce arrhythmias. Some patients may require amiodarone or lidocaine infusions. Almost all patients should be evaluated for automated internal cardiac defibrillators.

Outcomes

The usefulness of SVR has recently been examined by the STICH trial.[26,27] One thousand patients with LV ejection fraction less than 35% were enrolled in the STICH trial and were randomized to receive either CABG alone or CABG with concomitant

SVR. The follow-up for this portion of the study was at 48 months with the primary end points of death (all causes) and cardiac rehospitalization. Surprisingly, both groups (CABG alone and CABG + SVR) experienced a relative low procedural mortality (<5%) and both groups demonstrated improvement in their heart failure symptoms. There was no difference between the two groups with regards to the primary end points of death and cardiac rehospitalization. These results will probably limit the application of the SVR procedure to patients with dyskinetic or aneurismal segments of LV. The second part of the STICH trial will evaluate the benefits of CABG revascularization relative to medical therapy alone as a treatment of heart failure in patients with ischemic cardiomyopathy.

DESTINATION THERAPY LVAD
Overview of Mechanical Circulatory Support

A variety of mechanical devices have been used to support the circulation and replace ventricular function in the setting of heart failure. Most commonly these devices are mechanical pumps, which achieve complete ventricular unloading and replacement; these devices are termed VADs. The first VAD designs were extracorporeal and connected to the heart by way of canulae and blood tubing.[13,14,42] Most commonly, VAD support is used to replace LV function (LVAD), but isolated RV support is possible, as well as biventricular support.[42,43] Early designs used pneumatic actuation but during the last 2 decades electrically powered designs have become more common. Electrical powering enabled more compact designs in which the entire pump can be implanted in the body, usually inferior to the heart in the abdomen or in a preperitoneal pocket. **Fig. 4** illustrates a typical implanted LVAD with drainage of the LV by way of an apical cannula. Blood is then pumped out of the device into a graft attached to the ascending aorta. The pump is electrically driven and a driveline (power cord) exits the patient's right upper abdominal wall, attaching to small, portable, external batteries enabling untethered activity.

Application of LVADs can be broadly categorized into three groups. First, patients for whom recovery of ventricular function is anticipated and the VAD is used to bridge the patient to recovery. Typically, the duration of support for the recovery strategy is days or weeks. Perhaps the most impressive cases of bridge-to-recovery are patients with acute viral myocarditis. This condition is believed to result from viral myocardial infection and secondary inflammation resulting in profound ventricular dysfunction. Small case series have described patients with viral myocarditis progressing to cardiogenic shock requiring VAD support.[44,45] In a large percentage of these cases inflammation subsides and ventricular functional recovery occurs, enabling device explantation.[46] Duration of VAD support for viral myocarditis ranges from days to weeks. Other acute conditions, in which ventricular functional recovery may occur during VAD support, include myocardial infarction associated with cardiogenic shock, and profound ventricular dysfunction following heart surgery (postcardiotomy failure). Importantly, for all three of these conditions, a certain subset of patients will not experience recovery and will require long-term support and possibly transplantation.[45]

The second and perhaps most traditional application of LVAD support is for bridging patients with either acute or chronic heart failure, until cardiac transplantation can be performed.[47] These patients are considered to have irreversible ventricular failure and are evaluated and deemed suitable for cardiac transplantation. Before considering LVAD support, patients generally are supported with less invasive therapies such as continuous intravenous inotropes. Implantable LVADs have been used to bridge

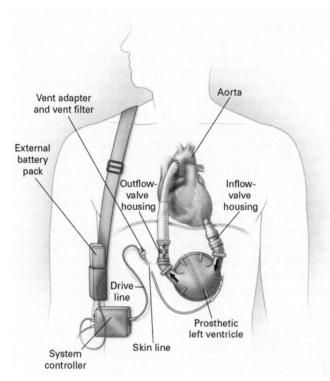

Fig. 4. The HeartMate XVE LV assist device is an implantable LVAD. The main pumping chamber is housed in the abdomen (either preperitoneally or intraperitoneally). Blood exits the apex of the left ventricle and fills the pump chamber. It is then ejected from the LVAD through the outflow cannula into the ascending aorta. The pump is electrically powered and externally vented. The system can operate on a battery pack, a standard electrical outlet, or a hand pump. (*From* Rose EA, Gelijns AC, Moskowitz AJ, et al. Long-term use of a left ventricular assist device for end-stage heart failure. N Engl J Med 2001;345(20):1435–43; with permission.)

patients to transplant since the late 1980s.[48] Positive outcomes with this application have been important in expanding the field of mechanical circulatory support. Functional recovery, as well as improvement in end-organ function, while on VAD support has been impressive and has served to better prepare candidates for heart transplantation relative to bridging with continuous intravenous inotropes.[49] Transition from the initial, pneumatically driven, implantable LVADs to electrically powered devices led to reduction in the external components for the VAD system, and improved mobility.[50] This advancement enabled patients to be discharged from the hospital while awaiting cardiac transplantation. Discharged patients enjoyed an improved quality of life and in some cases demonstrated an ability to return to employment.[50–52] Typical waiting periods for cardiac transplantation on VAD support varies due to patient size, blood type and presence of anti-HLA antibodies, but typically ranges from 3 to 6 months.[53] For this duration of support, device malfunction is uncommon and often remedied by replacement of external components. Infection rates ranged from 5% to 10% with the driveline exit site being the most common site of infection.[53] Finally, thromboembolic complications that historically have comprised an important limiting factor for mechanical circulatory support in general have been acceptable, particularly with devices featuring a textured, blood contacting surface.[54]

These favorable outcomes using implantable LVADs to bridge patients to transplant have led to several important developments. First, more patients are being bridged to heart transplant with LVADs relative to using continuous intravenous inotropes **Fig. 5**. The second development seen during the last decade is that patients with end-stage heart failure, who fail to qualify for transplant, are being considered for permanent LVAD support as a substitute for cardiac transplant, so-called destination therapy LVAD (DT LVAD).[4] This third application consists of patients who have chronic and severe heart failure that has failed standard medical therapies and who are not candidates for transplant. Thus, permanent LVAD treatment has evolved from the bridge-to-transplant experience as a result of positive and encouraging outcomes. Furthermore, permanent or destination LVAD application is often not entirely distinct from the bridge-to-transplant application because a patient's eligibility for transplant may change over time. For example, a patient who is felt to be inappropriate for transplant due to obesity may achieve dieting and weight reduction on LVAD support, enabling reconsideration of transplant therapy; the patient may have started as a destination implant but ultimately can be offered transplant.[55] Nevertheless, the emergence of destination LVAD therapy for end-stage heart failure has important impact over and above transplant. Cardiac transplant is limited by suitable donors to approximately 2000 patients per year in this country.[56] Unfortunately, there are an estimated 100,000 end-stage heart failure patients; therefore, destination LVAD may address a much larger group for whom there are essentially no other therapeutic options.[1]

Indications for DT LVAD

In 2003, as a result of the REMATCH trial, the Food and Drug Administration (FDA) approved the HeartMate XVE (Thoratec Corporation, Pleasanton, California, USA) implantable LVAD for DT.[4] Importantly, federal and private insurers have acknowledged the survival and quality-of-life benefits and have agreed to provide reimbursement for this product as DT. Nevertheless, the complexity and cost of the therapy is great and, therefore, indications for treatment are strictly defined. Importantly, the therapy is currently indicated for chronic heart failure; acute heart failure such as post-infarction or acute viral myocarditis is not an indication. Another important mandate is

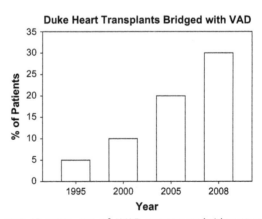

Fig. 5. During the past 13 years, use of LVAD systems as bridge to transplantation has increased more than sixfold at our institution.

that patients must have received and essentially failed conventional therapies including medical and potential surgical options. Standard medical therapies included β-blockers, angiotensin-converting enzyme inhibitors, and diuretics. These therapies have all been demonstrated to enhance survival in heart failure patients; FDA guidelines for DT LVAD require that these drugs have been trialed for at least 60 of the last 90 days. As patients progress to end-stage heart failure, they often are unable to tolerate these oral medications owing to the development of a low-output state manifested by hypotension, secondary renal insufficiency, and refractory volume overload including pulmonary edema. At this point, standard oral medications are discontinued and patients are stabilized with intravenous inotropic infusions such as dobutamine (β-adrenergic receptor agonist) or milrinone (phosphodiesterase inhibitor). These inotropic drugs clearly may provide transient symptomatic improvement but they have not been shown to improve survival in any cohort of heart failure patients.[57] Therefore, although failure of oral medical therapy is required before consideration of DT LVAD, prolonged continuous inotropic infusions before referral should be avoided. In addition, other conventional surgical therapies should be considered, if appropriate, before DT LVAD. For example, some patients with ischemic cardiomyopathy may benefit from revascularization. Other patients with end-stage heart failure may have important aortic or mitral valvular dysfunction that can be addressed with surgery. If there is significant hope for recovery of functional capacity, and the procedural risk is acceptable, then these conventional surgical options should be attempted.

Another important treatment option for end-stage heart failure is biventricular pacing for ventricular resynchronization.[58] In select patients with prolonged QRS duration, this pacing therapy has been shown to improve symptoms and functional class.[59,60] Therefore, given the relative noninvasive nature of this option, patients with the appropriate indications should first undergo a trial of biventricular pacing. Practically, most patients who are referred for DT LVAD have failed biventricular pacing.

TRANSPLANT INELIGIBILITY

An additional important requirement for DT LVAD consideration is that patients be evaluated and found ineligible for transplant. When a medical center offering DT LVAD therapy does not offer cardiac transplant evaluation, a special relationship with a transplant center needs to be established so that patients can be evaluated for transplant before being considered for permanent, implantable LVAD. Perhaps the most common reason why DT LVAD patients are considered ineligible for transplant is advanced age. Typically, many transplant centers have established age 65 or 70 to be the upper limit. This limit is consistent with International Society of Heart & Lung Transplantation (ISHLT) registry data, which demonstrate reduced outcomes with transplant in this older subset. Other common reasons for transplant ineligibility include obesity or increased body mass index (BMI, calculated as weight in kilograms divided by the square of height in meters). Importantly, these patients may achieve weight reduction during LVAD support and be reconsidered for transplant.[61] Other reasons for transplant ineligibility include extremely high levels for anti-HLA antibodies, which preclude adequate donor matching. Also history of recent malignancy and severe heart failure is an important factor that makes patients ineligible for transplant due to risks of reactivation of malignancy with immunosuppression. An example is the patient who receives adriamycin chemotherapy and suffers secondary cardiac toxicity. Furthermore, other end-organ dysfunction, such as some degree of primary pulmonary disease or renal insufficiency, may make heart failure patients ineligible for transplant but still suitable for LVAD consideration. In addition, severe pulmonary hypertension or increased pulmonary vascular resistance may disqualify patients from consideration of transplant, but they may still be suitable for DT LVAD.

Importantly, common to the evaluation for transplant and DT LVAD, is the psychological and social screening. Included in this assessment is an evaluation for medical compliance. Patients who are found to be psychologically unstable are not eligible for either therapy. Similarly, lack of social support or demonstration of active substance abuse makes a patient ineligible for either therapy. In summary, the needs for social support, psychological stability, and medical compliance are similar for transplant and LVAD therapy.

Determination of Severity of Heart Failure

Given the procedural risks of LVAD therapy, it is important that stable heart failure patients with life expectancy greater than 1 or 2 years not be offered this therapy. On the other hand, patients who have progressed to secondary end-organ dysfunction may have missed the optimal treatment window, as studies have shown markedly increased procedural risk.[62] Therefore, proper timing is critical; unfortunately, predicting survival is challenging for advanced heart failure. Workup should include exercise testing whenever possible; the maximal oxygen consumption less than 14 mL/kg/min has been associated with high 1-year mortality and should serve as an indication of heart failure severity warranting DT LVAD.[63] Other markers for high heart failure mortality include repeated hospitalizations for decompensation, cardiorenal syndrome, and clinical need for continuous inotropic infusions. Poor hemodynamics also predict negative outcomes and should be obtained routinely by right-heart catheterization. Evaluation and intervention before secondary end-organ dysfunction, malnutrition, or complicating infection is critical to successful outcomes and requires a multidisciplinary advanced heart failure team.

Preoperative Assessment and Optimization

There is a trend toward more elective implants for DT LVADs. This strategy has emerged from the observation that so-called crash-and-burn patients have high procedural mortality, which is probably unacceptable given the cost and complexity of this treatment.[62] Thus, hemodynamic optimization and improvement of end-organ function is an important focus before taking the patient to the operating room. Patients who are unstable may be optimized with intravenous inotropes and invasive monitoring. Those who fail these measures may benefit from temporary mechanical support before the implantable LVAD. Usually, this consists of intraaortic balloon pump to improve hemodynamics. Although typically employed for ischemic heart conditions, our experience suggests patients with advanced myopathies of any cause derive benefit from periods of intraaortic balloon pump (IABP) support. Other types of temporary support include percutaneous LVADs such as the Tandem Heart (Cardiac Assist, Inc., Pittsburgh, Pennsylvania, USA) or the Impella (AbioMed, Inc., Danvers, Massachusetts, USA) devices. These are capable of LV unloading and achieve flows up to 4 L/min. With these temporary devices, many patients will show evidence for improvement in end-organ perfusion such as resolution of oliguria, improvement in serum creatinine and normalization of serum hepatocellular enzyme levels. Patients who fail to respond to these temporary support measures are probably at high procedural risks for the implantable LVAD.[62,64]

Another important element of the preoperative evaluation is to rule out, and treat any signs of, infection. In general, any fever in the preoperative period warrants pan-culturing and in some instances empiric antibiotics. This aggressive course is indicated because infection is an important cause of heart failure, decompensation, and death. In addition, infection represents a common morbidity and cause of death post-LVAD implant. In general, old lines should be replaced before the implant procedure. Preprocedural prophylactic antibiotics should include vancomycin, as well as an agent effective for gram-negative organisms and an antifungal agent.[65] All 3 should be administered before the skin incision.

Intraoperative Procedure

Intraoperative transesophageal echocardiogram is performed after initiation of anesthesia. It is important to exclude the presence of a patent foreman ovale or any other septal defect. With LV unloading, such defects can allow significant right-to-left shunting and systemic desaturation. Any identified defect should be repaired. Competency of the aortic valve is also evaluated: significant aortic insuffiency (AI) leads to regurgitant volume and reduced systemic output. Severe AI warrants replacement or repair (although need for this additional intervention substantially increases the risk of the procedure).[66] Severe tricuspid insufficiency is often surgically addressed and probably does not add significant additional risk. Most surgeons agree that mitral insufficiency does not need to be corrected because the LV becomes unloaded after LVAD placement.[66]

Most implantable LVADs are placed by way of a median sternotomy, which affords good exposure of the ascending aorta for outflow graft attachment and of the LV apex, which is typically canulated for inflow to the pump. Typically, the incision is extended downward onto the upper abdomen, enabling placement of the pump just inferior to the heart in either a preperitoneal pocket or directly into the abdominal cavity. As LVAD pump designs have become smaller, extension of the median sternotomy may not be necessary. The dissection of the pump pocket should be performed first, before heparin administration; the driveline is usually tunneled out of the right upper abdomen, again before heparin administration.

The next step of the procedure typically involves attachment of the pump to the native heart. There are two sites of attachment that consist of the apical LV cannula and the outflow graft to the ascending aorta. The order in which these steps are performed is not critical and some surgeons prefer one attachment before the other. Furthermore, although CPB is typically employed for these attachments, the placement of the apical canula and the outflow graft can be performed without CPB. CPB provides an element of safety and control, but proponents of reducing the use of CPB argue that bleeding and coagulapathy are reduced when CPB is avoided.

The apical canula is placed after removal of a core of LV apical myocardium. Usually, a series of felt-pledget reinforced 2-0 sutures are used to secure a synthetic ring to which the apical canula is attached. Care is taken to resect any trabeculations in the LV apex that might interfere with drainage of the LV into the canula. Similarly, any LV thrombus, which commonly develops with end-stage heart failure, must be removed. Typically, the apical left anterior descending coronary artery is preserved. Furthermore, care is taken to direct the apical canula away from the septum toward the mitral valve orifice. Occasionally, particularly in smaller LVs, the apical canula can become pushed into the heart, leading to obstruction of drainage by either the septum or the lateral free wall. The remedy consists of repositioning the canula and retracting it away from the ventricular apex. The attachment of the outflow graft consists of an end-to-side anastamosis to the ascending aorta; typically this is accomplished with a running 4-0 propylene suture. Many cases may be reoperative with the patient having had prior coronary bypass grafts; in these instances care must be taken to avoid injury to these grafts that may result in regions of myocardial ischemia, ischemic ventricular arrhythmias, and, in some cases, RV dysfunction.

Following placement of the canulae, the next steps consist of deairing, pump activation, and weaning from CPB. Typically, these procedures should be performed in a field flooded with CO_2, thus reducing the negative impact of embolized air. In addition to conventional deairing strategies, submerging the pump in warm saline may be helpful. Initially, pump settings should be reduced to avoid complete emptying of the LV and creation of suction that could also lead to entrainment of air. Optimizing RV function also helps keep the LV filled and prevents entrainment of air. After the patient is safely weaned off bypass, the heparin is reversed and clots will form in the field and around the outside of the pump. After the protamine reversal, the risk of air entrainment is reduced and the pump speed can be more safely increased. An unfortunate scenario occurs when air is present and enters the aorta, leading to obstruction in the right coronary artery. If the air persists in the right coronary artery, RV ischemia and dysfunction will occur. This occurrence in turn results in underfilling of the LV, potential suction with further entrainment of air; thus, a negative cycle can lead to circulatory failure and the need to return to CPB. Attention to details and focus on maintaining good RV performance and avoiding air entrainment at the time the patient is weaned off CPB helps avoid this negative scenario.

Therefore, in initiating LVAD support, an important concern is RV performance. In general, LV unloading should reduce the afterload of the RV and improve RV output. Nevertheless, RV dysfunction is common after implantable LVAD procedures.[67] Adequate heart rate and an atrioventricular synchronous rhythm help to optimize RV performance. Inotropic support is typically employed in the form of low-dose epinephrine or dobutamine. Excessive leftward septal shift can occur if pump speed is too high; this should be avoided as it can lead to reduced RV function as well as worsening tricuspid insufficiency. Additional agents should be employed to reduce pulmonary vascular resistance; for example, inhaled nitric oxide has been shown to reduce pulmonary vascular resistance and increase LVAD output.[68] This agent is particularly useful because it does not have systemic effect. Iloprost (inhaled prostaglandin) has been similarly used and seems to have little systemic effect.[69] If these traditional strategies do not achieve adequate right-heart performance, a final option is mechanical support in the form of an RVAD. Usually, RVAD placement requires canulation of the right atrium and pulmonary artery. Temporary RVAD support is often all that is required and devices such as the CentriMag have been used at our institution.

Postoperative Care

Immediately after implant, bleeding is an important concern: many patients will have hepatic insufficiency and coagulapathy. In addition, temporary mechanical support, such as IABP before the LVAD, may have resulted in platelet dysfunction. Furthermore, recent studies have shown that LVAD support may affect von Willebrand factor and induce a form of acquired von Willebrand disease.[70] For all these reasons, an important initial focus is achieving normal platelet function.

RV performance remains an important issue in the early postoperative period. Some investigators have shown that many patients supported with implantable LVADs will have ongoing intravenous inotropic requirements for RV dysfunction.[71] Most of these patients will ultimately be weaned off inotropes and achieve normal hemodynamics, but support for 2 to 3 weeks is not uncommon in a small fraction of patients.[71] Furthermore, ongoing support with diuretics is not uncommon for peripheral edema. For patients with axial flow or centrifugal pumps, reassessment of pump speed should be performed to ensure complete LV unloading, which translates into reduced afterload for the RV. Ongoing attention to adequate heart rate and rhythm, and avoidance of arrhythmias, are also important to optimize RV performance. Pulmonary processes such as major effusions or atelectasis may have a negative impact on pulmonary vascular resistance leading to reduced RV output and elevated central venous pressures, therefore these pulmonary conditions should also be corrected.

Outcomes

The REMATCH study was a prospective randomized trial that compared optimal medical management to implantable LVAD in patients with end-stage heart disease, who were ineligible for cardiac transplantation. Most patients who were randomized to these two therapies were of ages greater than 65, dependent on continuous intravenous inotropes, and had evidence of secondary renal insufficiency.[4] The only device used in this trial was the vented electric HeartMate XVE. This device is a larger first-generation pump that provides pulsatile flow. The trial demonstrated improved survival and quality of life with the LVAD treatment relative to optimal medical management (**Fig. 6**). Unfortunately, mortality and morbidity remained high even in the LVAD treatment arm. Thus the trial supported permanent use of implantable LVADs for patients who are transplant ineligible, but also highlighted many of the limitations of the HeartMate XVE design.

The REMATCH trial led to FDA approval of the HeartMate XVE as a DT. Specific criteria for DT LVAD therapy have been defined by the FDA, and a postapproval registry was mandated to further evaluate outcomes. Furthermore, DT LVAD therapy was limited to designated hospitals, as controlled by the Joint Commission for Hospital Accreditation. The therapy has been slow to develop with the HeartMate XVE, but outcomes have generally improved post-REMATCH (**Fig. 7**).[72]

Despite improving outcomes, the broader application of the HeartMate XVE device was limited by the substantial morbidity as outlined in the REMATCH trial. The morbidity was in part due to the large size of the device, which prevented implantation

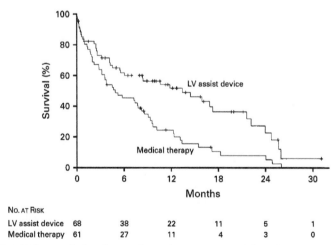

Fig. 6. Kaplan-Meier survival estimates from the REMATCH trial. Patients supported by the HeartMate XVE LVAD had significantly better survival compared with those on maximal medical therapy (P = .001). (*From* Rose EA, Gelijns AC, Moskowitz AJ, et al. Long-term use of a left ventricular assist device for end-stage heart failure. N Engl J Med 2001;345(20):1435–43; with permission.)

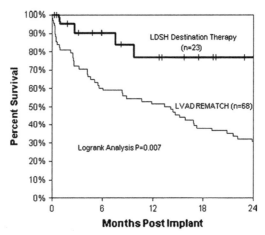

Fig. 7. Current-era DT LVAD at LDS Hospital in Salt Lake City, Utah, (LDSH DT) demonstrates significantly improved 2-year survival compared with the original REMATCH trial patients who received LVAD therapy (LVAD REMATCH) (*P* < .0001). (*From* Long JW, AH Healy, Rasmusson BY, et al. Improving outcomes with long-term "destination" therapy using left ventricular assist devices. J Thorac Cardiovasc Surg 2008;135(6):1353–61; with permission.)

in most female patients. The larger size required an extended incision, which probably also impacted postoperative recovery. Related to the increased size was a substantial risk for infection.[73] Device-related infections included driveline infections, infection of the pump pocket, and other infections involving blood-contacting elements of the device (so-called LVAD endocarditis). These different infections were difficult to treat and eradicate, and proved limiting. The most important limitation for this LVAD design, however, was durability. The HeartMate XVE seemed durable when used for several months as a bridge to transplant, but more prolonged use as a destination device revealed definite durability issues. The device predictably failed between 1 and 2 years.[73] Sites of failure included the bearings and the inflow valve. Although device replacement has been performed successfully, it represented another major procedure including the need for CPB support. Thus, as newer devices evolved, the most important goal was improved durability.

NEWER IMPLANTABLE LVAD DESIGNS

First-generation, implantable LVADs featured pulsatile delivery of blood to the systemic circulation with stroke volumes similar to those of the native heart. Newer-generation devices have progressed to continuous-flow designs. This design change offered several important theoretical advantages: first, in general, continuous-flow pumps could be electromagnetically driven, with fewer bearings and without valves; thus, theoretically they would have greater durability. Second, continuous-flow pumps lacked a diastolic phase during which blood would be stagnant within the device; this feature theoretically should reduce thromboembolic risk. Finally, because these devices do not have to accommodate the human stroke volume, the size is considerably reduced relative to pulsatile pumps. Potential limitations for continuous-flow devices also existed, including potential for greater blood agitation and hemolysis, particularly at higher pump revolutions per minute. Also, the lack of pulsatility may result in inadequate perfusion of certain end-organ beds. Fortunately, early clinical

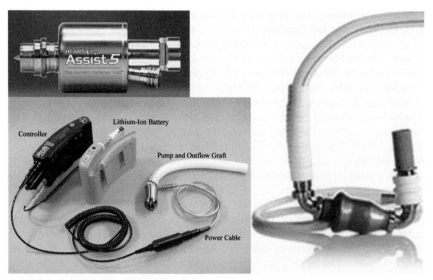

Fig. 8. Second-generation LVAD devices. (*Top left*) The Debakey Heart Assist 5 by Micromed Cardiovascular, Houston, Texas, USA. (*Bottom left*) The Jarvik 2000 by Jarvik Heart, New York, USA. (*Right*) The HeartMate II by Thoratec Corporation, Pleasanton, California, USA. (Jarvik *from* Frazier OH, Myers TJ, Westaby S, et al. Clinical experience with an implantable, intracardiac, continuous flow circulatory support device: physiologic implications and their relationship to patient selection. Ann Thorac Surg 2004;77:133–42; and Griffith BP, Kormos RL, Borovetz HS, et al. HeartMate II left ventricular assist system: from concept to first clinical use. Ann Thorac Surg 2001;71:S116–120S. http://www.jarvikheart.com.)

results with continuous-flow devices seem to support these theoretical advantages and have disproven some of the potential limitations. Two continuous-flow designs that have been clinically investigated are axial-flow and centrifugal pumps.

Axial-flow pumps feature an impellar that is support by a single central bearing. The impellar is driven by an overlying electromagnetic field. Examples of this design

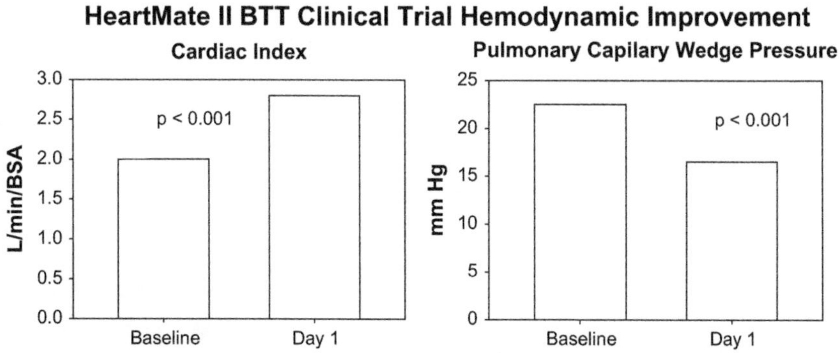

HeartMate II BTT Clinical Trial Hemodynamic Improvement

Cardiac Index

L/min/BSA — Baseline: 2.0, Day 1: 2.8 (p < 0.001)

Pulmonary Capilary Wedge Pressure

mm Hg — Baseline: 22.5, Day 1: 16.5 (p < 0.001)

Fig. 9. The HeartMate II bridge-to-transplant trial demonstrated an improvement in the hemodynamic profile of patients who received the device within 1 day of implant. Cardiac index improved by an average of more than 0.7 L/min/BSA (*left*) and pulmonary capillary wedge pressure (PCWP) decreased by more than 6 mmHG (*right*). (*Data from* John R, Kamdar F, Liao K, et al. Improved survival and decreasing incidence of adverse events with the Heartmate II left ventricular assist device as bridge-to-transplant therapy. Ann Thorac Surg 2008;86:1227.)

include the HeartMate II (Thoratec Corporation, Pleasanton, California, USA), Debakey HeartAssist 5 (Micromed Cardiovascular, Inc., Houston, Texas, USA) and the Jarvik 2000 (Jarvik Heart, Inc, New York, USA) (**Fig. 8**). The greatest clinical experience has been with the HeartMate II pump. This device was trialed in two phases: the first was with the pump used as a bridge to transplant. In this bridge study, outcomes with the HeartMate II were compared with historical performance measures obtained with the HeartMate XVE device. The HeartMate II bridge-to-transplant trial showed the device to be capable of restoring normal hemodynamics (**Fig. 9**). In addition, functional recovery with the HeartMate II was impressive, with most patients returning to New York Heart Association (NYHA) class I or II (**Fig. 10**). Furthermore, morbidity with the HeartMate II appeared reduced relative to historical outcomes with the Heart-Mate XVE. Based on these results, the HeartMate II device has been approved for the bridge-to-transplant indication.[74]

The second phase of investigation has examined the HeartMate II as DT. The DT trial randomized patients to either the HeartMate II or HeartMate XVE. This trial also included a small cohort who were not randomized because they were ineligible for the HeartMate XVE because of low BSA. Another group consisted of patients who required device replacement, and these again were not randomized. The single most important observation from this study was the improved durability of the Heart-Mate II relative to HeartMate XVE. There were few reports of HeartMate II pump failure or wear-out; the most common serious device failure related to driveline malfunctions that were generally caused by trauma. These driveline failures occasionally required device replacement, although many of the leads could be repaired.[75] The device durability seems to be greater than 3 or 4 years.

The thromboembolic profile for the HeartMate II device also seems to be favorable, and equivalent to that of the HeartMate XVE.[76] Although initial anticoagulation guidelines included coumadin, aspirin, and dipyridimole, bleeding complications appeared to be the more frequent and concerning adverse event. Patients appeared to have increased incidence of gastrointestinal bleeds; these observations led to progressive reduction in target international normalized ratio (INR) levels as well as reduced use of antiplatelet agents. Other investigators have shown reduced von Willebrand factor function, which may be related to loss of high–molecular-weight multimers that are

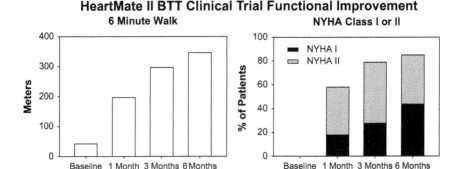

HeartMate II BTT Clinical Trial Functional Improvement

Fig. 10. The HeartMate II bridge-to-transplant trial also demonstrated an improvement in the functional status of patients who received the device. Six-minute walking distance (*left*) and the proportion of patients with NYHA class I or II heart failure (*right*) increased steadily during the course of LVAD therapy. (*Data from* John R, Kamdar F, Liao K, et al. Improved survival and decreasing incidence of adverse events with the Heartmate II left ventricular assist device as bridge-to-transplant therapy. Ann Thorac Surg 2008;86:1227.)

normally responsible for binding to platelets and collagen.[70] It is unclear if this acquired von Willebrand condition is device-specific.

Implantable LVADs with a centrifugal design have also undergone clinical testing. These designs feature an electromagnetically driven rotor that is magnetically levitated. This design therefore lacks bearings and, theoretically, may be the most durable (**Fig. 11**). Examples of this design are the VentrAssist (Ventracor, Inc, Foster City, California, USA), the Levacor (AbioMed, Inc), and the HeartWare HVAD (Thoratec Corporation, Pleasanton, California, USA), which are similarly undergoing testing for the bridge-to-transplant indication as well as for DT.

DESTINATION LVAD THERAPY, FUTURE FRONTIERS

The balance of thromboembolism and bleeding will always remain an important challenge for mechanical circulatory support. Pump designs and blood contacting materials remain an important focus for LVADs. Textured surfaces seem to show reduced thrombosis risk relative to smooth surfaces. Textured titanium is now commonly employed for blood-contacting elements. Another potentially important area of research involves development of biocompatible surfaces or coatings. For example, some devices have employed heparin coating for blood-contacting surfaces, but this strategy has not proven clinically beneficial. Another experimental strategy involves expansion of endothelial progenitor cells and seeding of LVAD materials to create a monolayer of endothelium lining the inside of the pump. This strategy would require a preprocedure incubation of the pump surfaces with endothelial progenitor cells. Preliminary studies suggest that these cells can become seated and withstand expected shear forces.

Another important limitation for current LVAD systems is infection. Infections may involve the driveline or be more complex, with involvement of the pump pocket or of blood-contacting elements of the device. Infection rates seem much higher for LVADs with drivelines exiting the body relative to other implants in which there is no exiting part. For example, pacemakers or automatic implanted cardiac defibrillators have long-term infection rates of less than 1%; unfortunately, implantable LVADs with exiting drivelines may have long-term major infection rates closer to 10%. Strategies to rectify these higher rates have included attempts at completely implanted

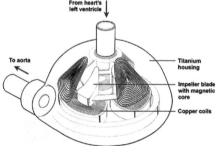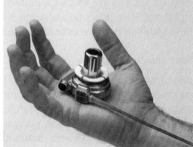

Fig. 11. Third generation LVAD devices, like the VentrAssist by Ventracor, Foster City, California, USA (*left*), and the HeartWare by Thoratec Corporation, Pleasanton, California, USA (*right*), have magnetically levitated impellers so there are no points of physical contact and therefore, theoretically, no possibility for wear. (*From* Aggarwal S, Cheema F, Oz MC, et al. Long-term mechanical circulatory support. Card Surg Adult 2008;3:1609–28; *Courtesy of* Ventracor, Inc, Foster City, California; with permission. Heartware: http://www.heartware.com.au.)

systems that are driven by transcutaneous energy transmission. Another effort has focused on reducing the size of the driveline.

An important frontier involves efforts to achieve recovery of ventricular function even for chronic heart failure patients supported on LVADs. Theoretically, this might convert permanent LVAD patients into patients who receive device support for months or years until sufficient reverse remodeling is achieved, such that device weaning and removal would be possible. Indeed, multiple basic studies have shown that LVAD mechanical unloading results in positive cellular and molecular changes, which constitute the process of reverse remodeling. The clinical results that are most supportive for this potential strategy are from the Harefield group in England.[77] This group has reported on almost two dozen chronic heart failure patients who underwent treatment with LVAD unloading in combination with standard oral heart failure medications. In addition, patients were treated with the experimental agent clembuterol, which acts as a β-2 adrenergic receptor and has anabolic steroid properties. This group has developed a complex LVAD-weaning protocol. Many of the patients achieved LVAD-explantation with long-term freedom from significant heart failure symptoms. Other investigators have introduced the concept of stem cell or gene therapy modification of the native heart during LVAD support.[78]

In summary, as smaller and more durable LVAD designs have developed, other frontiers of research are focused on improved biocompatibility and developing adjuvant treatment strategies to enable recovery of the native heart. With these ongoing efforts, implantable LVAD therapy should play an expanding role in the future treatment of end-stage heart failure.

CARDIAC ALLOGRAFT TRANSPLANTATION

Cardiac allograft transplantation is indicated in patients with symptomatic end-stage heart failure whose life expectancy is considered to be less than 1 or 2 years. Allocation of donor organs is coordinated by local organ procurement organizations (OPOs) under the oversight of the United Network for Organ Sharing (UNOS). UNOS maintains a prioritized waiting list of all patients in the country who need transplantation. Donated hearts are first allocated to the highest priority (status 1A and 1B) local (within the same OPO) recipients who are size- and ABO blood-group compatible. If no high priority local recipients accept the organ, then the organ is offered regionally to status 1A and 1B patients in a stepwise pattern before it is offered to local and regional status two patients. This allocation scheme was last modified in July of 2006 to redistribute organ allocation to more critically ill recipients (**Fig. 12**).

Patient Selection

Cardiac transplantation can be offered to patients with end-stage heart failure due to many disease etiologies, the most common of which are coronary artery disease and nonischemic (idiopathic) dilated cardiomyopathy. Other less common causes that require transplantation include congenital conditions, valvular heart disease, and retransplantation. The general distribution of these causes for heart transplantation has not changed significantly during the past 10 to 20 years.[79]

Probably the single most important component impacting survival after cardiac transplantation is recipient selection. This procedure can provide considerable improvements in mortality and quality of life in appropriate patients. To better delineate which patients will benefit the most, there are specific inclusion and exclusion criteria for transplantation. Stable patients who are being considered for cardiac transplantation should undergo cardiopulmonary exercise stress testing. Patients whose

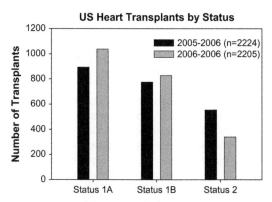

Fig. 12. Allocation changes in July 2006 resulted in an increase in transplants for status 1A and 1B patients compared with status 2 patients. (*Data from* 2007 annual report of the U.S. organ procurement and transplantation network and the scientific registry of transplant recipients: transplant data 1997–2006. H. S. B. Health Resources and Services Administration, Division of Transplantation. Rockville, Maryland, USA.)

peak VO_2 is less than or equal to 14 mL/kg/min off β-blockade or less than or equal to 12 mL/kg/min on β-blockade are felt to have increased 1-year mortality and should be considered as candidates for cardiac transplantation (**Fig. 13**).[80,81] Patients with VO_2 less than or equal to 10 mL/kg/min seem to benefit the most from cardiac transplantation.[80] For patients with borderline VO_2, the use of a heart failure survival score may help guide the selection of appropriate transplantation candidates. In addition, patients being evaluated for transplantation should undergo right-heart catheterization. Because most donor right ventricles are not accustomed to elevated resistance within the pulmonary vasculature, right-heart failure after cardiac transplantation represents a significant morbidity and mortality. Patients with pulmonary vascular resistance of more than five Wood units or transpulmonary gradient of greater than 20 mm Hg that does not respond to LV unloading (either with a vasodilator or by mechanical means) are at increased risk for mortality after transplantation.[80] This

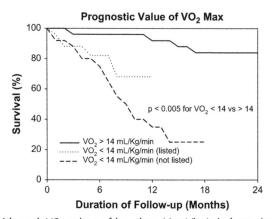

Fig. 13. Patients with peak VO_2 values of less than 14 mL/kg/min have significantly reduced mortality. These patients would likely benefit most from cardiac transplantation. (*Data from* Mancini D, Eisen H, Kussmaul W, et al. Value of peak exercise oxygen consumption for optimal timing of cardiac transplantation in ambulatory patients with heart failure. Circulation 1991;83:778–86.)

risk is augmented if, in the setting of one or more of the above risk factors, the pulmonary artery systolic pressure exceeds 60 mm Hg. Another study has suggested that if the patient's pulmonary vascular resistance can be decreased to less than 2.5 Wood units, but, in doing so, the systemic systolic blood pressure drops to less than 85 mm Hg, then the patient remains at a high risk for early post-transplant right-heart failure and death.[80]

Aside from hemodynamic considerations, the patient's comorbidity profile must be considered before listing for transplantation. Ideal candidates have isolated heart failure with preservation of other end-organ function. Other noncardiac end-organ dysfunction and systemic medical conditions often exclude patients from cardiac transplantation. Specific contraindications are listed in **Box 1**. In addition to these contraindications, special consideration should be made to the patient's immune response to a panel of reactive antibodies (PRA). Recently, predetermination of anti-HLA antibody specificity has enabled virtual crossmatches between these recipients and prospective donors.[82] Still, severely elevated PRA may practically preclude successful transplantation.

Donor Selection

Potential heart donors are declared brain dead by 2 local physicians who are not part of the transplant team. After brain-death declaration, organ-procurement agents interview the potential donor's family and care-givers to obtain data regarding cause of death, previous medical and surgical history, social history (including any high-risk behaviors), body size, blood type, and viral serologies (including HIV and hepatitis). Additional donor studies are obtained to examine cardiac structure and function; these include ECG, cardiac enzymes, echocardiography, and Swan-Ganz catheterization with hemodynamic measurements. Assessment of intravenous inotropic requirements should also be reviewed. Coronary angiography is obtained selectively in older (age >40 years) or high-risk donors, but this may not be available at all institutions. Donors who are HIV positive, have severe ventricular dysfunction, or severe coronary artery disease

---

Box 1
Relative contraindications to cardiac allograft transplantation

Age > 70 years

BMI > 30 kg/m^2

Diabetes with end-organ damage (other than retinopathy)

Poor glycemic control (HbA$_{1c}$ > 7.5)

Primary severe renal insufficiency (eGFR < 40 mL/min)

Primary severe pulmonary insufficiency

Active infection

Severely symptomatic cerebrovascular disease that cannot be revascularized

Peripheral vascular disease that will limit postoperative rehabilitation and is not amenable to revascularization

Ongoing active tobacco, alcohol, or illicit substance abuse

Mental retardation or dementia

Demonstrated inability to comply with drug therapy

Lack of sufficient social support

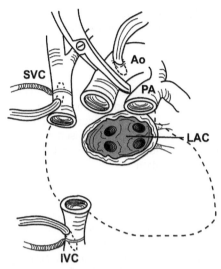

Fig. 14. After recipient cardiectomy, there should be sufficient cuffs of SVC, IVC, LA, aorta, and PA to perform the necessary anastamoses without tension. (*From* Miniati DN, Robbins RC. Heart transplantation: a thirty-year perspective. Annu Rev Med 2002;53(1):189; with permission.)

should not be used for transplantation. Donors with positive hepatitis serologies, history of cancer, mildly to moderately depressed cardiac function, and noncritical coronary disease may not be ideal for use in standard list transplant patients, but may be used for critically ill recipients or those in alternate list programs (see below). In addition to

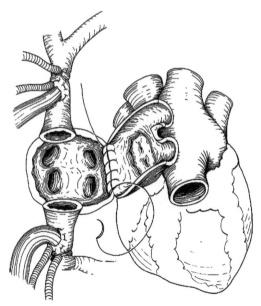

Fig. 15. The left atrial anastamosis is performed with a single running suture that secures the donor left atrial cuff to the recipient. (*From* Gamel AE, Yonan NA, Rahman AN, et al. Alternative heart transplantation technique. Ann Thorac Surg 1995;59(1):258–60; with permission.)

consideration of the donor features, the transplant surgeon must match donor-recipient factors such as size, ABO compatibility, and HLA-antibody compatibility as well as logistic factors including ischemic time.[83]

Organ Preservation

Most donor hearts are currently preserved with specialized cold colloid solutions and placed in cold storage at 2°C These colloid solutions are designed to prevent myocardial edema; examples include University of Wisconsin and Celsior solutions. This cold-storage technique yields good results for total ischemic times less than 4 hours. Recently, studies using warm perfused storage have been undertaken with hopes of improving and extending preservation.

Procedure

Orthotopic cardiac transplantation is performed through a median sternotomy using total CPB, achieved with bicaval snaring and cross-clamping of the aorta. The recipient cardiectomy is performed leaving sufficient lengths of aorta, pulmonary artery, and right and left atrial cuffs (**Fig. 14**). Next, the donor heart is removed from its storage solution, inspected, and prepared for implant. The donor left atrial cuff is anastamosed to the recipient's left atrial cuff using a running 3-0 polypropylene suture (**Fig. 15**). The right atrium is then anastamosed using either an atrial level (**Fig. 16**) or a bicaval (**Fig. 17**) technique. In recent years, there has been increasing use of bicaval anastamoses.[84] In the bicaval technique, the inferior and superior vena cavae of the recipient and donors are individually anastamosed. Proponents of the bicaval attachment have argued that, relative to an atrial level anastamosis, this technique preserves sinoatrial (SA) node function, results in less tricuspid insufficiency, and better RV function.

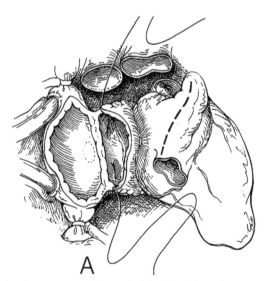

Fig. 16. If an atrial-level anastamosis is intended for the right atrium, an appropriate cuff of RA should be left during recipient cardiectomy. The donor right atrium is prepared with ligation of the SVC and opening of the right atrium along an imaginary line connecting the IVC to the tip of the right atrial appendage. (*From* Schnoor M, Schäfer T, Lühmann D, et al. Bicaval versus standard technique in orthotopic heart transplantation: a systematic review and meta-analysis. J Thorac Cardiovasc Surg 2007;134(5):1322–31; with permission.)

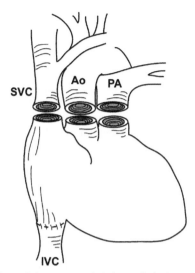

Fig. 17. If a caval-level right atrial anastamosis is intended, the recipient cardiectomy is performed, leaving cuffs of atrium at the tips of the SVC and IVC. The donor IVC and SVC are then reanastamosed to these cuffs. (*From* Miniati DN, Robbins RC. Heart transplantation: a thirty-year perspective. Annu Rev Med 2002;53(1):189; with permission.)

Finally, end to end pulmonary artery and aortic anastamoses are created, completing the transplant procedure.

Postoperative Management

After heart transplant, patients need to be monitored closely for right-heart dysfunction. In fact, nearly 20% of early postoperative deaths after cardiac transplantation occur due to RV failure.[85] Typically, right-heart dysfunction is managed by providing adequate heart rate and atrioventricular synchrony. Inotropic support with low-dose epinephrine, dobutamine and milrinone is common.[86] Agents that increase pulmonary vascular constriction should be avoided.[85] For severe right heart failure (decreasing cardiac output in the setting of increasing central venous pressure and decreasing pulmonary artery pressures), inhaled nitric oxide, temporary right VADs, or even extracorporeal membrane oxygenation are used.[42,43,87–90]

Immune Suppression

The role of induction therapy for cardiac transplantation is controversial. Although some have argued that induction therapy decreases the incidence of rejection, there are data that show that this decrease in rejection does not improve overall survival.[91–93] Moreover, advocates of induction therapy tout its safety, but those opposed refer to studies that describe increased risk of infection and malignancy.[94–96] Many programs use induction therapy as a "renal sparing" strategy that allows for delaying the administration of calcineurin inhibitors postoperatively.[97] Zenapax, thymoglobulin, and simulect, which are monoclonal anti-interleukin-2 receptor antibodies, have been used more frequently for induction therapy in recent years, whereas OKT3 and antithymocyte globulin, which were previously used as induction therapy in the 1990s, have lost considerable popularity.[56]

Regardless of the use of induction therapy, most cardiac transplant patients receive methylprednisilone 1000 mg IV before reperfusion of the heart along with a dose of an antimetabolite. A randomized, double-blind trial comparing azathioprine (AZA) to mycophenolate mofetil (MMF) demonstrated increased survival and decreased graft loss for patients treated with MMF.[98] Therefore, the antimetabolite agent of choice has transitioned from AZA to MMF.[56] A corticosteroid taper is then instituted during the following week and calcineurin inhibitors are started either immediately postoperatively or after a 24- to 48-hour delay (depending on the use of induction therapy). Again, in recent years, the favored calcineurin inhibitor has transitioned from cyclosporine to tacrolimus.[56] Although, historically, most patients were maintained on corticosteroids for many years after the transplant, in recent years there has been increasing use of corticosteroid withdrawal protocols at 1 and 2 years postoperatively.[56] Studies suggest that earlier weaning of steroids in select patients has not resulted in greater rejection. Limiting corticosteroids should reduce a variety of complications, most importantly infections.[56]

Management of immunosuppression is a balance between over-immunosuppression, which can result in infection, malignancy, bone marrow suppression, or other toxicities versus under-immunosuppression, which can lead to rejection. Ideally, patients are kept within the appropriate range, in which they avoid rejection and the complications of over-immunosuppression. This balance has traditionally been achieved by following blood levels of the calcineurin inhibitors and performing endomyocardial biopsy (**Fig. 18**). Endomyocardial biopsies are performed at routine intervals and with any change in clinical status, providing direct information on immune-cell infiltration in the allograft. Based on these results, patients' immunosuppression can be appropriately modified.

Unfortunately, endomyocardial biopsy is time-consuming and expensive. Moreover, it can be limited by sampling error and interobserver variability. Finally, because it is an invasive procedure, there is an associated major morbidity of approximately 1%.[99] For these reasons, a noninvasive method for detection of rejection has been an active area of investigation. Recently, the Cardiac Allograft Gene Expression Observational (CARGO) Study developed a microarray gene expression map (the AlloMap) to distinguish between ISHLT grade 0 and grade 3A acute cellular rejection based on mononuclear cell mRNAs in peripheral blood. This methodology examines the gene-expression profiles of peripheral blood mononuclear cells (PBMCs) and generates a score (between 0 and 40) based on the relative expression of a set of 20 genes. Some of these genes gauge the immune response process, whereas others serve to normalize the score. The score has been shown to have a positive predictive value of 6.8% and a negative predictive value of 99.6% for grade 3A rejection (**Fig. 19**).[99] Many centers use AlloMap testing after the first postoperative year. A low score effectively rules out grade 3A rejection, eliminating the need for invasive biopsy. On the other hand, a high AlloMap score requires a biopsy. After the first postoperative year, the incidence of rejection is low and the AlloMap score helps significantly reduce unnecessary biopsies.

Complications

During the immediate postoperative period and during the first post-transplant year, primary graft failure is an important cause of morbidity and mortality. In this time period, the incidence of profound graft dysfunction necessitating mechanical support is between 5% and 10%.[100] Moreover, during the first post-transplant year, infection and rejection are also important causes of death.[56] After the fifth year, cardiac graft vasculopathy represents the most common cause of death, accounting for

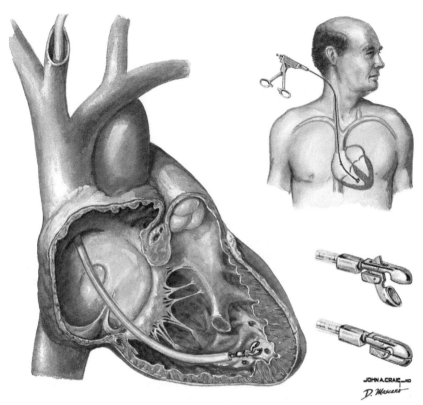

Fig. 18. Surveillance RV endomyocardial biopsy is performed by passing a biotome through the right internal jugular vein using a modified Seldinger method into the apex of the right ventricle. A biopsy is then obtained using fluoroscopic guidance and the specimen is then removed for pathologic analysis. (*Reprinted with permission from* Netter Anatomy Illustration Collection, © Elsevier Inc. All rights reserved.)

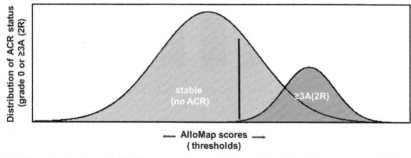

Fig. 19. The distribution of AlloMap scores is predictive of the risk of 3A rejection. If AlloMap score exceeds the cutoff value, confirmatory endomyocardial biopsy is required. (*From* Fang KC. Clinical utilities of peripheral blood gene expression profiling in the management of cardiac transplant patients. J Immunotoxicol 2007;4(3):209–17; with permission.)

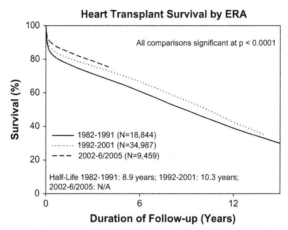

Fig. 20. US heart transplant survival divided by era of transplant procedure. Patients transplanted in since 2002 have improved survival compared with those transplanted in the prior 2 decades. (*Data from* Taylor DO, Edwards LB, Boucek MM, et al. Registry of the International Society for Heart and Lung Transplantation: twenty-fourth official adult heart transplant report–2007. J Heart Lung Transplant 2007;26:769–81.)

approximately 30% of late deaths. Similarly, after the fifth year, malignancy accounts for approximately 20% of deaths.[79]

Outcomes

Despite the limitations of rejection and infection, cardiac transplantation remains the single most effective therapy for end-stage heart failure. Although mortality is greatest within the first postoperative year (approximately 10%), annual mortality falls to less

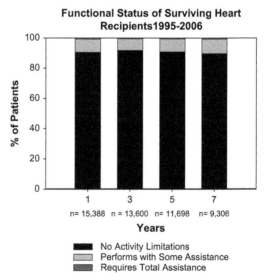

Fig. 21. After cardiac transplantation, many patients regain full function and have no limitations. This result is maintained over time. (*Data from* Taylor DO, Edwards LB, Boucek MM, et al. Registry of the International Society for Heart and Lung Transplantation: twenty-fourth official adult heart transplant report–2007. J Heart Lung Transplant 2007;26:769–81.)

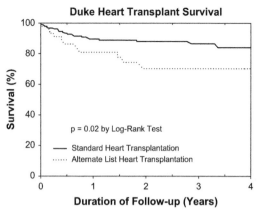

Fig. 22. Survival after alternate list heart transplantation is acceptable compared with historical optimal medical management data, but survival after standard list heart transplantation is significantly better.

than 5% for subsequent years. Furthermore, improvements in immunosuppressive management have resulted in steadily improving outcomes during the past 2 decades (**Fig. 20**).[79] The benefits of cardiac allograft transplantation are not isolated to a mortality advantage. Those patients who survive cardiac transplantation also have significant functional benefit. Most of these patients, who preoperatively had NYHA class III and IV heart failure, will function without limitation postoperatively (**Fig. 21**). A small fraction of patients are actually able to return to employment.

MARGINAL DONOR ORGAN, ALTERNATE LIST TRANSPLANTATION

Occasionally, otherwise well-suited patients may not be eligible for cardiac transplantation based on one or more of the traditional contraindications (see **Box 1**). These patients, who otherwise would fare well with transplantation, may be offered enrollment in an alternate list transplantation program. Most commonly, these patients are ineligible due to advanced age, but those who are ineligible due to other relative contraindications can also be considered for such programs.[101] Alternate list patients are listed with UNOS, but are offered nonideal organs that have been turned down by standard list recipients.[100,101] Once an organ has been turned down for all other standard list recipients, it can be considered for alternate list recipients. Usually, alternate list patients receive organs with mild coronary artery disease, positive hepatitis serology, or some degree of LV dysfunction. Because of the secondary risks associated with these marginal donors, it is imperative that these patients be counseled and specifically consented to the alternate list program. Survival after alternate list cardiac transplantation is inferior to standard transplantation, but it is far superior to medical management.[4,101] These programs enable greater use of donor organs and offer cardiac transplant to recipients who would otherwise be deemed ineligible (**Fig. 22**).

REFERENCES

1. Rosamond W, Flegal K, Furie K, et al. Heart disease and stroke statistics–2008 update: a report from the American Heart Association Statistics Committee and Stroke Statistics Subcommittee. Circulation 2008;117:e25–146.
2. Lloyd-Jones DM, Larson MG, Leip EP, et al. Lifetime risk for developing congestive heart failure: the Framingham Heart Study. Circulation 2002;106:3068–72.

3. O'Connor C, Gattis W, Zannad F, et al. Beta-blocker therapy in advanced heart failure: clinical characteristics and long-term outcomes. Eur J Heart Fail 1999;1:81–8.

4. Rose EA, Gelijns AC, Moskowitz AJ, et al. Long-term use of a left ventricular assist device for end-stage heart failure. N Engl J Med 2001;345:1435–43.

5. Califf RM, Adams KF, McKenna WJ, et al. A randomized controlled trial of epoprostenol therapy for severe congestive heart failure: the Flolan International Randomized Survival Trial (FIRST). Am Heart J 1997;134:44–54.

6. Effect of enalapril on survival in patients with reduced left ventricular ejection fractions and congestive heart failure. The SOLVD Investigators. N Engl J Med 1991;325:293–302.

7. Packer M, Coats AJS, Fowler MB, et al. Effect of carvedilol on survival in severe chronic heart failure. N Engl J Med 2001;344:1651–8.

8. Barnard C. The operation. A human cardiac transplant: an interim report of a successful operation performed at Groote Schuur hospital, Cape Town. S Afr Med J 1967;41:1271–4.

9. Dong E, Lower RR, Hurley EJ, et al. Transplantation of the heart. Dis Chest 1965; 48:455–7.

10. Shumway NE, Lower RR, Angell WW. Present status of cardiac transplantation. Angiology 1966;17:289–91.

11. Cooley DA, Bloodwell RD, Hallman GL, et al. Transplantation of the human heart. Report of four cases. JAMA 1968;205:479–86.

12. Cooley DA. The first implantation of an artificial heart: reflections and observations. Transplant Proc 1973;5:1135–7.

13. DeBakey ME. Left ventricular bypass pump for cardiac assistance. Clinical experience. Am J Cardiol 1971;27:3–11.

14. DeBakey ME, Kennedy JH. Mechanical circulatory support: current status. Am J Cardiol 1971;27:1–2.

15. Batista RJ, Santos JL, Takeshita N, et al. Partial left ventriculectomy to improve left ventricular function in end-stage heart disease. J Card Surg 1996;11:96–7 [discussion 98].

16. McCarthy M. Batista procedure proves its value in the USA. Lancet 1997;349: 855.

17. McCarthy JF, McCarthy PM, Starling RC, et al. Partial left ventriculectomy and mitral valve repair for end-stage congestive heart failure. Eur J Cardiothorac Surg 1998;13:337–43.

18. McCarthy PM, Starling RC, Young JB, et al. Left ventricular reduction surgery with mitral valve repair. J Heart Lung Transplant 2000;19:564–7.

19. Starling RC, McCarthy PM, Buda T, et al. Results of partial left ventriculectomy for dilated cardiomyopathy - hemodynamic, clinical and echocardiographic observations. J Am Coll Cardiol 2000;36:2098–103.

20. Franco-Cereceda A, McCarthy PM, Blackstone EH, et al. Partial left ventriculectomy for dilated cardiomyopathy: is this an alternative to transplantation? J Thorac Cardiovasc Surg 2001;121:879–93.

21. Batista RJV, Verde J, Nery P, et al. Partial left ventriculectomy to treat end-stage heart disease. Ann Thorac Surg 1997;64:634–8.

22. Dor V, Saab M, Coste P, et al. Left ventricular aneurysm: a new surgical approach. Thorac Cardiovasc Surg 1989;37:11–9.

23. Dor V. Left ventricular restoration by endoventricular circular patch plasty (EVCPP). Z Kardiol 2000;89:70–5.

24. Dor V, Montiglio F, Sabatier M, et al. Left ventricular shape changes induced by aneurysmectomy with endoventricular circular patch plasty reconstruction. Eur Heart J 1994;15:1063–9.

25. Athanasuleas CL, Buckberg GD, Stanley AWH, et al. Surgical ventricular restoration: the RESTORE Group experience. Heart Fail Rev 2005;9:287–97.

26. Velazquez EJ, Lee KL, O'Connor CM, et al. The rationale and design of the Surgical Treatment for Ischemic Heart Failure (STICH) trial. J Thorac Cardiovasc Surg 2007;134:1540–7.

27. Jones RH, Velazquez EJ, Michler RE, et al. Coronary bypass surgery with or without surgical ventricular reconstruction. N Engl J Med 2009;360:1705–17.

28. Harrison J, Califf R, Woodlief L, et al. Systolic left ventricular function after reperfusion therapy for acute myocardial infarction. Analysis of determinants of improvement. The TAMI Study Group. Circulation 1993;87:1531–41.

29. Dor V. Surgical remodeling of left ventricle. Surg Clin North Am 2004;84:27–43.

30. Gaudron P, Eilles C, Kugler I, et al. Progressive left ventricular dysfunction and remodeling after myocardial infarction. Potential mechanisms and early predictors. Circulation 1993;87:755–63.

31. Diwan A, Krenz M, Syed FM, et al. Inhibition of ischemic cardiomyocyte apoptosis through targeted ablation of Bnip3 restrains postinfarction remodeling in mice. J Clin Invest 2007;117:2825–33.

32. Hayakawa Y, Chandra M, Miao W, et al. Inhibition of cardiac myocyte apoptosis improves cardiac function and abolishes mortality in the peripartum cardiomyopathy of G{alpha}q transgenic mice. Circulation 2003;108:3036–41.

33. Dor V, Civaia F, Alexandrescu C, et al. The post-myocardial infarction scarred ventricle and congestive heart failure: the preeminence of magnetic resonance imaging for preoperative, intraoperative, and postoperative assessment. J Thorac Cardiovasc Surg 2008;136:1405–12.

34. Ailawadi G, Kron IL. New strategies for surgical management of ischemic cardiomyopathy. Expert Rev Cardiovasc Ther 2008;6:521–30.

35. Patel ND, Williams JA, Nwakanma LU, et al. Surgical ventricular restoration for advanced congestive heart failure: should pulmonary hypertension be a contraindication? Ann Thorac Surg 2006;82:879–88.

36. Williams J, Patel N, Nwakanma L, et al. Outcomes following surgical ventricular restoration in elderly patients with congestive heart failure. Am J Geriatr Cardiol 2007;16:67–75.

37. Menicanti L, Donato MD, Castelvecchio S, et al. Functional ischemic mitral regurgitation in anterior ventricular remodeling: results of surgical ventricular restoration with and without mitral repair. Heart Fail Rev 2005;9:317–27.

38. Lee S, Chang B-C, Youn Y-N, et al. Changes in left ventricular function and dimension after surgical ventricular restoration with or without concomitant mitral valve procedure. Circ J 2007;71:1516–20.

39. Di Donato M, Castelvecchio S, Brankovic J, et al. Effectiveness of surgical ventricular restoration in patients with dilated ischemic cardiomyopathy and unrepaired mild mitral regurgitation. J Thorac Cardiovasc Surg 2007;134:1548–53.

40. Milano CA, Daneshmand MA, Rankin JS, et al. Survival prognosis and surgical management of ischemic mitral regurgitation. Ann Thorac Surg 2008;86:735–44.

41. Maxey TS, Reece TB, Ellman PI, et al. The beating heart approach is not necessary for the Dor procedure. Ann Thorac Surg 2003;76:1571–5.

42. Icenogle TB, Williams RJ, Smith RG, et al. Extracorporeal pulsatile biventricular support after cardiac transplantation. Ann Thorac Surg 1989;47:614–6.

43. Esmore D, Spratt P, Branch J, et al. Right ventricular assist and prostacyclin infusion for allograft failure in the presence of high pulmonary vascular resistance. J Heart Transplant 1990;9:136–41.
44. Grinda J-M, Chevalier P, D'Attellis N, et al. Fulminant myocarditis in adults and children: bi-ventricular assist device for recovery. Eur J Cardiothorac Surg 2004;26:1169–73.
45. Farrar DJ, Holman WR, McBride LR, et al. Long-term follow-up of Thoratec ventricular assist device bridge-to-recovery patients successfully removed from support after recovery of ventricular function. J Heart Lung Transplant 2002;21:516–21.
46. Acker MA. Mechanical circulatory support for patients with acute-fulminant myocarditis. Ann Thorac Surg 2001;71:S73–6.
47. Hill J, Farrar D, Hershon J, et al. Use of a prosthetic ventricle as a bridge to cardiac transplantation for postinfarction cardiogenic shock. N Engl J Med 1986;314:626–8.
48. Starnes V, Oyer P, Portner P, et al. Isolated left ventricular assist as bridge to cardiac transplantation. J Thorac Cardiovasc Surg 1988;96:62–71.
49. Aaronson KD, Eppinger MJ, Dyke DB, et al. Left ventricular assist device therapy improves utilization of donor hearts. J Am Coll Cardiol 2002;39:1247–54.
50. Omoto R, Kyo S, Nishimura M, et al. Japanese multicenter clinical evaluation of the HeartMate vented electric left ventricular assist system. J Artif Organs 2005;8: 34–40.
51. Holmes E. Outpatient management of long-term assist devices. Cardiol Clin 2003;21:93–9.
52. Kherani AR, Oz MC. Ventricular assistance to bridge to transplantation. Surg Clin North Am 2004;84:75–89.
53. Monkowski DH, Axelrod P, Fekete T, et al. Infections associated with ventricular assist devices: epidemiology and effect on prognosis after transplantation. Transpl Infect Dis 2007;9:114–20.
54. Oz M, Argenziano M, Catanese KA, et al. Bridge experience with long-term implantable left ventricular assist devices: are they an alternative to transplantation? Circulation 1997;95:1844–52.
55. Felker GM, Rogers JG. Same bridge, new destinations: rethinking paradigms for mechanical cardiac support in heart failure. J Am Coll Cardiol 2006;47:930–2.
56. 2007 Annual Report of the U.S. organ procurement and transplantation network and the scientific registry of transplant recipients: transplant data 1997–2006 , in Health Resources and Services Administration HSB, Division of Transplantation (ed). Rockville (MD), 2007.
57. Investigators TE, ESCAPE Study Coordinators. Evaluation study of congestive heart failure and pulmonary artery catheterization effectiveness: The ESCAPE Trial. JAMA 2005;294:1625–33.
58. Klein M, Gold M. Use of traditional and biventricular implantable cardiac devices for primary and secondary prevention of sudden death. Cardiol Clin 2008;26: 419–31.
59. Albright C, Quinn T, Berberian G, et al. Measurement of QRS duration for biventricular pacing optimization. ASAIO J 2008;54:335–40.
60. Reuter S, Garrigue S, Bordachar P, et al. Intermediate-term results of biventricular pacing in heart failure: correlation between clinical and hemodynamic data. Pacing Clin Electrophysiol 2000;23:1713–7.
61. Daneshmand MA, Blue L, Farrar DJ, et al. BMI does not affect outcomes in destination therapy LVAD. ASAIO J 2008;54:42.

62. Lietz K, Long JW, Kfoury AG, et al. Outcomes of left ventricular assist device implantation as destination therapy in the post-REMATCH era: implications for patient selection. Circulation 2007;116:497–505.
63. Mancini DM, Beniaminovitz A, Levin H, et al. Low incidence of myocardial recovery after left ventricular assist device implantation in patients with chronic heart failure. Circulation 1998;98:2383–9.
64. Lietz K, Miller LW. Destination therapy: current results and future promise. Semin Thorac Cardiovasc Surg 2008;20:225–33.
65. HeartMate best practice guidelines. Pleasanton (CA): Thoratec Corporation; 2008.
66. Pal JD, Klodell CT, John R, et al. Abstract 5857: low operative mortality with implantation of a continuous flow LVAD and impact of concurrent cardiac procedures. Circulation 2008;118:S1017.
67. Fukamachi K, McCarthy PM, Smedira NG, et al. Preoperative risk factors for right ventricular failure after implantable left ventricular assist device insertion. Ann Thorac Surg 1999;68:2181–4.
68. Argenziano M, Choudhri AF, Moazami N, et al. Randomized, double-blind trial of inhaled nitric oxide in LVAD recipients with pulmonary hypertension. Ann Thorac Surg 1998;65:340–5.
69. Yin N, Kaestle S, Yin J, et al. Inhaled nitric oxide versus aerosolized iloprost for the treatment of pulmonary hypertension with left heart disease. Crit Care Med 2009;37:980–6.
70. Geisen U, Heilmann C, Beyersdorf F, et al. Non-surgical bleeding in patients with ventricular assist devices could be explained by acquired von Willebrand disease. Eur J Cardiothorac Surg 2008;33:679–84.
71. Ogletree-Hughes ML, Stull LB, Sweet WE, et al. Mechanical unloading restores {beta}-adrenergic responsiveness and reverses receptor downregulation in the failing human heart. Circulation 2001;104:881–6.
72. Long JW, Healy AH, Rasmusson BY, et al. Improving outcomes with long-term "destination" therapy using left ventricular assist devices. J Thorac Cardiovasc Surg 2008;135:1353–61.
73. Martin J, Friesewinkel O, Benk C, et al. Improved durability of the HeartMate XVE left ventricular assist device provides safe mechanical support up to 1 year but is associated with high risk of device failure in the second year. J Heart Lung Transplant 2006;25:384–90.
74. John R, Kamdar F, Liao K, et al. Improved survival and decreasing incidence of adverse events with the HeartMate II left ventricular assist device as bridge-to-transplant therapy. Ann Thorac Surg 2008;86:1227–35.
75. Frazier O, Gemmato C, Myers T, et al. Initial clinical experience with the Heart-Mate II axial-flow left ventricular assist device. Tex Heart Inst J 2007;34:275–81.
76. John R, Kamdar F, Liao K, et al. Low thromboembolic risk for patients with the HeartMate II left ventricular assist device. J Thorac Cardiovasc Surg 2008;136:1318–23.
77. Birks EJ, Tansley PD, Hardy J, et al. Left ventricular assist device and drug therapy for the reversal of heart failure. N Engl J Med 2006;355:1873–84.
78. Yaoita H, Maruyama Y. Intervention for apoptosis in cardiomyopathy. Heart Fail Rev 2008;13:181–91.
79. Taylor DO, Edwards LB, Boucek MM, et al. Registry of the International Society for Heart and Lung Transplantation: twenty-fourth official adult heart transplant report–2007. J Heart Lung Transplant 2007;26:769–81.
80. Mehra MR, Kobashigawa J, Starling R, et al. Listing criteria for heart transplantation: International Society for Heart and Lung Transplantation Guidelines for

the care of cardiac transplant candidates – 2006. J Heart Lung Transplant 2006; 25:1024–42.

81. Mancini D, Eisen H, Kussmaul W, et al. Value of peak exercise oxygen consumption for optimal timing of cardiac transplantation in ambulatory patients with heart failure. Circulation 1991;83:778–86.

82. Yang J, Schall C, Smith D, et al. HLA sensitization in pediatric pre-transplant cardiac patients supported by mechanical assist devices: the utility of luminex. J Heart Lung Transplant 2009;28:123–9.

83. Baldwin J, Anderson J, Boucek M, et al. 24th Bethesda conference: cardiac transplantation. Task Force 2: donor guidelines. J Am Coll Cardiol 1993;22: 15–20.

84. Weiss ES, Nwakanma LU, Russell SB, et al. Outcomes in bicaval versus biatrial techniques in heart transplantation: an analysis of the UNOS database. J Heart Lung Transplant 2008;27:178–83.

85. Stobierska-Dzierzek B, Awad H, Michler RE. The evolving management of acute right-sided heart failure in cardiac transplant recipients. J Am Coll Cardiol 2001; 38:923–31.

86. Miniati DN, Robbins RC. Heart transplantation: a thirty-year perspective. Annu Rev Med 2002;53:189.

87. Carrier M, Blaise G, Bélisle S, et al. Nitric oxide inhalation in the treatment of primary graft failure following heart transplantation. J Heart Lung Transplant 1999;18:664–7.

88. George S, Boscoe M. Inhaled nitric oxide for right ventricular dysfunction following cardiac transplantation. Br J Clin Pract 1997;51:53–5.

89. Whyte RI, Deeb GM, McCurry KR, et al. Extracorporeal life support after heart or lung transplantation. Ann Thorac Surg 1994;58:754–8.

90. Barzaghi N, Olivei M, Minzioni G, et al. ECMO and inhaled nitric oxide for cardiopulmonary failure after heart retransplantation. Ann Thorac Surg 1997;63:533–5.

91. Zhang R, Haverich A, Strüber M, et al. Delayed onset of cardiac allograft vasculopathy by induction therapy using anti-thymocyte globulin. J Heart Lung Transplant 2008;27:603–9.

92. Goland S, Czer LSC, Coleman B, et al. Induction therapy with thymoglobulin after heart transplantation: impact of therapy duration on lymphocyte depletion and recovery, rejection, and cytomegalovirus infection rates. J Heart Lung Transplant 2008;27:1115–21.

93. Chou NK, Wang SS, Chen YS, et al. Induction immunosuppression with basiliximab in heart transplantation. Transplant Proc 2008;40:2623–5.

94. Baran DA. Induction therapy in cardiac transplantation: when and why? Heart Fail Clin 2007;3:31–41.

95. Mattei MF, Redonnet M, Gandjbakhch I, et al. Lower risk of infectious deaths in cardiac transplant patients receiving basiliximab versus anti-thymocyte globulin as induction therapy. J Heart Lung Transplant 2007;26:693–9.

96. Crespo-Leiro MG, Alonso-Pulpón L, Arizón JM, et al. Influence of induction therapy, immunosuppressive regimen and anti-viral prophylaxis on development of lymphomas after heart transplantation: data from the Spanish post-heart transplant tumour registry. J Heart Lung Transplant 2007;26:1105–9.

97. McLean MK, Barr ML. Current state of heart transplantation. Transplantation Updates 2008;2:3–10.

98. Eisen HJ, Kobashigawa J, Keogh A, et al. Three-year results of a randomized, double-blind, controlled trial of mycophenolate mofetil versus azathioprine in cardiac transplant recipients. J Heart Lung Transplant 2005;24:517–25.

99. Deng MC, Eisen HJ, Mehra MR, et al. Noninvasive discrimination of rejection in cardiac allograft recipients using gene expression profiling. Am J Transplant 2006;6:150–60.
100. Lima B, Rajagopal K, Petersen RP, et al. Marginal cardiac allografts do not have increased primary graft dysfunction in alternate list transplantation. Circulation 2006;114:I27–32.
101. Felker GM, Milano CA, Yager JEE, et al. Outcomes with an alternate list strategy for heart transplantation. J Heart Lung Transplant 2005;24:1781–6.

The Surgical Treatment of Atrial Fibrillation

Anson M. Lee, MD, Spencer J. Melby, MD, Ralph J. Damiano Jr, MD*

KEYWORDS

- Atrial fibrillation • Maze procedure • Cardiac ablation
- Arrhythmia surgery • Pulmonary vein isolation

Atrial fibrillation (AF) affects 2.2 million Americans, making it the most common form of sustained cardiac arrhythmia.[1,2] Admissions for inpatient care associated with AF have risen dramatically over the last several years, and are expected to increase further. AF annual hospitalizations in the United States are predicted to rise from 376,000 in 1999 to more than 3.3 million by 2025.[3] Furthermore, an estimated 5% of all patients undergoing cardiac surgery have AF, making it an important surgical problem.

AF is associated with significant morbidity and mortality because of its three detrimental sequelae: (1) palpitations, causing patient discomfort and anxiety; (2) loss of synchronous atrioventricular (AV) contraction, compromising cardiac hemodynamics and resulting in ventricular dysfunction; and (3) stasis of blood flow in the left atrium, leading to increased risk for thromboembolism and stroke.[4–8] AF confers a three- to fivefold increased risk for stroke, and is responsible for an estimated 15% to 20% of all strokes.[1] AF independently increases mortality rates. Using data from the Framingham Heart Study, Benjamin and colleagues[9] established the risk factor-adjusted odds ratio for death in men and women with AF as 1.5 and 1.9, respectively. In a separate population-based study, investigators observed a threefold increased risk of death over a relatively short mean follow-up of 3.6 years.[10]

CLASSIFICATION OF AF

The nomenclature used to classify AF in the medical literature is variable and inconsistent across investigators, but the classification system published jointly by the American Heart Association, the American College of Cardiology, and the Heart Rhythm Society is the most widely used.[11] This system defines AF as either

---

This work was supported in part by National Institutes of Health grants 5R01HL32257, R01HL085113, and T32HL0776.

Financial Disclosures: Dr. Damiano receives consultant fees from AtriCure and Medtronic.

Division of Cardiothoracic Surgery, Washington University School of Medicine, Barnes-Jewish Hospital, 660 South Euclid, Campus Box 8234, St. Louis, MO 63110, USA

* Corresponding author.

E-mail address: damianor@wustl.edu (R.J. Damiano).

Surg Clin N Am 89 (2009) 1001–1020

doi:10.1016/j.suc.2009.06.001

surgical.theclinics.com

paroxysmal or persistent. When a patient has had two or more episodes, AF is considered recurrent. If recurrent AF terminates spontaneously, it is designated as paroxysmal; but if it is sustained beyond 7 days, it is termed persistent. Pharmacologic or electrical cardioversion before expected spontaneous termination does not change the persistent designation. The Heart Rhythm Society recently released a consensus statement to aid in the uniform reporting of trials for the clinical management of AF. The term "permanent" was eliminated and replaced with the term "long-standing AF" when the duration is greater than 1 year.[12]

ELECTROPHYSIOLOGY OF AF

AF is characterized by irregular activation of the atria. Electrical activity in the atria during AF can exhibit two different patterns. One pattern consists of a stable source, either a focal trigger or a small reentrant circuit, with fibrillatory conduction away from the source. The other pattern is characterized by multiple changing sources or reentrant circuits. These patterns are not mutually exclusive in any particular patient. Data obtained from almost half of the patients who had undergone intraoperative mapping before arrhythmia surgery revealed that the source of AF was not stable and was capable of moving from one atrium to the other.[13] As such, any surgical treatment to restore sinus rhythm is not complete without consideration of the substrate for AF in any particular patient.

Four factors contribute to the electrophysiological substrate that determines whether AF is initiated and/or sustained. These are:

1. A trigger – usually a premature depolarization or runs of focal ectopic depolarizations
2. Atrial refractory period – both its magnitude and spatial distribution
3. Conduction velocity – its magnitude and anisotropic spread
4. Atrial geometry and anatomy – both macroscopic and microscopic.

These four factors interact to create a substrate capable of sustaining AF. A nonreentrant trigger can spread away from a point with differing conduction velocities in differing directions, interacting with an inhomogeneous distribution of refractory periods. Unidirectional block occurs in this setting of anisotropy, leading to the traditional reentrant circuits associated with AF. Any pathology of the heart can affect the atrial myocardium and change its physiology through one or more of these four factors.[14] For any given atria, there exists a critical mass as determined by the tissue geometry, the magnitude of refractory periods, and the conduction velocity. This is the amount of tissue required to support a reentrant circuit, and is defined by the equation WL = CV × RP (wavelength = conduction velocity × refractory period). If either CV or RP decreases, the amount of tissue needed to sustain AF decreases and the probability of a patient having AF increases.[15] The surgical treatment of AF is directed at altering the geometry and anatomy of the atrium to render the electrophysiological substrate unable to support AF.

There has been a great deal of emphasis placed on the role of the pulmonary veins (PVs) in triggering AF. Haissaguerre found in a clinical study that paroxysmal AF often originates in the PVs.[16] Intraoperative mapping studies have shown rapid firing originating from the region of the PVs.[14] Although variable between patients, electrically excitable cardiac muscle extends 1 to 4 cm beyond the ostium of the PVs.[17] Pacemaker tissue may even be present in the PVs during development.[18] Because of their unique physiology, successful cure of AF is achieved in some patients by the isolation of the PVs.[16] Furthermore, if triggers of AF were outside the PVs, and other substrates that sustain AF were within the veins, AF would be prevented with PV isolation. Thus, pulmonary vein isolation (PVI) is the mainstay of interventional electrophysiology catheter-based techniques.

Despite these successes, it is important to note that PVI fails to cure AF in many patients, especially those with long-standing AF. More recent studies have shown that up to a third of patients with paroxysmal AF have triggers other than the PVs. This occurs more frequently in women and in patients with large atria.[19] In patients with persistent AF, the mechanism of AF is usually more complex and often not dependent on focal triggers to sustain the rhythm.[20]

Caution should be taken in interpreting interventional studies, whether catheter ablation or surgery, as to whether they imply an underlying mechanism for AF. Most intraoperative and catheter mapping systems do not have the spatial resolution to separate reentrant from non-reentrant mechanisms. Therefore even though focal trigger-based fibrillation may be reported from investigational mapping, the underlying mechanism of AF may be more complex. Claims of cure by PVI alone must be tempered by the knowledge that the PVI intervention often incorporates more than just the PVs. Commonly the PVs, adjacent atrial muscle, and the muscle in the oblique sinus between the veins are ablated during a catheter-based PVI, accounting for over one-third of the left atrium. This large area of ablation substantially reduces the critical mass available to sustain AF and may incorporate other non-PV substrates of AF.

The classifications of paroxysmal, persistent, and long-standing AF do not imply a specific mechanism. Even though clinical results have shown that in paroxysmal AF, PVI is effective 70% to 80% of the time, it is clear that 20% to 30% of the time the PVs are not the only substrate driving AF.[13] Furthermore, human mapping data from the authors' laboratory did not show any significant difference in mechanism between paroxysmal and persistent AF.[13]

Because AF is a complex arrhythmia, cardiac mapping requires a high density of closely placed electrodes and a sophisticated mapping and signal processing system. Intraoperative mapping has not been useful in providing real-time information during surgery. The traditional surgical algorithm of obtaining preoperative or intraoperative mapping data and using that information to guide surgical technique, as was done with arrhythmias like Wolf-Parkinson-White syndrome, has not been feasible for AF.

Map-guided techniques to treat AF are an area of continued research. Mapping techniques are being developed that may allow interventionalists to customize the incision set to the specific underlying mechanism.[21–23] One particularly promising technique is ECG imaging.[24] This noninvasive technique involves recording signals from the body surface of awake patients and mathematically fitting these potentials onto the surface of the heart with anatomic data obtained from computed tomography. If performed preoperatively, this would allow for the delineation of the mechanism of AF before the proposed intervention, allowing physicians to triage patients to the most effective procedure.

MEDICAL TREATMENT

Medical therapy for AF in restoring sinus rhythm has had poor results. Antiarrhythmic drugs generally have low therapeutic indices and limited long-term efficacy.[25,26] As a consequence, medical therapy is often aimed at *rate* control rather than *rhythm* control. Drugs are given to reduce the ventricular response rate, which reduces palpitations and avoids tachycardia-induced cardiomyopathy. The justification for this strategy arises from the Atrial Fibrillation Follow-up Investigation of Rhythm Management (AFFIRM) study.[27] The results of this study showed that management with rhythm control did not have any more survival benefit than a rate control strategy in anticoagulated patients with AF.[28,29] Rate control may have potential advantages over rhythm control, such as a lower risk for adverse side effects that are seen with aggressive rhythm control.[29]

Catheter fulguration of the His bundle is an extreme form of ventricular rate control. First described by Scheinman and colleagues[30] in 1982, the ablation of the AV node–His bundle complex effectively controlled the irregular cardiac rhythm in AF and other supraventricular arrhythmias. Unfortunately, ablation of the AV node requires permanent pacemaker insertion. Despite this drawback, AV node ablation is currently a common treatment of medically refractory AF, especially for those patients who cannot tolerate pharmacologic rate control.

Rate control alone does not address all the pathophysiological effects of AF. Although the ventricular response rate can often be controlled pharmacologically or with AV node ablation, the atria are still in fibrillation. The absence of atrial "kick" can result in worsening symptoms of congestive heart failure. More importantly, patients with AF remain at risk for developing thromboembolism, requiring indefinite anticoagulation with warfarin. Warfarin has a significant side effect profile, with a major complication rate of approximately 2% per year.[31–33]

Although the AFFIRM trial showed no difference in long-term outcome between rhythm versus rate control, there are clinically meaningful advantages of normal sinus rhythm. These advantages include increased exercise tolerance, freedom from anticoagulation medications, decreased palpitations, and prevention of atrial remodeling.[27,34] The presence of sinus rhythm was also associated with a significantly decreased risk of death (HR = 0.53, $P<.0001$) in a post hoc analysis of the AFFIRM trial.[35] This beneficial effect on mortality from sinus rhythm is also borne out in the surgical literature.[36–39]

DEVELOPMENT OF THE COX-MAZE PROCEDURE

In the 1980s, several groups began developing procedures for the surgical treatment of AF. The majority of these have only historical significance now because they were unable to address all 3 detrimental sequelae of AF simultaneously. The left atrial isolation procedure, introduced by Williams and colleagues[40] isolated AF to the left atrium, restoring regular rhythm and hemodynamics in patients with left-sided fibrillation. However, patients were still at risk for thromboembolism. In 1985, Guiraudon and colleagues introduced the corridor procedure, which isolated a strip of atrial septum containing the SA and AV nodes. This restored a regular ventricular response, but left both atria fibrillating, leading to hemodynamic inadequacy and a persistent risk for thromboembolism.[41] In 1985, Cox described an atrial transection procedure that involved a long incision across both atria and down into the septum. This procedure cured AF in a canine model, but was ineffective in humans.[42] Although unsuccessful, these techniques laid the groundwork for the subsequent development of the Cox-Maze procedure.

The team led by Dr. James Cox at Washington University in St. Louis developed the Maze procedure in 1987.[43–45] The Cox-Maze procedure was an empiric operation designed to interrupt the macro-reentrant circuits thought to be responsible for AF at the time. Unlike earlier procedures, the Maze procedure addressed all three detrimental sequelae of AF, restoring AF synchrony, a regular ventricular response, and decreasing the risk of thromboembolism and stroke.[46] The operation involved creating multiple incisions across the right and left atria. In effect, these incisions directed the electrical impulses from the SA node while preventing reentrant circuits from forming.

It also allowed all of the atrial myocardium to be activated, preserving atrial transport function in most patients.[47] After two iterations addressing late complications and technical difficulty, the Cox-Maze III emerged (**Fig. 1**).[48,49]

The Cox-Maze III procedure has become the gold standard for the surgical treatment of AF. In a long-term study of patients who had the Cox-Maze III procedure, 97% of the patients at late follow-up were free of symptomatic AF.[50] Similar results have been reproduced by other institutions around the world.[51–53]

SURGICAL ABLATION TECHNOLOGY

Although several groups have reported excellent results with the Cox-Maze III, the procedure did not gain widespread acceptance because of its complexity and technical difficulty. During the last 10 years, most groups have replaced the traditional cut-and-sew lesions of the Cox-Maze III with ablations using various energy sources in an effort to make the procedure technically simpler and faster to perform.[54] These linear lines of ablation have been created using a variety of energy sources including radio frequency (RF) energy, microwave, cryoablation, laser and high-frequency ultrasound.[55–59] The development of ablation technologies has revolutionized the surgical treatment of AF. Although very few patients (<1%) with AF undergoing cardiac surgery before 2000 underwent a Cox-Maze procedure, over 40% of patients with AF undergoing cardiac surgery had a concomitant ablation procedure in 2006.[60]

The safe and effective use of these new ablation devices requires a thorough understanding of the biophysics of the energy source and their behavior on atrial tissue. Most importantly, a device must reliably produce conduction block to prevent AF. An ablation device must have the capability to reliably make transmural lesions from either the epicardial or endocardial surface. Experimental work has shown that even small gaps in ablation lines can conduct fibrillatory wavefronts.[61] Surgeons must also understand the safety profile of ablation devices. This requires a precise definition of dose-response curves to limit excessive or inadequate ablation and knowledge of the effect of the device on surrounding vital cardiac structures, such as coronary

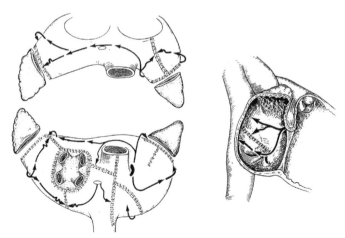

Fig. 1. The incisions of the Cox-Maze III procedure with the propagation of the sinus impulse represented by arrows. (*From* Cox JL. Evolving applications of the Maze procedure for atrial fibrillation [invited editorial]. Ann Thorac Surg 1993;55:578–80. *Reprinted with permission from* The Society of Thoracic Surgeons.)

arteries and valves. A device should also make AF surgery simpler and require less time to perform than a traditional case. This requires features such as rapidity of lesion formation, simplicity of use, and adequacy of length and flexibility. A device should be amenable to minimally invasive approaches. A brief discussion of cryoablation and RF ablation, the most used ablation technologies, follows. Microwave and laser devices are no longer on the market and are not discussed.

Cryoablation

Cryoablation has been used in arrhythmia surgery for decades. There are currently two commercially available sources of cryothermal energy. The original technology uses nitrous oxide and is manufactured by Atricure (Cincinnati, Ohio). The nitrous oxide devices use rigid reusable probes, although there are flexible probes in development. CryoCath Technologies (Montreal, Quebec, Canada) introduced a device using argon, which is now distributed by ATS (Minneapolis, Minnesota). The original device used a disposable flexible catheter, and newer iterations have included a clamp device. At one atmosphere of pressure, nitrous oxide is capable of achieving a temperature of $-89.5°C$, whereas argon has a minimum temperature of $-185.7°C$.

Cryoablation causes tissue injury through the freezing and rewarming process. Acutely, ice crystals disrupt cell membranes, whereas, chronically, microvascular damage leads to local tissue ischemia. Apoptosis plays a clear, but incompletely understood role in lesion formation.[62,63] The size and depth of cryolesions are determined by numerous factors, including probe temperature, tissue temperature, probe size, the duration and number of ablations, and the particular liquid used as the cooling agent.[64–67]

Cryoablation has the distinct advantage of preserving collagen structure.[68] Thus, it preserves the fibrous skeleton of the heart, making it safe for use around valvular tissue. Furthermore, cryoablation has a proven track record in the treatment of arrhythmias. Nitrous oxide cryoablation has had extensive clinical use and an excellent safety profile. A European randomized trial comparing mitral valve surgery to mitral valve surgery with concomitant left atrial cryoablation showed increased freedom from AF for the cryoablation group (43% versus 73% at 12 months).[69] Ad and Cox developed a less invasive Maze procedure using cryoablation that reduced the number of atriotomies from 12 to 4 using cryoablation with preserved efficacy.[70]

Despite a proven track record, cryoablation does have some drawbacks. It is largely ineffective on the beating heart. Because of the heat sink provided by circulating endocardial blood, epicardial cryolesions on the beating heart have not been uniformly transmural. In one study, investigators were only able to create transmural lesions 62% of the time around the PVs and only two out of eight (25%) ablations on the left atrial appendage were transmural.[71] Experimental studies have shown late intimal hyperplasia of coronary arteries after cryoablation, and these structures should be avoided.[63]

In summary, cryoablation is unique among the currently available ablation technologies in that it destroys tissue by freezing rather than heating. The important advantage is its ability to preserve tissue architecture. The nitrous oxide technology has a well-defined efficacy and safety profile and is generally safe except around the coronary arteries. The potential disadvantages of cryoablation technology include the relatively long time necessary to create a lesion (1–3 minutes). There is also difficulty in creating lesions on the beating heart because of the heat sink of the circulating blood volume. Furthermore, if blood is frozen during epicardial ablation on the beating heart, it coagulates, creating a potential risk for thromboembolism.

RF Energy

In the electrophysiology laboratory, RF energy has been used for cardiac ablation for many years.[72] RF energy uses an alternating current in the range of 100 to 1000 kHz which is high enough to prevent rapid myocardial depolarization and the induction of ventricular fibrillation yet low enough to prevent tissue vaporization and perforation. A lesion is created through thermal injury. As the RF radiation passes through tissue, resistive heating occurs within a narrow rim of tissue in direct contact with the electrode. Passive conduction continues from this interface to create the lesion on deeper tissue.

RF ablation devices can be unipolar or bipolar. With unipolar catheters, the energy is dispersed between the electrode tip and an indifferent electrode, usually the grounding pad applied to the patient. In bipolar clamp devices, alternating current is generated between two closely approximated electrodes, which results in a more focused ablation. The lesion size depends on tissue-electrode contact area, the interface temperature, the current and voltage (power), and the duration of delivery. An obstacle to deeper tissue penetration is char formation at the tissue-electrode interface. Irrigated devices have been developed that reduce charring and allow for deeper penetration of radiation. These irrigated catheters were shown to create larger volume lesions than dry RF devices.[73,74]

There are numerous unipolar RF devices available. Estech (San Ramon, California) has marketed several Cobra catheters, both dry and irrigated unipolar catheters, which are segmented and flexible. These devices can create variable lesion lengths of 10 mm to 95 mm. The electrodes can be individually selected and temperature controlled. Medtronic has developed a unipolar RF device, the Cardioblate catheter. This is an irrigated unipolar RF catheter used to make point-by-point ablations by dragging it across the tissue to make a linear lesion.

The most widely used devices are bipolar RF clamps. With two electrodes instead of one, the path of energy is more focused. This allows for faster ablation (usually less than 20 s), while limiting destruction to tissue that is in close proximity to the electrodes. With bipolar devices, the electrodes are clamped over the targeted atrial tissue. The first bipolar RF device was introduced by Atricure, Inc. The isolator was a specially designed clamp with 1-mm wide and 5-cm long electrodes embedded in the jaws of the clamp. The device was unique in that it had an algorithm created to detect real-time measurement of lesion transmurality. The conductance between the electrodes was measured during ablation. When the conductance dropped to a stable minimum level, this was well correlated experimentally and clinically to histologically transmural lesions.[75–77] More recent iterations have introduced more uniform clamp strength and a unique dual electrode designed to achieve wider and more consistent lesions. The Medtronic bipolar clamp, the Cardioblate BP, has an irrigated, flexible jaw along with an articulating head, with 5-cm long electrodes. This device has an algorithm, like the Atricure device, that predicts transmurality of lesions. This device was shown to be effective in the experimental setting.[78,79]

Newer RF ablation devices have been released by other manufacturers, and these are all variations of the same themes of earlier devices.[80,81] The Cobra Adhere and Cobra Adhere XL (Estech) devices are unipolar devices with suction to aid in minimally invasive applications, such as port access or thoracoscopic approaches. The VisiTrax device (nContact Surgical, Morrisville, North Carolina) is another unipolar device coupled with suction for minimally invasive applications.

Dose-response curves for unipolar RF have been described.[82–84] Although these studies show reliable lesion formation in animals with ablation times of 1 to 2 minutes, these devices have not performed well in humans. In one study, after 2-minute endocardial ablations during mitral valve surgery, only 20% of the in vivo lesions were transmural.[85] Epicardial ablation was even more difficult. Both animal and human studies have consistently shown that unipolar RF is incapable of creating epicardial transmural lesions on the beating heart.[84,85] In contrast, bipolar RF ablation, was capable of creating transmural lesions on the beating heart in animals and humans.[55,76,77]

Like cryoablation, RF ablation is a well-developed technology, and much is known about its safety profile. A number of clinical complications of unipolar RF devices have been described, including coronary artery injuries, cerebrovascular accidents, and esophageal perforation leading to atrioesophageal fistula.[86–89] Use of the bipolar RF devices has eliminated virtually all of the collateral damage seen with the unipolar devices, and there have been no clinical complications reported in the literature. One drawback of the bipolar devices is the requirement for the tissue to be clamped in the jaws of the device. This has limited the potential lesion set, particularly on the beating heart, and requires the use of adjunctive unipolar technology to create a complete Cox-Maze lesion set.

INDICATIONS FOR SURGICAL TREATMENT OF AF

The principal indication for surgery for AF is intolerance of the arrhythmia in patients who have failed medical management. Patients with paroxysmal atrial flutter or fibrillation are often more symptomatic than those with persistent or long-standing AF. Major symptoms include dyspnea on exertion, easy fatigability, lethargy, palpitations, and a general sense of unease.

The Heart Rhythm Society created a task force to evaluate indications for catheter and surgical ablation of AF.[12] The recommendations were developed in partnership with the European Heart Rhythm Association, the European Cardiac Arrhythmia Society, the American College of Cardiology, the American Heart Association, and the Society of Thoracic Surgeons. Because the treatment of AF is complex, they recommended that a team-based approach, including electrophysiologists and surgeons, is used to appropriately select patients for stand-alone surgical treatment of AF. The consensus of the Task Force established the following indications for surgical ablation of AF:[12]

1. Symptomatic AF patients undergoing other cardiac surgical procedures
2. Selected asymptomatic AF patients undergoing cardiac surgery in whom the ablation can be performed with minimal risk
3. Stand-alone AF surgery should be considered for symptomatic AF patients who have failed medical management and prefer a surgical approach, or have failed one or more attempts at catheter ablation, or are not candidates for catheter ablation.

Another important group of patients who should be considered for surgery are those who cannot take warfarin or those who have had a stroke while adequately anticoagulated. The Cox-Maze procedure significantly reduces the risk for stroke in these patients. About 20% of patients who had the original cut-and-sew procedure at the authors' institution experienced at least one episode of cerebral thromboembolism that resulted in a temporary or permanent neurologic deficit. At a mean follow-up of 5.4 years, less than 1% of patients (1/178) had a late stroke following the Cox-Maze procedure.[50]

SURGICAL TECHNIQUE: THE COX-MAZE PROCEDURE

The final version of the standard cut-and-sew technique to cure AF was the Cox-Maze III procedure.[43–45] The complexity of the cut-and-sew technique led many surgeons to replace the incisions with linear ablations. Bipolar RF energy has been used successfully by the authors' group to replace the majority of the surgical incisions of the Cox-Maze III procedure. The authors' current procedure incorporates most of the lesions of the Cox-Maze III procedure, and has been named the Cox-Maze IV (**Fig. 2**).[55,90] Midterm follow-up has shown that this modification has significantly shortened the operative time without compromising the success rate of the traditional cut-and-sew Cox-Maze III procedure.[91]

The Cox-Maze IV procedure is performed with the patient on cardiopulmonary bypass either through a median sternotomy or a right mini thoracotomy. The right and left PVs are bluntly dissected to prepare for isolation. If the patient is in AF, an intravenous bolus of amiodarone is given and the patient is cardioverted. This allows for determination of pacing thresholds on both sets of PVs before ablation. The bipolar ablations are then performed on a cuff of atrial tissue surrounding the right and left PVs separately. After isolation, exit block is verified with pacing from all of the PVs.

The right atrial lesions are performed with the heart beating through a single vertical atriotomy and a small purse-string suture at the base of the right atrial appendage (**Fig. 3**). A unipolar energy source (cryoablation, RF, and so forth) is used to complete the ablation lines at the tricuspid valve.

After completion of the right-sided lesions, the left-sided lesions are performed through a standard left atriotomy with the heart arrested. This is illustrated schematically in **Fig. 4**. The atriotomy is extended inferiorly around the right inferior PV and superiorly onto the dome of the left atrium. Care is taken to connect this incision to the RF ablation line surrounding the right PVs. A lesion is made with the bipolar RF device, connecting the left atrium incision inferiorly to the ablation line encircling the left PVs. Another ablation is performed from the superior aspect of the left atriotomy, across the dome of the left atrium, and into the left superior PV. A bipolar RF lesion is

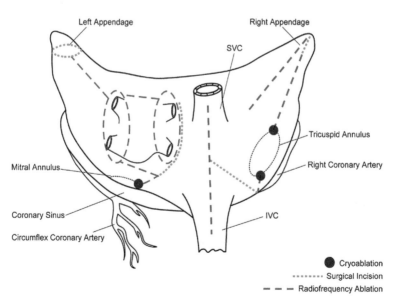

Fig. 2. Cox-Maze IV procedure lesion set. Most of the incisions of the Cox-Maze III have been replaced with ablation. Modifications included independent isolation of PVs with connecting lesion, and no atrial septal incision (originally used for exposure). *Abbreviations:* IVC, inferior vena cava; SVC, superior vena cava.

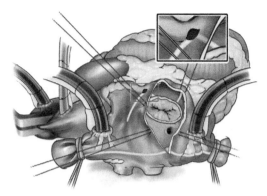

Fig. 3. The surgeon's view of the right atrium through the vertical atriotomy used to create the right-sided lesions of the Cox-Maze IV procedure. Note the pale demarcations of the lines of ablation created with the bipolar RF clamps on the atrial wall. Unipolar energy, like cryothermy, is used to finish the ablation lines at the tricuspid annulus.

then created up to the mitral valve annulus. This lesion is performed from the inferior aspect of the left atrial incision across the posterior left atrium, AV groove, and the coronary sinus. The ablation is performed in the space between the circumflex and right coronary artery circulation to avoid damage to the coronary arteries.

To complete the Cox-Maze, a unipolar energy source (cryoablation, RF, and so forth) is used to connect the last ablation line to the mitral valve annulus. To reduce the risk for systemic thromboembolism, the left atrial appendage is amputated. A final ablation is performed through the amputated left atrial appendage into one of the left PVs. The left atrial appendage is oversewn. In patients undergoing a mitral valve replacement, amputation of the left atrial appendage before performing the other left atrial lesions is recommended to avoid excessive traction.

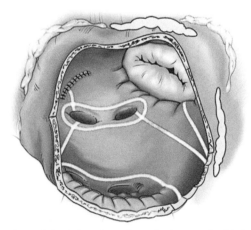

Fig. 4. The surgeon's view of the left atrium through the standard left atriotomy. Note the pale demarcations of the lines of ablation created with the bipolar RF clamps on the atrial wall. On the left atrium, the line toward the mitral valve is also finished with a unipolar energy source, most often cryothermy.

SURGICAL RESULTS: COX-MAZE PROCEDURE

The long-term results of the Cox-Maze III procedure have been excellent. The experience encompassing 198 patients at Washington University showed that 97% of patients at a mean follow-up of 5.4 years were in sinus rhythm with no difference between patients undergoing lone versus concomitant procedures. The cure rates off antiarrhythmic medications were 80% and 73% in patients undergoing lone and concomitant Cox-Maze procedures, respectively, at late follow-up.[50]

The results with the ablation-based Cox-Maze IV have been similar. In a prospective, single-center trial from the authors' institution, 91% of patients at 6-months follow-up were free from AF, and operative mortality was 0%.[55] These results were later validated in a multicenter trial.[58] Moreover, the adaptation of bipolar RF has shortened the operation considerably, dropping mean cross-clamp times for patients undergoing a lone Cox-Maze III procedure from 92 ± 26 minutes to 44 ± 21 minutes for patients undergoing a Cox-Maze IV.[92] A propensity analysis comparing the Cox-Maze IV patients with a historical cohort of patients undergoing the Cox-Maze III showed that the Cox-Maze IV had statistically identical outcomes at 1-year follow-up.[91]

The Cox-Maze procedure has been effective at decreasing the risk for late stroke in this patient population. Nineteen percent (58/306) of patients undergoing Cox-Maze III at Washington University had experienced a neurologic event before surgery, and there were only two minor strokes during long-term follow-up (mean 3.9 ± 2.7 years). The long-term stroke rate after the Cox-Maze procedure has been 0.1% per year, despite the fact that the majority of patients were able to discontinue anticoagulation medication.[46] Other centers have reported similar results. In a series from Japan, patients with chronic AF who had a concomitant Cox-Maze procedure with their mitral valve replacement were 99% stroke-free at a follow-up of 8 years, whereas the group with mitral valve replacement alone were 89% stroke-free.[93]

OTHER AF PROCEDURES

More limited procedures have been proposed for the surgical treatment of AF. These fall into two broad groups, left atrial lesion sets and operations that isolate the PVs.

PVI

Based on the original reports of Hassaiguerre,[16] it has been well documented that the triggers for paroxysmal AF originate from the PVs in most cases. However, over 30% of triggers originate outside the PVs.[19] A number of surgeons have published the technique of PVI as a procedure to treat AF.[94–97] PVI as a therapeutic strategy is attractive because this procedure can be often done without cardiopulmonary bypass through small incisions, or endoscopically. To increase efficacy, some investigators have added ablation of the ganglionic plexi (GP).[98–100]

The results of PVI have been variable. In a series by Wolf and colleagues,[97] 91% of patients undergoing a video-assisted bilateral PVI and left atrial appendage exclusion were free from AF at 3-months follow-up. Edgerton and colleagues[101] reported on 57 patients undergoing PVI with GP ablation with more thorough follow-up and found 82% of their patients with paroxysmal AF to be free from AF at 6 months, with 74% off antiarrhythmic drugs. In a study involving 21 patients undergoing PVI with GP ablation, McClelland and colleagues[99] reported 88% procedural success in patients with paroxysmal AF, with procedural success defined as freedom from AF at 1 year without antiarrhythmic drugs. A recent multicenter trial reported 87% normal sinus rhythm in a more diverse patient population including patients with long-standing persistent AF, although this subset had only 71% normal sinus rhythm rate.[102] Results from the authors' institution are similar, with 83% freedom from AF and 67% off drugs at a mean follow-up of 24 ± 37 months using data from 24-hour Holter monitoring.

However, the success of PVI is largely dependent on patient selection. Patients with long-standing or persistent AF had very poor results. Fifty-six percent of patients in Edgerton's group were free from AF at 6 months (35% were off antiarrythmics).[103] In patients undergoing concomitant procedures, the results were even worse. Of 23 patients undergoing mitral valve surgery or coronary revascularization with concomitant PVI, only 50% of patients were free from AF at a mean follow-up of 57 ± 37 months.[92] In a randomized trial, Gaita and colleagues[104] reported similar poor results with 29% freedom from AF in patients undergoing concomitant PVI with valve surgery. In the setting of mitral valve disease Tada and colleagues[96] reported 61% freedom from AF and only 17% freedom from antiarrythmic drugs in their series of 66 patients undergoing PVI.

These results of PVI emphasize the importance of understanding the electrophysiological substrate in patients with AF.

Ganglionated Plexus Ablation

The addition of ganglionated plexus ablation by some authors is based on experimental data showing that autonomic ganglia in these plexi play a role in the initiation and maintenance of AF.[105,106] However, the authors' practice is not to ablate the ganglia, as experimental evidence in their laboratory and others have shown recovery of autonomic function as early as 4 weeks after GP ablation.[107–109] Furthermore, long-term follow-up regarding the effects of GP ablation is lacking. Thus, GP ablation should be reserved for centers participating in clinical trials.

Left Atrial Lesion Sets

The left atrial lesion set generally involves creating PVI and a lesion to the mitral annulus and removal of the left atrial appendage. A multitude of ablation devices have been used in the formation of these lesions sets, with varying techniques and varying degrees of success.[88,104,110–116] A meta-analysis by Barnett and Ad in 2006 showed a 73% success for left atrial lesion sets versus 87% for biatrial lesion sets (P = .05).[117] The only randomized control trial comparing the efficacy of left atrial lesion set versus no ablation procedure was reported by Doukas and colleagues.[118] For a cohort of patients undergoing mitral valve surgery, 44% had normal sinus rhythm 1 year after undergoing RF ablation of the left atrium versus only 4.5% in the patients undergoing valve surgery alone.

Although the results of Barnett and Ad's meta-analysis showed that left atrial lesion sets are not as effective as biatrial lesion sets, left atrial lesion sets are better than no treatment at all. There is evidence in the literature that some of the lesions on the left atrium are important to include regardless of surgical approach. One in particular is the isthmus lesion down to the mitral valve annulus (see **Fig. 4**). In a report on differing left atrial lesion sets by Gillinov and colleagues,[119] patients with long-standing persistent AF had a greater chance of recurrent AF if their lesion set did not include a line down to the mitral annulus. Furthermore, data from the authors' institution show the importance of isolating the entire posterior atrium around the PVs as a single unit (**Fig. 5**). Freedom from AF, off antiarrhythmic drugs was significantly higher for patients who had a "box" lesion around the PVs than those who had a single ablation connecting the islands of atrial tissue around the left and right PVs. At 6 months, 79% of patients with the "box" lesion were free from AF, off antiarrhythmic drugs versus 54% of the patients without it (P = .011).[120]

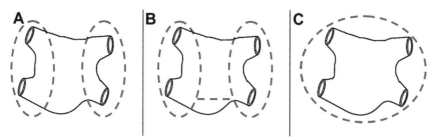

Fig. 5. Isolation of the pulmonary veins: (A) Isolation of the PVs separately, (B) Isolation of the PVs separately with a bridging ablation. (C) Isolation of the entire posterior left atrium as a unit, including the PVs. The practice of the authors' institution in performing the Cox-Maze IV is to isolate the entire posterior atrium by connecting the PVs with a superior and inferior ablation, creating a "box" lesion (not shown).

SUMMARY

AF is a complex disease affecting a significant portion of the general population. In the last decade, interventional therapy (catheter and surgical ablation) has emerged to play an ever increasing role for patients with symptomatic, medically refractory arrhythmia. The introduction of ablation devices has revolutionized the surgical treatment of AF making procedures available to a wider patient population.

There have been few randomized trials comparing the different surgical procedures, but conclusions can be drawn from two decades of surgical experience and retrospective series. In patients with lone AF, PVI had good early results for paroxysmal AF.[99,101] At the authors' institution, this procedure is performed in patients who have paroxysmal AF and a left atrial size of 4 cm or less. In patients with large atria, the authors prefer a full Cox-Maze lesion set, because of the high incidence of nonpulmonary vein triggers in this population.[19] They also prefer a full lesion set in patients with long-standing, persistent lone AF as a result of the poor results of PVI in this group.

If a patient fails a catheter ablation, the surgeon needs to accurately diagnose the recurrent arrhythmia. A number of these patients will have atypical atrial flutter that cannot be treated with PVI alone and requires either a complete biatrial or left atrial lesion set including the isthmus lesion. Patients may also have atrial tachycardia, which is better treated by catheter ablation or medication. To determine the precise arrhythmia, these patients should be evaluated by an electrophysiologist and a surgeon before an operation. At the authors' institution, noninvasive ECG imaging is used to help define the mechanism of recurrence.[121,122]

In patients with AF undergoing concomitant procedures and requiring cardiopulmonary bypass, a Cox-Maze procedure is the procedure of choice. For patients undergoing mitral valve procedures, this adds 10 to 15 minutes of cross-clamp time. In most patients, the authors prefer a biatrial lesion set. The right atrial lesions can be performed with the heart beating (see **Fig. 3**). In selected patients, with left-sided pathology and a normal size right atrium, a left atrial lesion set alone has been performed with good results. In patients undergoing coronary bypass grafting, the high success rate of the Cox-Maze lesion set has been documented by the authors' group.[123] However, there have been no randomized comparisons of lesion sets in this population.

More limited lesion sets have a more limited role. In patients with paroxysmal AF undergoing off-pump coronary bypass grafting, our policy had been to perform PVI with removal of the left atrial appendage. Poor results in patients with long-standing AF have led the authors to abandon this procedure in those patients.

REFERENCES

1. Lloyd-Jones D, Adams R, Carnethon M, et al. Heart disease and stroke statistics – 2009 update: a report from the American Heart Association Statistics Committee and Stroke Statistics Subcommittee. Circulation 2009;119(3):480–6.
2. Lloyd-Jones DM, Wang TJ, Leip EP, et al. Lifetime risk for development of atrial fibrillation: the Framingham Heart Study. Circulation 2004;110(9):1042–6.
3. Wattigney WA, Mensah GA, Croft JB. Increasing trends in hospitalization for atrial fibrillation in the United States, 1985 through 1999: implications for primary prevention. Circulation 2003;108(6):711–6.
4. Benjamin EJ, Levy D, Vaziri SM, et al. Independent risk factors for atrial fibrillation in a population-based cohort. The Framingham Heart Study. JAMA 1994; 271(11):840–4.
5. Cairns JA. Stroke prevention in atrial fibrillation trial. Circulation 1991;84(2): 933–5.
6. Hart RG, Halperin JL, Pearce LA, et al. Lessons from the stroke prevention in atrial fibrillation trials. Ann Intern Med 2003;138(10):831–8.
7. Wolf PA, Abbott RD, Kannel WB. Atrial fibrillation as an independent risk factor for stroke: the Framingham Study. Stroke 1991;22(8):983–8.
8. Wolf PA, Benjamin EJ, Belanger AJ, et al. Secular trends in the prevalence of atrial fibrillation: the Framingham Study. Am Heart J 1996;131(4):790–5.
9. Benjamin EJ, Wolf PA, D'Agostino RB, et al. Impact of atrial fibrillation on the risk of death: the Framingham Heart Study. Circulation 1998;98(10):946–52.
10. Vidaillet H, Granada JF, Chyou PH, et al. A population-based study of mortality among patients with atrial fibrillation or flutter. Am J Med 2002;113(5):365–70.
11. Fuster V, Ryden LE, Asinger RW, et al. ACC/AHA/ESC Guidelines for the management of patients with atrial fibrillation: executive summary a report of the American College of Cardiology/American Heart Association Task Force on Practice Guidelines and the European Society of Cardiology Committee for Practice Guidelines and Policy Conferences (Committee to Develop Guidelines for the Management of Patients With Atrial Fibrillation) developed in collaboration with the North American Society of Pacing and Electrophysiology. Circulation 2001;104(17):2118–50.
12. Calkins H, Brugada J, Packer DL, et al. HRS/EHRA/ECAS expert Consensus Statement on catheter and surgical ablation of atrial fibrillation: recommendations for personnel, policy, procedures and follow-up. A report of the Heart Rhythm Society (HRS) Task Force on catheter and surgical ablation of atrial fibrillation. Heart Rhythm 2007;4(6):816–61.
13. Schuessler RB, Kay MW, Melby SJ, et al. Spatial and temporal stability of the dominant frequency of activation in human atrial fibrillation. J Electrocardiol 2006;39(4 Suppl):S7–12.
14. Boineau JP, Schuessler RB, Canavan TE, et al. The human atrial pacemaker complex. J Electrocardiol 1989;22(Suppl):189–97.
15. Byrd GD, Prasad SM, Ripplinger CM, et al. Importance of geometry and refractory period in sustaining atrial fibrillation: testing the critical mass hypothesis. Circulation 2005;112(9 Suppl):I7–13.

16. Haissaguerre M, Jais P, Shah DC, et al. Spontaneous initiation of atrial fibrillation by ectopic beats originating in the pulmonary veins. N Engl J Med 1998;339(10): 659–66.

17. Spach MS, Barr RC, Jewett PH. Spread of excitation from the atrium into thoracic veins in human beings and dogs. Am J Cardiol 1972;30(8):844–54.

18. Blom NA, Gittenberger-de Groot AC, DeRuiter MC, et al. Development of the cardiac conduction tissue in human embryos using HNK-1 antigen expression: possible relevance for understanding of abnormal atrial automaticity. Circulation 1999;99(6):800–6.

19. Lee SH, Tai CT, Hsieh MH, et al. Predictors of non-pulmonary vein ectopic beats initiating paroxysmal atrial fibrillation: implication for catheter ablation. J Am Coll Cardiol 2005;46(6):1054–9.

20. Nattel S. New ideas about atrial fibrillation 50 years on. Nature 2002;415(6868): 219–26.

21. Nitta T, Ishii Y, Miyagi Y, et al. Concurrent multiple left atrial focal activations with fibrillatory conduction and right atrial focal or reentrant activation as the mechanism in atrial fibrillation. J Thorac Cardiovasc Surg 2004;127(3):770–8.

22. Nitta T, Ohmori H, Sakamoto S, et al. Map-guided surgery for atrial fibrillation. J Thorac Cardiovasc Surg 2005;129(2):291–9.

23. Schuessler RB. Do we need a map to get through the maze? J Thorac Cardiovasc Surg 2004;127(3):627–8.

24. Ghosh S, Avari JN, Rhee EK, et al. Hypertrophic cardiomyopathy with preexcitation: insights from noninvasive electrocardiographic imaging (ECGI) and catheter mapping. J Cardiovasc Electrophysiol 2008;19(11):1215–7.

25. Fuster V, Ryden LE, Asinger RW, et al. ACC/AHA/ESC guidelines for the management of patients with atrial fibrillation: executive summary. A Report of the American College of Cardiology/American Heart Association Task Force on Practice Guidelines and the European Society of Cardiology Committee for Practice Guidelines and Policy Conferences (Committee to Develop Guidelines for the Management of Patients With Atrial Fibrillation): developed in collaboration with the North American Society of Pacing and Electrophysiology. J Am Coll Cardiol 2001;38(4):1231–66.

26. Miller MR, McNamara RL, Segal JB, et al. Efficacy of agents for pharmacologic conversion of atrial fibrillation and subsequent maintenance of sinus rhythm: a meta-analysis of clinical trials. J Fam Pract 2000;49(11):1033–46.

27. Waldo AL. Management of atrial fibrillation: the need for AFFIRMative action. AFFIRM investigators. Atrial Fibrillation Follow-up Investigation of Rhythm Management. Am J Cardiol 1999;84(6):698–700.

28. Van Gelder IC, Hagens VE, Bosker HA, et al. A comparison of rate control and rhythm control in patients with recurrent persistent atrial fibrillation. N Engl J Med 2002;347(23):1834–40.

29. Wyse DG, Waldo AL, DiMarco JP, et al. A comparison of rate control and rhythm control in patients with atrial fibrillation. N Engl J Med 2002;347(23):1825–33.

30. Scheinman MM, Morady F, Hess DS, et al. Catheter-induced ablation of the atrioventricular junction to control refractory supraventricular arrhythmias. JAMA 1982;248(7):851–5.

31. Copland M, Walker ID, Tait RC. Oral anticoagulation and hemorrhagic complications in an elderly population with atrial fibrillation. Arch Intern Med 2001; 161(17):2125–8.

32. DiMarco JP, Flaker G, Waldo AL, et al. Factors affecting bleeding risk during anticoagulant therapy in patients with atrial fibrillation: observations from the

Atrial Fibrillation Follow-up Investigation of Rhythm Management (AFFIRM) study. Am Heart J 2005;149(4):650–6.

33. Levine MN, Raskob G, Landefeld S, et al. Hemorrhagic complications of anticoagulant treatment. Chest 2001;119(1 Suppl):108S–21S.

34. Maintenance of sinus rhythm in patients with atrial fibrillation: an AFFIRM substudy of the first antiarrhythmic drug. J Am Coll Cardiol 2003;42(1):20–9.

35. Corley SD, Epstein AE, DiMarco JP, et al. Relationships between sinus rhythm, treatment, and survival in the Atrial Fibrillation Follow-Up Investigation of Rhythm Management (AFFIRM) Study. Circulation 2004;109(12):1509–13.

36. Bando K, Kasegawa H, Okada Y, et al. Impact of preoperative and postoperative atrial fibrillation on outcome after mitral valvuloplasty for nonischemic mitral regurgitation. J Thorac Cardiovasc Surg 2005;129(5):1032–40.

37. Bando K, Kobayashi J, Kosakai Y, et al. Impact of Cox maze procedure on outcome in patients with atrial fibrillation and mitral valve disease. J Thorac Cardiovasc Surg 2002;124(3):575–83.

38. Itoh A, Kobayashi J, Bando K, et al. The impact of mitral valve surgery combined with maze procedure. Eur J Cardiothorac Surg 2006;29(6):1030–5.

39. Melo J, Santiago T, Aguiar C, et al. Surgery for atrial fibrillation in patients with mitral valve disease: results at five years from the International Registry of Atrial Fibrillation Surgery. J Thorac Cardiovasc Surg 2008;135(4):863–9.

40. Williams JM, Ungerleider RM, Lofland GK, et al. Left atrial isolation: new technique for the treatment of supraventricular arrhythmias. J Thorac Cardiovasc Surg 1980;80(3):373–80.

41. Leitch JW, Klein G, Yee R, et al. Sinus node-atrioventricular node isolation: long-term results with the "corridor" operation for atrial fibrillation. J Am Coll Cardiol 1991;17(4):970–5.

42. Smith PK, Holman WL, Cox JL. Surgical treatment of supraventricular tachyarrhythmias. Surg Clin North Am 1985;65(3):553–70.

43. Cox JL. The surgical treatment of atrial fibrillation. IV. Surgical technique. J Thorac Cardiovasc Surg 1991;101(4):584–92.

44. Cox JL, Canavan TE, Schuessler RB, et al. The surgical treatment of atrial fibrillation. II. Intraoperative electrophysiologic mapping and description of the electrophysiologic basis of atrial flutter and atrial fibrillation. J Thorac Cardiovasc Surg 1991;101(3):406–26.

45. Cox JL, Schuessler RB, D'Agostino HJ Jr, et al. The surgical treatment of atrial fibrillation. III. Development of a definitive surgical procedure. J Thorac Cardiovasc Surg 1991;101(4):569–83.

46. Cox JL, Ad N, Palazzo T. Impact of the maze procedure on the stroke rate in patients with atrial fibrillation. J Thorac Cardiovasc Surg 1999;118(5):833–40.

47. Feinberg MS, Waggoner AD, Kater KM, et al. Restoration of atrial function after the maze procedure for patients with atrial fibrillation. Assessment by Doppler echocardiography. Circulation 1994;90(5 Pt 2):II285–92.

48. Cox JL. The minimally invasive Maze-III procedure. Oper Tech Thorac Cardiovasc Surg 2000;5:79–92.

49. Cox JL, Boineau JP, Schuessler RB, et al. Modification of the maze procedure for atrial flutter and atrial fibrillation. I. Rationale and surgical results. J Thorac Cardiovasc Surg 1995;110(2):473–84.

50. Prasad SM, Maniar HS, Camillo CJ, et al. The Cox maze III procedure for atrial fibrillation: long-term efficacy in patients undergoing lone versus concomitant procedures. J Thorac Cardiovasc Surg 2003;126(6):1822–8.

51. McCarthy PM, Gillinov AM, Castle L, et al. The Cox-Maze procedure: the Cleveland Clinic experience. Semin Thorac Cardiovasc Surg 2000;12(1):25–9.
52. Raanani E, Albage A, David TE, et al. The efficacy of the Cox/maze procedure combined with mitral valve surgery: a matched control study. Eur J Cardiothorac Surg 2001;19(4):438–42.
53. Schaff HV, Dearani JA, Daly RC, et al. Cox-Maze procedure for atrial fibrillation: Mayo Clinic experience. Semin Thorac Cardiovasc Surg 2000;12(1):30–7.
54. Khargi K, Hutten BA, Lemke B, et al. Surgical treatment of atrial fibrillation; a systematic review. Eur J Cardiothorac Surg 2005;27(2):258–65.
55. Gaynor SL, Diodato MD, Prasad SM, et al. A prospective, single-center clinical trial of a modified Cox maze procedure with bipolar radiofrequency ablation. J Thorac Cardiovasc Surg 2004;128(4):535–42.
56. Gillinov AM, Smedira NG, Cosgrove DM 3rd. Microwave ablation of atrial fibrillation during mitral valve operations. Ann Thorac Surg 2002;74(4):1259–61.
57. Lee JW, Choo SJ, Kim KI, et al. Atrial fibrillation surgery simplified with cryoablation to improve left atrial function. Ann Thorac Surg 2001;72(5):1479–83.
58. Mokadam NA, McCarthy PM, Gillinov AM, et al. A prospective multicenter trial of bipolar radiofrequency ablation for atrial fibrillation: early results. Ann Thorac Surg 2004;78(5):1665–70.
59. Reddy VY, Houghtaling C, Fallon J, et al. Use of a diode laser balloon ablation catheter to generate circumferential pulmonary venous lesions in an open-thoracotomy caprine model. Pacing Clin Electrophysiol 2004;27(1):52–7.
60. Gammie JS, Haddad M, Milford-Beland S, et al. Atrial fibrillation correction surgery: lessons from the Society of Thoracic Surgeons National Cardiac Database. Ann Thorac Surg 2008;85(3):909–14.
61. Melby SJ, Lee AM, Zierer A, et al. Atrial fibrillation propagates through gaps in ablation lines: implications for ablative treatment of atrial fibrillation. Heart Rhythm 2008;5(9):1296–301.
62. Gage AA, Baust J. Mechanisms of tissue injury in cryosurgery. Cryobiology 1998;37(3):171–86.
63. Mikat EM, Hackel DB, Harrison L, et al. Reaction of the myocardium and coronary arteries to cryosurgery. Lab Invest 1977;37(6):632–41.
64. Ghalili K, Roth JA, Kwan SK, et al. Comparison of left ventricular cryolesions created by liquid nitrogen and nitrous oxide. J Am Coll Cardiol 1992;20(6):1425–9.
65. Holman WL, Ikeshita M, Douglas JM Jr, et al. Cardiac cryosurgery: effects of myocardial temperature on cryolesion size. Surgery 1983;93(2):268–72.
66. Hunt GB, Chard RB, Johnson DC, et al. Comparison of early and late dimensions and arrhythmogenicity of cryolesions in the normothermic canine heart. J Thorac Cardiovasc Surg 1989;97(2):313–8.
67. Markovitz LJ, Frame LH, Josephson ME, et al. Cardiac cryolesions: factors affecting their size and a means of monitoring their formation. Ann Thorac Surg 1988;46(5):531–5.
68. Gage AM, Montes M, Gage AA. Freezing the canine thoracic aorta in situ. J Surg Res 1979;27(5):331–40.
69. Blomstrom-Lundqvist C, Johansson B, Berglin E, et al. A randomized double-blind study of epicardial left atrial cryoablation for permanent atrial fibrillation in patients undergoing mitral valve surgery: the SWEDish Multicentre Atrial Fibrillation study (SWEDMAF). Eur Heart J 2007;28(23):2902–8.
70. Ad N, Cox JL. The Maze procedure for the treatment of atrial fibrillation: a minimally invasive approach. J Card Surg 2004;19(3):196–200.

71. Doll N, Kornherr P, Aupperle H, et al. Epicardial treatment of atrial fibrillation using cryoablation in an acute off-pump sheep model. Thorac Cardiovasc Surg 2003;51(5):267–73.

72. Viola N, Williams MR, Oz MC, et al. The technology in use for the surgical ablation of atrial fibrillation. Semin Thorac Cardiovasc Surg 2002; 14(3):198–205.

73. Khargi K, Deneke T, Haardt H, et al. Saline-irrigated, cooled-tip radiofrequency ablation is an effective technique to perform the maze procedure. Ann Thorac Surg 2001;72(3):S1090–5.

74. Nakagawa H, Wittkampf FH, Yamanashi WS, et al. Inverse relationship between electrode size and lesion size during radiofrequency ablation with active electrode cooling. Circulation 1998;98(5):458–65.

75. Gaynor SL, Ishii Y, Diodato MD, et al. Successful performance of Cox-Maze procedure on beating heart using bipolar radiofrequency ablation: a feasibility study in animals. Ann Thorac Surg 2004;78(5):1671–7.

76. Prasad SM, Maniar HS, Diodato MD, et al. Physiological consequences of bipolar radiofrequency energy on the atria and pulmonary veins: a chronic animal study. Ann Thorac Surg 2003;76(3):836–41 [discussion: 841–2].

77. Prasad SM, Maniar HS, Schuessler RB, et al. Chronic transmural atrial ablation by using bipolar radiofrequency energy on the beating heart. J Thorac Cardiovasc Surg 2002;124(4):708–13.

78. Hamner CE, Potter DD Jr, Cho KR, et al. Irrigated radiofrequency ablation with transmurality feedback reliably produces Cox maze lesions in vivo. Ann Thorac Surg 2005;80(6):2263–70.

79. Melby SJ, Gaynor SL, Lubahn JG, et al. Efficacy and safety of right and left atrial ablations on the beating heart with irrigated bipolar radiofrequency energy: a long-term animal study. J Thorac Cardiovasc Surg 2006;132(4):853–60.

80. Demazumder D, Mirotznik MS, Schwartzman D. Biophysics of radiofrequency ablation using an irrigated electrode. J Interv Card Electrophysiol 2001;5(4): 377–89.

81. Ruchat P, Schlaepfer J, Delabays A, et al. Left atrial radiofrequency compartmentalization for chronic atrial fibrillation during heart surgery. Thorac Cardiovasc Surg 2002;50(3):155–9.

82. Kress DC, Krum D, Chekanov V, et al. Validation of a left atrial lesion pattern for intraoperative ablation of atrial fibrillation. Ann Thorac Surg 2002;73(4):1160–8.

83. Santiago T, Melo JQ, Gouveia RH, et al. Intra-atrial temperatures in radiofrequency endocardial ablation: histologic evaluation of lesions. Ann Thorac Surg 2003; 75(5):1495–501.

84. Thomas SP, Guy DJ, Boyd AC, et al. Comparison of epicardial and endocardial linear ablation using handheld probes. Ann Thorac Surg 2003;75(2):543–8.

85. Santiago T, Melo J, Gouveia RH, et al. Epicardial radiofrequency applications: in vitro and in vivo studies on human atrial myocardium. Eur J Cardiothorac Surg 2003;24(4):481–6 [discussion: 486].

86. Demaria RG, Page P, Leung TK, et al. Surgical radiofrequency ablation induces coronary endothelial dysfunction in porcine coronary arteries. Eur J Cardiothorac Surg 2003;23(3):277–82.

87. Gillinov AM, Pettersson G, Rice TW. Esophageal injury during radiofrequency ablation for atrial fibrillation. J Thorac Cardiovasc Surg 2001;122(6):1239–40.

88. Kottkamp H, Hindricks G, Autschbach R, et al. Specific linear left atrial lesions in atrial fibrillation: intraoperative radiofrequency ablation using minimally invasive surgical techniques. J Am Coll Cardiol 2002;40(3):475–80.

89. Laczkovics A, Khargi K, Deneke T. Esophageal perforation during left atrial radiofrequency ablation. J Thorac Cardiovasc Surg 2003;126(6):2119–20 [author reply: 2120].

90. Damiano RJ Jr, Gaynor SL. Atrial fibrillation ablation during mitral valve surgery using the Atricure device. Oper Tech Thorac Cardiovasc Surg 2004; 9(1):24–33.

91. Lall SC, Melby SJ, Voeller RK, et al. The effect of ablation technology on surgical outcomes after the Cox-maze procedure: a propensity analysis. J Thorac Cardiovasc Surg 2007;133(2):389–96.

92. Melby SJ, Zierer A, Bailey MS, et al. A new era in the surgical treatment of atrial fibrillation: the impact of ablation technology and lesion set on procedural efficacy. Ann Surg 2006;244(4):583–92.

93. Bando K, Kobayashi J, Hirata M, et al. Early and late stroke after mitral valve replacement with a mechanical prosthesis: risk factor analysis of a 24-year experience. J Thorac Cardiovasc Surg 2003;126(2):358–64.

94. Geidel S, Lass M, Boczor S, et al. Monopolar and bipolar radiofrequency ablation surgery: 3-year experience in 90 patients with permanent atrial fibrillation. Heart Surg Forum 2004;7(5):E398–402.

95. Salenger R, Lahey SJ, Saltman AE. The completely endoscopic treatment of atrial fibrillation: report on the first 14 patients with early results. Heart Surg Forum 2004;7(6):E555–8.

96. Tada H, Ito S, Naito S, et al. Long-term results of cryoablation with a new cryoprobe to eliminate chronic atrial fibrillation associated with mitral valve disease. Pacing Clin Electrophysiol 2005;28(Suppl 1):S73–7.

97. Wolf RK, Schneeberger EW, Osterday R, et al. Video-assisted bilateral pulmonary vein isolation and left atrial appendage exclusion for atrial fibrillation. J Thorac Cardiovasc Surg 2005;130(3):797–802.

98. Doll N, Pritzwald-Stegmann P, Czesla M, et al. Ablation of ganglionic plexi during combined surgery for atrial fibrillation. Ann Thorac Surg 2008;86(5):1659–63.

99. McClelland JH, Duke D, Reddy R. Preliminary results of a limited thoracotomy: new approach to treat atrial fibrillation. J Cardiovasc Electrophysiol 2007; 18(12):1289–95.

100. Mehall JR, Kohut RM Jr, Schneeberger EW, et al. Intraoperative epicardial electrophysiologic mapping and isolation of autonomic ganglionic plexi. Ann Thorac Surg 2007;83(2):538–41.

101. Edgerton JR, Jackman WM, Mack MJ. Minimally invasive pulmonary vein isolation and partial autonomic denervation for surgical treatment of atrial fibrillation. J Interv Card Electrophysiol 2007;20(3):89–93.

102. Beyer E, Lee R, Lam BK. Point: minimally invasive bipolar radiofrequency ablation of lone atrial fibrillation: early multicenter results. J Thorac Cardiovasc Surg 2009;137(3):521–6.

103. Edgerton JR, Edgerton ZJ, Weaver T, et al. Minimally invasive pulmonary vein isolation and partial autonomic denervation for surgical treatment of atrial fibrillation. Ann Thorac Surg 2008;86(1):35–8 [discussion: 39].

104. Gaita F, Riccardi R, Caponi D, et al. Linear cryoablation of the left atrium versus pulmonary vein cryoisolation in patients with permanent atrial fibrillation and valvular heart disease: correlation of electroanatomic mapping and long-term clinical results. Circulation 2005;111(2):136–42.

105. Po SS, Scherlag BJ, Yamanashi WS, et al. Experimental model for paroxysmal atrial fibrillation arising at the pulmonary vein-atrial junctions. Heart Rhythm 2006;3(2):201–8.

106. Scherlag BJ, Nakagawa H, Jackman WM, et al. Electrical stimulation to identify neural elements on the heart: their role in atrial fibrillation. J Interv Card Electrophysiol 2005;13(Suppl 1):37–42.

107. Mounsey JP. Recovery from vagal denervation and atrial fibrillation inducibility: effects are complex and not always predictable. Heart Rhythm 2006;3(6):709–10.

108. Oh S, Zhang Y, Bibevski S, et al. Vagal denervation and atrial fibrillation inducibility: epicardial fat pad ablation does not have long-term effects. Heart Rhythm 2006;3(6):701–8.

109. Sakamoto S, Schuessler RB, Lee AM, et al. Focal ablation of epicardial ganglionated plexus: electrophysiological modification and regeneration of vagal tone in canine atria. Innov Technol Tech Cardiothorac Vasc Surg 2008;3(3):67.

110. Benussi S, Nascimbene S, Agricola E, et al. Surgical ablation of atrial fibrillation using the epicardial radiofrequency approach: mid-term results and risk analysis. Ann Thorac Surg 2002;74(4):1050–6 [discussion: 1057].

111. Fasol R, Meinhart J, Binder T. A modified and simplified radiofrequency ablation in patients with mitral valve disease. J Thorac Cardiovasc Surg 2005;129(1):215–7.

112. Imai K, Sueda T, Orihashi K, et al. Clinical analysis of results of a simple left atrial procedure for chronic atrial fibrillation. Ann Thorac Surg 2001;71(2):577–81.

113. Knaut M, Spitzer SG, Karolyi L, et al. Intraoperative microwave ablation for curative treatment of atrial fibrillation in open heart surgery–the MICRO-STAF and MICRO-PASS pilot trial. MICROwave application in surgical treatment of atrial fibrillation. MICROwave application for the treatment of atrial fibrillation in bypass-surgery. Thorac Cardiovasc Surg 1999;47(Suppl 3):379–84.

114. Kondo N, Takahashi K, Minakawa M, et al. Left atrial maze procedure: a useful addition to other corrective operations. Ann Thorac Surg 2003;75(5):1490–4.

115. Schuetz A, Schulze CJ, Sarvanakis KK, et al. Surgical treatment of permanent atrial fibrillation using microwave energy ablation: a prospective randomized clinical trial. Eur J Cardiothorac Surg 2003;24(4):475–80 [discussion: 480].

116. Sie HT, Beukema WP, Misier AR, et al. Radiofrequency modified maze in patients with atrial fibrillation undergoing concomitant cardiac surgery. J Thorac Cardiovasc Surg 2001;122(2):249–56.

117. Barnett SD, Ad N. Surgical ablation as treatment for the elimination of atrial fibrillation: a meta-analysis. J Thorac Cardiovasc Surg 2006;131(5):1029–35.

118. Doukas G, Samani NJ, Alexiou C, et al. Left atrial radiofrequency ablation during mitral valve surgery for continuous atrial fibrillation: a randomized controlled trial. JAMA 2005;294(18):2323–9.

119. Gillinov AM, McCarthy PM, Blackstone EH, et al. Surgical ablation of atrial fibrillation with bipolar radiofrequency as the primary modality. J Thorac Cardiovasc Surg 2005;129(6):1322–9.

120. Voeller RK, Bailey MS, Zierer A, et al. Isolating the entire posterior left atrium improves surgical outcomes after the Cox maze procedure. J Thorac Cardiovasc Surg 2008;135(4):870–7.

121. Wang Y, Schuessler RB, Damiano RJ, et al. Noninvasive electrocardiographic imaging (ECGI) of scar-related atypical atrial flutter. Heart Rhythm 2007;4(12):1565–7.

122. Wang Y, Cuculich PS, Woodard PK, et al. Focal atrial tachycardia after pulmonary vein isolation: noninvasive mapping with electrocardiographic imaging (ECGI). Heart Rhythm 2007;4(8):1081–4.

123. Damiano RJ Jr, Gaynor SL, Bailey M, et al. The long-term outcome of patients with coronary disease and atrial fibrillation undergoing the Cox maze procedure. J Thorac Cardiovasc Surg 2003;126(6):2016–21.

Congenital Heart Disease Surgery in the Adult

Bret A. Mettler, MD[a], Benjamin B. Peeler, MD[a,b,*]

KEYWORDS

- Adult congenital heart disease surgery • Palliative
- Hypoplast • Bicuspid • Detect

As a result of improved treatment of congenital heart disease (CHD) over the last half century, the number of patients reaching adulthood with CHD continues to grow. During the advent of surgical treatment in the 1950s, surgical mortality rates greater than 50% to 60% were usual, whereas 50 years later, the rate of survival is greater than 90% in most modern units. More than 80% of children born with CHD are now expected to survive into adulthood. Since the year 2000, the number of adults with CHD has exceeded the number of children with CHD.

With increased success in treating CHD, a challenging group of adults with unique anatomy and physiology in addition to the usual effects of aging has been created. Although in some cases surgical treatment of CHD in children has been "curative" with an appropriately connected 2-ventricle circulation without septal defects, a large proportion of patients have been treated with "palliative" operations as their best treatment option. Because of the significant evolution in the understanding of CHD and its surgical treatment in the last 50 years, there are many patients who are now reaching adulthood having had repairs that by current practice would be considered "historical," as they are rarely performed.[1] Additionally, another 10% of congenital heart defects are not discovered until adulthood. All of these patients present unique and fascinating challenges, and their best care requires bridging pediatric and adult medical and surgical care. A timely and appropriate debate regarding the creation of the best system and environment for the growing population of adults with CHD is underway. The review that follows is a discussion of some of the more common surgical issues arising in this evolving group of patients.

[a] Department of Surgery, Division of Thoracic and Cardiovascular Surgery, University of Virginia Medical Center, PO Box 800679, Charlottesville, VA 22908-0679, USA
[b] Virginia Children's Heart Center, University of Virginia Medical Center, Charlottesville, VA 22908, USA
* Corresponding author.
E-mail address: BP2T@virginia.edu (B.B. Peeler).

Surg Clin N Am 89 (2009) 1021–1032
doi:10.1016/j.suc.2009.05.008
0039-6109/09/$ – see front matter © 2009 Published by Elsevier Inc.
surgical.theclinics.com

THE SINGLE VENTRICLE PATIENT

The diverse groups of patients falling under the category of single ventricle lesions are currently treated using the Fontan pathway. Originally described for patients with tricuspid atresia, the Fontan procedure has now been extended to nearly all forms of single ventricle circulation. The Fontan pathway describes a gradual, multistep redirection of blood flow from a single ventricle, connected to the systemic outflow, with the venous inflow passively into the pulmonary arteries. In many cases, the Fontan pathway involves neonatal palliation in addition to an intervening Glenn procedure (superior vena cava [SVC] to pulmonary artery) before a Fontan connection (inferior vena cava [IVC] to pulmonary artery). There have been several variations in the surgical approach since inception. Classically, the right atrial appendage was directly connected to the pulmonary artery with the atrial septal defect (ASD) closed. Since that time, the lateral tunnel and extracardiac Fontan have shown to have superior long-term outcomes.[2]

Several long-term problems can occur in these patients. Patients who have had a Fontan operation are at risk for arrhythmias, with the incidence of atrial flutter or fibrillation increasing as the duration of follow-up increases. When arrhythmias are present, an underlying hemodynamic cause should always be sought, and in particular, obstruction of the Fontan circuit needs to be excluded. In many cases, chronic right atrial distension in a "classic Fontan" is present. Systemic and pulmonary thromboembolism may be associated with dysrhythmia secondary to sluggish circulation. Protein-losing enteropathy occurs in up to 10% of patients and is associated with ascites, peripheral edema, pleural and pericardial effusions, and chronic diarrhea. Hepatic dysfunction may also occur secondary to venous congestion. Right pulmonary vein obstruction has been documented because of compression from an enlarged right atrium or bulging atrial baffle. Over time, patients may develop progressive cyanosis representing worsening ventricular function, venous collateral channels draining directly into the left atrium, or pulmonary arteriovenous malformation.

Reintervention in patients who have had a Fontan operation is considered if a residual ASD persists, resulting in a significant right-to-left shunt, symptoms, or cyanosis. A persistent residual shunt secondary to a previous palliative surgical shunt or residual ventricle-to-pulmonary artery connection may also require surgical revision. Atrioventricular (AV) valve regurgitation can cause increased pulmonary pressures, and often repair is required to improve passive flow. The development of venous collateral channels or pulmonary arteriovenous malformations with worsening cyanosis may require catheter-based embolism. Pulmonary venous obstruction also requires surgical intervention. The development of sustained atrial flutter or fibrillation requires an immediate attempt to restore sinus rhythm once right atrial thrombus has been excluded, whereas a high degree AV block or sick sinus syndrome necessitates pacemaker insertion.

Valve repair or replacement is required in patients with systemic AV valve regurgitation, leading to elevated pulmonary artery pressures. Patients with residual shunts of significance may require closure of the residual shunt, whereas those with obstruction at the Fontan anastomosis may be candidates for balloon angioplasty, stenting, or surgical revision. With the development of venous collateral channels or arteriovenous malformations, transcatheter occlusion or conversion of a classic Glenn shunt to a bidirectional Glenn shunt is necessary. Patients with poorly controlled atrial flutter may be candidates for catheter ablation. Conversion of a classical Fontan to a lateral tunnel or external conduit with concomitant atrial maze procedure may be considered for the treatment of serious refractory atrial arrhythmias.[3,4] An impressive experience with Fontan conversion coupled with arrhythmia surgery has been gained by Deal and colleagues,[3] and it has been well described in the literature. Patients with protein-losing enteropathy may be candidates for fenestration in the atrial septum or revision of the Fontan. Medical therapy with subcutaneous heparin, octreotide, and prednisone has been tried with little success. At this time, neither surgical nor medical therapy has been shown to be more effective, and the choice needs to be approached on a per case basis. Transplantation may be necessary for systemic ventricular failure or intractable protein-losing enteropathy.

The Fontan operation remains a palliative yet highly successful procedure, with a reported 10-year survival between 60% and 80%. If protein-losing enteropathy develops, the 5-year survival decreases to 50%.[5] Despite the stated shortcomings, the Fontan pathway is the best option at this point for patients with a functional single ventricle.

ASD

There are 4 types of ASDs: ostium primum, ostium secundum, sinus venosus, and coronary sinus. Clinically significant ASDs have a Qp:Qs ratio greater than 1.5:1 and should be closed. A certain number of ASDs escape detection and account for most of the congenital heart lesions discovered in adulthood. Most patients with "symptomatic" ASDs present with symptoms of dyspnea and fatigue, but these symptoms may be associated with palpitations caused by atrial arrhythmias. Less often, patients with an ASD may permit a paradoxical embolism and present with an ischemic cerebral event. Although the timing of symptom development is unpredictable, smaller ASDs become apparent after the fifth decade of life whereas larger ASDs usually present in the third decade.

Initial evaluation includes documenting the presence, type, and size of the ASD.[6] Echocardiography is the initial modality used for evaluating patients suspected of having an ASD. Heart catheterization may be required to evaluate pulmonary artery pressures, assess pulmonary vascular reactivity, and delineate anomalous pulmonary venous connections. Coronary angiography is performed in patients at high risk of coronary artery disease or in patients who are older than 40 years and planning surgical repair. Magnetic resonance imaging (MRI) has been used as a primary mode of evaluation or as an adjunct to catheterization when results are equivocal for patients suspected of having an ASD. Lung biopsy may be required when the reversibility of the pulmonary hypertension is uncertain from the hemodynamic data.

Consensus statements regarding timing and necessity of closure have been published. Most clinicians believe that the presence of a "significant" ASD would warrant intervention in the setting of a significant shunt, determined by a Qp:Qs ratio greater than 2:1. If pulmonary artery pressures are greater than two-thirds of systemic blood pressure, a left-to-right shunt of at least 1.5:1 would be present, and closure would be indicated. Other indications include evidence of pulmonary vascular reactivity when challenged with pulmonary vasodilators or a lung biopsy with pulmonary arterial changes being potentially reversible. A history of a cryptogenic cerebrovascular event in the presence of a small ASD with right-to-left shunting is also recommended for closure.

Device closure may be offered as an alternative to surgical closure in patients with secundum ASD up to 38 mm in diameter. At the University of Virginia, 95% of secundum ASDs are closed with a percutaneous device; indications for surgical closure include especially large defects with poor tissue rims.[7-10] Surgical closure may also be offered, and it may be especially attractive, should the patient prefer the time-honored surgical approach or if atrial arrhythmia surgery is planned. The availability of an inframammary, right mini thoracotomy or mini sternotomy approach to a typical secundum ASD should be described to interested patients considering surgery. In patients with a sinus venosus ASD or ostium primum ASD, closure using percutaneous devices is not possible at this time, and they require surgical repair. Coronary sinus ASDs are characterized by a communication between the coronary sinus and the left atrium. Coronary sinus ASDs are often associated with a left-sided SVC, and they require baffling between the coronary sinus and right atrium.

Early and intermediate follow-up is excellent after device closure. The intermediate results are comparable to those of surgery, with a high rate of shunt closure and few major complications. Long-term outcome is unknown. Longer follow-up is needed to determine the incidence of arrhythmias and thromboembolic complications late after device closure. For secundum ASD without pulmonary hypertension, surgical closure should result in a very low (<1%) operative mortality. Early and long-term follow-up is excellent. After surgical repair, preoperative symptoms, if any, should decrease or abate. The presence of preoperative atrial flutter or fibrillation may warrant surgical closure of the defect with concomitant ablative therapy or an atrial maze procedure.

Likewise, atrial flutter and/or fibrillation may arise de novo after repair, but they are better tolerated and often more responsive to antiarrhythmic therapy. Late atrial fibrillation may occur in up to one-third of patients, especially in adults older than 40 years or if atrial arrhythmias were present preoperatively. Some surgeons may elect to anticoagulate high-risk patients with warfarin for the first 6 postoperative months, as they are at risk of atrial fibrillation and stroke. Anticoagulation can likely be discontinued thereafter, if they remain arrhythmia-free.

The sinus venosus ASD represents a defect in the sinus venarum portion of the atrial septum. The superior sinus venosus defect lies adjacent to the SVC and is almost always associated with anomalous return of at least the right upper pulmonary veins into the SVC or right atrium.[11] The inferior sinus venosus defect lies closer to the IVC and can be associated with anomalous drainage of the lower right pulmonary veins into the right atrium. The authors prefer the more anatomic "double patch closure" repair, which baffles the anomalous veins into the left atrium while closing the ASD and patches the right atriotomy–superior vena cavotomy widely open to decrease the possibility of SVC stenosis. The authors have had no incidence of pulmonary vein or SVC stenosis and have not required postoperative pacemaker placement for iatrogenic rhythm problems. The alternative "Warden repair" involves transection of the SVC with reimplantation into the right atrial appendage and closure of the ASD.

By definition, the ostium primum ASD, or partial AV canal, is accompanied by a cleft in the anterior leaflet of the mitral valve. Repair of this defect requires repair of the cleft mitral leaflet in addition to ASD closure in all cases. Depending on the chronicity of the defect and the severity of mitral regurgitation, repair of the mitral valve may involve merely simple interrupted suture repair of the cleft or the addition of a mitral annuloplasty for annular reduction and stabilization.[12–14] It is unusual for these patients to require mitral valve replacement at initial surgery.

COARCTATION OF THE AORTA

Currently, the vast majority of aortic coarctations are repaired in the neonatal period. The risk of early repair is quite low and may avoid many of the cardiovascular complications associated with maturation, including systemic hypertension with ensuing left ventricular hypertrophy.[15] Aortic coarctation is most often treated with excision of the coarcted segment with an extended end-to-end anastomosis or with a subclavian flap angioplasty. Historically, most aortic coarctations were fixed with prosthetic patch angioplasty of the coarcted area, in many cases using Dacron, Gore-Tex (Gore Medical, Flagstaff, AZ), or homograft. The Dacron patch repair has been particularly morbid, with pseudoaneurysms developing in 40% of cases at the site of use. Open repair of these pseudoaneurysms has been associated with significant morbidity and mortality, especially when associated complications, including aortobronchial fistula, have occurred.[16,17] Endovascular repair of these lesions has provided a safe and effective alternative in these high-risk patients.

TETRALOGY OF FALLOT/PULMONARY VALVE REPLACEMENT

Tetralogy of Fallot is one of the most common and successfully treated congenital heart defects. The survival curves for patients undergoing complete repairs now nearly approximate that of the general population. Before the era of effective treatment, 95% mortality was expected by the fourth decade of life. The large and growing numbers of adults with complete repairs, though generally doing quite well, are subject to potential limitations in life expectancy because of the nature of their lesion and future repair requirements. Most indications for reintervention involve the right ventricular outflow tract, as the detrimental effect of free pulmonary insufficiency is now more clearly understood. Currently, annulus-sparing repairs are favored when possible, whereas patients repaired in a previous era often underwent a transannular patching, leading to pulmonary insufficiency. Over time, this results in right ventricular volume overload, with progressive ventricular dysfunction, leading to supraventricular and ventricular arrhythmias, left ventricular dysfunction, and tricuspid insufficiency. Patients may be relatively asymptomatic until severe right ventricular dysfunction develops. Once arrhythmias develop, multiple reports have shown a 6% risk of late sudden cardiac death at 30-year follow-up. Risk factors for ventricular arrhythmias and sudden death include older age at repair, transannular patch repair, severe pulmonary insufficiency, left ventricular dilatation and dysfunction, right ventricular outflow tract aneurysm, and prolonged QRS duration.

Pulmonary valve replacement has been shown to result in decreased right ventricular dilatation, improved right ventricular function, and improvement in symptoms. Despite these advancements, it is unclear if pulmonary valve replacement decreases the incidence of ventricular tachycardia or sudden death. Although timing of pulmonary valve replacement after previous tetralogy repair has been controversial, data suggest that an aggressive stance toward replacement leads to better outcomes.[18] In a review of patients undergoing pulmonary valve replacement before or after age 17 years, valve replacement led to normalization of right ventricular volumes, improvement in biventricular function, and increased exercise capacity. Leaving strict age criteria aside, most clinicians advocated for earlier replacement, based on data indicating a better maintenance of right ventricular contractility.[19]

At the University of Virginia, the authors have experienced no major morbidity or mortality from pulmonary valve replacement in more than 75 cases since 2000. For pulmonary valve replacement, a standard approach is used to redo sternotomy in an adult. The authors have a femoral arterial line in all cases to facilitate femoral cannulation, should this be required. If major difficulty with reentry is expected, axillary access is often gained before beginning the sternotomy . After right axillary artery exposure is completed, an 8-mm Dacron graft is attached in an end-to-side manner. The arterial cannula is then inserted into the graft only after successful sternal reentry or if cardiopulmonary bypass is required emergently. The heart is not arrested for these cases. The use of a bioprosthetic valve for pulmonary valve replacement is favored because of the observation of some early pulmonary insufficiency with pulmonary homografts.

EBSTEIN ANOMALY

Ebstein anomaly is a malformation of the tricuspid valve, involving apical displacement of the septal and posterior leaflets leading to "atrialization" of a portion of the right ventricle. The annular circumference is usually enlarged. There may also be varying degrees of malformation of the anterior leaflet, often described as "sail-like." Most often, a varying degree of tricuspid regurgitation and an enlarged right atrium are observed. In patients with Ebstein anomaly, an atrial level shunt is present in 50%, and 1 or more accessory conduction pathways are present in 25%, increasing the risk of atrial arrhythmias. Other identified commonalities with variable clinical significance include anatomic and physiologic right ventricular inflow and outflow obstruction, impaired left ventricular function, and varying degrees of cyanosis. The lesions most often associated with Ebstein anomaly are ventricular septal defects and pulmonary stenoses, with less frequent associations with aortic coarctation and mitral valve prolapse.[20]

Patients with severe Ebstein anomaly are usually discovered in utero or at birth, but patients with mild malformation may be asymptomatic with no functional limitation. Patients with moderate Ebstein anomaly may become symptomatic during late adolescence or young adult life, most commonly presenting with exercise intolerance, fatigue, and symptomatic supraventricular arrhythmias. If an atrial defect is present, patients may be cyanotic, particularly with exercise, and are at risk of a paradoxical embolus. Alternatively, they may have a left-to-right shunt at rest that reverses with effort. End-stage disease with severe tricuspid regurgitation and right ventricular dysfunction may manifest as right-sided cardiac failure and is often precipitated by an arrhythmia, such as atrial flutter or fibrillation. Although sudden death may occur at any age, it is more likely if an accessory pathway is present.

Echocardiography is used in evaluating the anatomic severity, and it shows the degree of right-sided enlargement, right ventricular dysfunction, and tricuspid regurgitation. The size of the anterior leaflet should be specifically evaluated, including the quality of the leaflet-free edge and the amount of tethering observed when surgical repair is considered. The quality of the anterior leaflet is crucial to the success of any type of attempted valve repair. The size and function of the persistent right ventricle is also needed. Echocardiography is used to document the presence of an atrial communication and the degree of shunting, to estimate the left ventricular function, and to determine mitral valve competence. Preoperative Holter monitor is performed to determine if accessory pathways are present. Exercise testing may be required to evaluate shunting and severity of pulmonary hypertension in the presence of atrial communication. Finally, coronary angiography is recommended in patients at risk for coronary artery disease or in patients older than 40 years, if surgical repair is considered.

Current indications for intervention include a deteriorating exercise capacity, with class II congestive heart failure, increasing heart size, cyanosis with resting oxygen saturation less than 90%, severe tricuspid regurgitation with symptoms, paradoxical transient ischemic attack or stroke, and sustained atrial arrhythmias.

In the repair of Ebstein anomaly, double venous cannulation is used. In the usual case of a markedly enlarged right atrium, a large swath of right atrial free wall can be removed. After the tricuspid valve is exposed, the leaflets are evaluated with particular attention to the morphology and quality of the anterior leaflet. Less satisfactory results are predicted by the presence of a thickened, muscularized anterior leaflet with fused or indistinct chordae. The Danielson and Carpentier methods of repair have been used successfully; however, the Carpentier repair has been found to be most useful.

The Danielson repair involves vertical plication of the atrialized portion of the right ventricle and creates a functional monocusp valve based on the anterior leaflet.[21] The displaced tricuspid leaflets are drawn up to the "true" tricuspid annulus, using horizontal mattress sutures with pledgets, obliterating the atrialized portion of the right ventricle. Performing a posterior annuloplasty with a polypropylene (Prolene) mattress suture also reduces the annular circumference.

The Carpentier repair uses a longitudinal plication of the right ventricle and tricuspid annulus, with resultant reduction in annular circumference. The anterior leaflet is detached along most of its annular circumference with a sliding plasty performed using a continuous polypropylene (Prolene) suture. Redistribution of the anterior leaflet around the refashioned annulus creates a monocusp valve spanning the tricuspid orifice. Finally, a tricuspid ring is used to support the repair.

It should not be understated that all attempts to repair the tricuspid valve should be considered, as replacement of the tricuspid valve is less desirable.[22] If the valve is not repairable, then replacement is required. If an atrial communication is present, it should be closed at the time of surgery. For patients who have normal pulmonary artery pressures with an inadequate right ventricle due to size or function, severe tricuspid regurgitation, and chronic supraventricular arrhythmias, a bidirectional cavopulmonary connection, also known as a $1\frac{1}{2}$ ventricle, may be required.

If a satisfactory repair is achieved, with or without a bidirectional cavopulmonary anastomosis, the prognosis is excellent. Late arrhythmias, most commonly atrial in origin, and seldom complete heart block, may occur. Valve re-replacement may be necessary with a failing bioprosthetic or a thrombosed mechanical valve. There is a high incidence of complete heart block with tricuspid valve re-replacement. Endocarditis prophylaxis is recommended for 6 months after Ebstein repair.[23]

LEFT VENTRICULAR OUTFLOW TRACT OBSTRUCTION AND BICUSPID AORTIC VALVE

Left ventricular outflow tract obstructions (LVOTOs) in the setting of concordant AV and ventriculoarterial connections can occur at several levels. Supravalvular obstruction is rarely an isolated stenosis of the ascending aorta, and it usually involves the major arteries and the distal sinuses of Valsalva. Supravalvular LVOTO is usually progressive, and aortic regurgitation is common. Supravalvular stenosis often manifests as part of Williams syndrome, with the constellation of systemic arterial, peripheral pulmonary, and coronary ostial stenoses. Systemic hypertension is also common.

Valve-level obstruction is most often associated with a bicuspid aortic valve. Although this obstruction is often an isolated abnormality, common associations include coarctation of the aorta, patent ductus arteriosus, or an ascending aortopathy. A bicuspid aortic valve is the most common congenital cardiac abnormality, occurring in 1% to 2% of the population, with a 4:1 male predominance.[24] Valve-level LVOTO progresses at a variable rate with somatic growth. Some patients with a bicuspid aortic valve will not experience any problems, although there is the lifelong risk of endocarditis. Others will develop calcific aortic stenosis or aortic insufficiency. These patients also have a higher incidence of aortic dissection and aneurysm formation.

Subvalvular obstruction presents as a discrete fibromuscular ridge, which partially or completely encircles the left ventricular outflow tract, or as a long fibromuscular narrowing beneath the base of the aortic valve.[25] Subvalvar LVOTO progresses at a variable rate, and low gradients may remain for many years. It is often associated with aortic regurgitation through an otherwise normal valve that has been damaged by the subvalvar jet of blood.[26] Although the aortic insufficiency may progress, it seldom becomes more than moderate when classified with echocardiography. Patients with subvalvar LVOTO associated with a small ventricular septal defect are particularly prone to endocarditis and should receive prophylaxis. Occasionally, there is tunnel-like narrowing of the entire left ventricular outflow tract with a small aortic root requiring surgical repair for relief of obstruction. Rarely, an abnormal insertion of the mitral valve or an accessory mitral leaflet may cause significant obstruction. The concurrence of left ventricular inflow tract obstruction and LVOTO is known as Shone syndrome.

Diagnostic evaluation should be performed to document the level, to quantitate the severity, and to define the anatomy of the obstruction and to identify associated abnormalities. Echocardiography is required on all patients. Often, a heart catheterization with provocative testing is used to assess the hemodynamics and severity of obstruction. Coronary angiography and aortography is required, if surgery is being planned. MRI is often helpful to assess for associated pulmonary artery stenoses or aortic coarctation.

Supravalvular LVOTO requires intervention for a catheterization gradient or mean echo gradient of greater than 50 mm Hg if the obstruction is discrete. Criteria to intervene for diffuse obstruction are not well defined, but they should be considered with similar parameters, as the end effects on the coronary arteries and myocardium are similar.[27–29] Valvar LVOTO requires intervention for symptoms including dyspnea, angina, or syncope. Most surgeons would also consider repair for "critical" aortic stenosis defined as an aortic valve surface area less than 0.6 cm^2. Intervention has also been entertained in patients with a lesser degree of obstruction who wish to play vigorous sports or become pregnant. Bicuspid aortic valves should be considered for intervention when moderate or severe regurgitation is associated with exertional symptoms, when the left ventricular end systolic dimension is greater than 55 mm or when the ejection fraction is less than 55%. Aortic root replacement is required for ascending aortic dissection and should be considered prophylactic for proximal aortic dilation greater than 55 mm. Subvalvar LVOTO should be considered for surgical repair when a resting catheterization or a mean echocardiography gradient is greater than 50 mm Hg, when symptoms develop, or when combined with more than mild aortic regurgitation.[29,30] If there is an associated ventricular septal defect, the gradient may be underestimated, and important subvalvar LVOTO may become manifest only after ventricular septal defect closure.

Repair of supravalvar LVOTO most often requires patch aortoplasty or, rarely, replacement of the proximal ascending aorta. Valve-level LVOTO may be treated using balloon valvuloplasty (if noncalcific), open aortic valvotomy, or valve replacement using either a pulmonary autograft or a prosthetic valve. Aortic valve disease, either isolated or in combination with supravalvar or subvalvar stenosis, has been increasingly treated using pulmonary autografts, especially in young adults. Discrete subvalvar LVOTO requires surgical intervention with either a myomectomy or a myotomy. In older patients, the aortic valve may also need to be replaced or repaired in the presence of aortic regurgitation. Tunnel-like subvalvar LVOTO may require augmentation of the LVOTO using the Konno procedure.[31] Historically, a left ventricular apicoaortic valved conduit was implanted to relieve the LVOTO; but the long-term durability was less than ideal, and the procedure has mostly been abandoned. Subvalvar LVOTO associated with repair of an AV septal defect often recurs if the fibromuscular tissue alone is excised. In this setting, patch enlargement of the infundibular septum is required. Patch enlargement of the superior bridging leaflet of the left AV valve or valve replacement may also be required.

Supravalvar LVOTO has a low operative mortality, and recurrence is uncommon. The long-term durability of patches and conduits used to relieve the obstruction requires surveillance to assess for endocarditis or aneurysm formation. Valve-level LVOTO treated by valvotomy or valvuloplasty may be associated with recurrent stenosis, calcification, or regurgitation and may require future valve replacement. Recurrent fibromuscular subvalvar LVOTO develops in 20% of patients, particularly if the aortic root is small, and it requires echocardiograph surveillance. Surgically treated tunnel-like subvalvar LVOTO, with or without aortic valve replacement, has a high recurrence rate and requires yearly surveillance.[32]

TRANSPOSITION OF THE GREAT ARTERIES

Transposition of the great arteries is defined as AV concordance with ventriculoarterial discordance. Two-thirds of patients have no associated abnormalities. The remaining third have abnormalities, including ventricular septal defects, with pulmonary or sub-pulmonary stenosis being most common. Simple transposition has a 90% mortality in the first year of life if not surgically repaired; thus patients seen as adults will have had an intervention. In such adults with transposition of the great vessels, the most common surgical procedure performed was the atrial switch. In the atrial switch, blood is redirected at the atrial level using a baffle (Mustard) or atrial flaps (Senning), achieving physiologic correction. In this setting, the right ventricle continues to support the systemic circulation. Presently, the atrial switch operation has been supplanted by the arterial switch operation (Jatene) in children, but few of these children have yet to reach adulthood. In a small proportion of patients who have a ventricular septal defect and pulmonary or subpulmonary stenosis, a Rastelli operation is required. In a Rastelli procedure, blood is redirected at the ventricular level by baffling left ventricular outflow to the aorta with a valved conduit placed from the right ventricle to the pulmonary artery. In this setting, the left ventricle supports the systemic circulation.

In the adult patient with complete transposition of the great vessels, the criteria for reintervention are continuing to evolve. In patients who have had an atrial level switch, reintervention may be indicated in patients with significant systemic (tricuspid) AV valve regurgitation, severe right or left ventricular dysfunction, and symptomatic arrhythmias. A baffle leak results in a left-to-right shunt (Qp:Qs > 1.5:1), and most right-to-left shunts with ventricular dysfunction require operative revision. If obstruction of either systemic or pulmonary venous return is present, balloon angioplasty of patch augmentation may be required to improve inflow.

Indications for reintervention in patients who have undergone an arterial switch operation include a right ventricular outflow tract obstruction determined by a gradient greater than 60 mm Hg on catheterization or echocardiography, a right ventricular to left ventricular pressure ratio greater than 0.6, myocardial ischemia from coronary artery obstruction, neoaortic valve insufficiency, and aortopulmonary collateral vessel. In patients who have undergone a Rastelli procedure, surgical revision is required with right ventricle-to-pulmonary artery conduit stenosis or symptomatic valve regurgitation.[33] Subaortic obstruction in the left ventricle-to-aorta tunnel, a residual ventricular septal defect, and branch pulmonary artery stensoses may also require surgical revision after the Rastelli operation.

Surgery may be necessary for baffle stenosis or leakage in patients who have had an atrial switch procedure.[34] Pathway obstruction is less common after the Senning operation and is usually amenable to balloon dilation. Balloon dilation of either an SVC or IVC stenosis may be attempted, but success is limited in adults. Whereas SVC stenosis is usually benign, IVC stenosis may be life threatening and should be treated expeditiously. Stent insertion has been described for baffle and caval stenoses and should be considered in patients refractory to dilation. In patients with an atrial switch procedure and severe systemic (tricuspid) AV valve regurgitation, valve repair or replacement is required. Patients with severe systemic (right) ventricular dysfunction and/or severe systemic (tricuspid) AV valve regurgitation after an atrial switch procedure should be evaluated for cardiac transplantation. A conversion procedure to an arterial switch following retraining of the left ventricle with a pulmonary artery band may also be contemplated. Atrial flutter occurs in 20% of atrial switch patients by age 20 years, and sinus node dysfunction or junctional rhythm is seen in half of these patients. Transvenous pacemaker insertion for symptomatic bradycardia or antitachycardia pacing is indicated in this setting. In patients who have had an atrial switch operation, transvenous pacing leads must traverse the upper limb of the atrial switch to enter the morphological left atrium and ventricle, with fixation required. Transvenous pacing for bradyarrhythmias is required in 15% of adult patients following intra-atrial repair and should be done by electrophysiologists with expertise in adult CHD. A baffle leak must be ruled out by transesophageal echocardiogram before pacemaker insertion (to reduce the risk of paradoxical embolism) and morphological assessment of the systemic venous pathway (to rule out a stenotic systemic channel). Epicardial leads are a surgical alternative when venous access is prohibitive. Transcatheter ablation procedures for intra-atrial reentry tachycardia, atrial flutter, and AV nodal reentry may be performed, with an initial rate of success in these patients being 60% to 70%. Ablation in these patients is more complex and associated with a lower cure rate due to both complex anatomy and previous surgical scars.

Patients who have had an arterial switch operation may require coronary artery bypass grafting for myocardial ischemia or augmentation of the right ventricular outflow tract for symptomatic obstruction. Patients who have had a Rastelli operation will most often require conduit replacement due to homograft calcification and stenosis or may require a left ventricle-to-aorta baffle revision if obstruction occurs.[35]

SUMMARY

Despite the obvious complexity of the surgical treatment of both children and adults with CHD, the current results are excellent in many centers. Improvements in not only cardiology and surgery, but also in anesthesia and critical care are responsible for these results. An important debate is underway regarding the most appropriate environment to care for these patients. Although excellent survival rates have been achieved with improvements in largely pediatric subspecialties, the development of comorbidities in adulthood mandates that ready access to adult specialist care be available. Select, large freestanding children's hospitals can easily provide this important adult subspecialist care readily, whereas adult hospitals are limited in many cases by a lack of experienced surgeons and cardiologists in the field of CHD. Medical centers with a "children's hospital within a hospital" or "free-leaning" children's hospitals are well suited to care for these patients at this point. The common features of the best centers will be the availability of a wide range of adult subspecialties in addition to experienced adult congenital cardiologists and surgeons, anesthesia, and critical care. Over the next decade, establishment of specialized units in several different practice environments will be required to continue to provide service to this increasing number of complex patients.

REFERENCES

1. Jenkins KJ, Newburger JW, Lock JE, et al. In-hospital mortality for surgical repair of congenital heart defects: preliminary observations of variation by hospital caseload. Pediatrics 1995;95(3):323–30.
2. Fernandez G, Costa F, Fontan F, et al. Prevalence of reoperation for pathway obstruction after Fontan operation. Ann Thorac Surg 1989;48:654–9.
3. Deal BJ, Mavroudis C, Backer CL, et al. Impact of arrhythmia circuit cryoablation during Fontan conversion for refractory atrial tachycardia. Am J Cardiol 1999;83:563–8.
4. Van Arsdell GS, Williams WG, Freedom RM. A practical approach to $1\frac{1}{2}$ ventricle repairs. Ann Thorac Surg 1998;66:678–80.
5. Driscoll DJ, Offord KP, Feldt RH, et al. Five- to fifteen-year follow up after Fontan operation. Circulation 1992;85:469–96.
6. Konstantinides S, Geibel A, Olschewski M, et al. A comparison of surgical and medical therapy for atrial septal defect in adults. N Engl J Med 1995;333(8):469–73.
7. Murphy JG, Gersh BJ, McGoon MD, et al. Long-term outcome after surgical repair of isolated atrial septal defect. Follow-up at 27 to 32 years. N Engl J Med 1990;323:1645–50.
8. Berger F, Vogel M, Alexi-Meskishvili V, et al. Comparison of results and complications of surgical and Amplatzer device closure of atrial septal defects. J Thorac Cardiovasc Surg 1999;118:674–80.
9. Moreno-Cabral RJ, Mamiya RT, Nakamura FF, et al. Ventricular septal defect and aortic insufficiency. Surgical treatment. J Thorac Cardiovasc Surg 1977;73(3):358–65.
10. Bridges ND, Perry SB, Keane JF, et al. Preoperative transcatheter closure of congenital muscular ventricular septal defects. N Engl J Med 1991;324:1312–7.
11. Meijboom F, Szatmari A, Utens E, et al. Long-term follow-up after surgical closure of ventricular septal defect in infancy and childhood. J Am Coll Cardiol 1994;24:1358–64.
12. Bergin ML, Warnes CA, Tajik AJ, et al. Partial atrioventricular canal defect: long-term follow-up after initial repair in patients > or = 40 years old. J Am Coll Cardiol 1995;25:1189–94.
13. King RM, Puga FJ, Danielson GK, et al. Prognostic factors and surgical treatment of partial atrioventricular canal. Circulation 1986;74:142–6.
14. Troost E, Gewillig M, Daenen W, et al. Behaviour of polyester grafts in adult patients with repaired coarctation of the aorta. Eur Heart J 2009;30(9):1136–41.
15. Campbell M. Natural history of coarctation of the aorta. Br Heart J 1970;32:633–40.
16. Gibbs JL. Treatment options for coarctation of the aorta. Heart 2000;84:11–3.
17. Ash R, Fischer D. Manifestations and results of treatment of patent ductus arteriosus in infancy and childhood. An analysis of 138 cases. Pediatrics 1955;16:695–703.

18. Murphy JG, Gersh BJ, Mair DD, et al. Long-term outcome in patients undergoing surgical repair of tetralogy of Fallot. N Engl J Med 1993;329:593–9.
19. Nollert G, Fischlein T, Bouterwek S, et al. Long-term survival in patients with repair of tetralogy of Fallot: 36-year follow-up of 490 survivors of the first year after surgical repair. J Am Coll Cardiol 1997;30:1374–83.
20. Celermajer DS, Bull C, Till JA, et al. Ebstein's anomaly: presentation and outcome from fetus to adult. J Am Coll Cardiol 1994;23:170–6.
21. Danielson GK, Driscoll DJ, Mair DD, et al. Operative treatment of Ebstein's anomaly. J Thorac Cardiovasc Surg 1992;104:1195–202.
22. Kiziltan HT, Theodoro DA, Warnes CA, et al. Late results of bioprosthetic tricuspid valve replacement in Ebstein's anomaly. Ann Thorac Surg 1998;66:1539–45.
23. Dajani AS, Taubert KA, Wilson W, et al. Prevention of bacterial endocarditis. Recommendations by the American Heart Association [see comments] [Review] [66 refs]. JAMA 1997;277:1794–801.
24. Keane JF, Driscoll DJ, Gersony WM, et al. Second natural history study of congenital heart defects: results of treatment of patients with aortic valvar stenosis. Circulation 1996;87(2):I16–27.
25. Choi JY, Sullivan ID. Fixed subaortic stenosis: anatomical spectrum and nature of progression. Br Heart J 1991;65:280–6.
26. Rohlicek CV, Pino SF, Hosking M, et al. Natural history and surgical outcomes for isolated discrete subaortic stenosis in children. Heart 1999;82:708–13.
27. Groenink M, Lohuis TAJ, Tijssen JPG, et al. Survival and complication free survival in Marfan's syndrome: implications of current guidelines. Heart 1999;82:499–504.
28. Gott VL, Greene PS, Alejo DE, et al. Replacement of the Aortic root in patients with Marfan's syndrome. N Engl J Med 1999;340:1307–13.
29. ACC/AHA guidelines for the management of patients with valvular heart disease. A Report of the American Collage of Cardiology/American Heart Association. Task Force on practice guidelines (Committee on management of patients with valvular heart disease). J Am Coll Cardiol 1998;32:1486–588.
30. Connelly MS, Webb GD, Somerville J, et al. Canadian Consensus Conference on Adult Congenital Heart Disease 1996. [Review] [106 refs]. Can J Cardiol 1998;14:395–452.
31. Roughneen PT, DeLeon SY, Cetta F, et al. Modified Konno-Rastan Procedure for subaortic stenosis: indications, operative techniques, and results. Ann Thorac Surg 1998;65:1368–76.
32. Serraf A, Zoghby J, Lacour-Gayet F, et al. Surgical treatment of subaortic stenosis: a seventeen-year experience. J Thorac Cardiovasc Surg 1999;117:669–78.
33. Vouhe PR, Tamisier D, Leca F, et al. Transposition of the great arteries, ventricular septal defect and right ventricular outflow tract obstruction: Rastelli or Lecompte procedure? J Thorac Cardiovasc Surg 1992;103:428–36.
34. Wilson NJ, Clarkson PM, Barratt-Boyes BG, et al. Long-term outcome after the mustard repair for simple transposition of the great arteries. 28-year follow-up. J Am Coll Cardiol 1998;32:758–65.
35. Connelly MS, Liu PP, Williams WG, et al. Congenitally corrected transposition in the adult: functional status and complications. J Am Coll Cardiol 1996;27(5):1238–43.

Index

Note: Page numbers of article titles are in **boldface** type.

A

Ablation, in atrial fibrillation management, 1005–1008
    cryoablation, 1006
    ganglionated plexus ablation, 1012
    RF, 1007–1008
    RF energy, 1007–1008
ACC. See *American College of Cardiology (ACC)*.
Activity(ies), energy requirements for, 751
Acute aortic dissection. See *Aortic dissection, acute.*
ß-Adrenergic blockade, in noncardiac surgery, 755–757
AHA. See *American Heart Association (AHA)*.
AMADEUS trial, 961
American College of Cardiology (ACC), 1008
American College of Cardiology (ACC)/American Heart Association (AHA), 2007
Perioperative Guidelines of, 750, 758
American Heart Association (AHA), 1008
Ample PS3 system, 962
Anesthesia/anesthetics
    in minimally invasive surgery of mitral valve, 925
    in minimally invasive valve surgery of aortic valve, 937
Aneurysm(s), aortic, thoracic. See *Thoracic aortic aneurysms.*
Angiography
    CT, in great vessel occlusive disease diagnosis, 825
    magnetic resonance, in great vessel occlusive disease diagnosis, 825
Antegrade transapical aortic valve implantation, 956–957
Aorta
    blunt injury of, **797–820.** See also *Blunt aortic injury (BAI).*
    chronic pseudoaneurysms of, 810
    coarctation of, surgery for, 1024–1025
    thoracic. See *Thoracic aorta.*
    traumatic injury of, TEVAR for, 907–909
Aortic aneurysms, thoracic. See *Thoracic aortic aneurysms.*
Aortic branch occlusion, intentional, TEVAR in, 909–910
Aortic disease, bicuspid, aortic dissection due to, 872–873
Aortic dissection
    acute
        classification of, 870–871
        clinical presentation of, 875–876
        described, 869

Surg Clin N Am 89 (2009) 1033–1045
doi:10.1016/S0039-6109(09)00103-0
0039-6109/09/$ – see front matter © 2009 Elsevier Inc. All rights reserved.

surgical.theclinics.com

Moving?

Make sure your subscription moves with you!

To notify us of your new address, find your **Clinics Account Number** (located on your mailing label above your name), and contact customer service at:

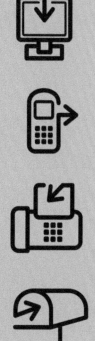

Email: journalscustomerservice-usa@elsevier.com

800-654-2452 (subscribers in the U.S. & Canada)
314-447-8871 (subscribers outside of the U.S. & Canada)

Fax number: 314-447-8029

Elsevier Health Sciences Division
Subscription Customer Service
3251 Riverport Lane
Maryland Heights, MO 63043